AF528619

Handbook of Veterinary Preventive Medicine

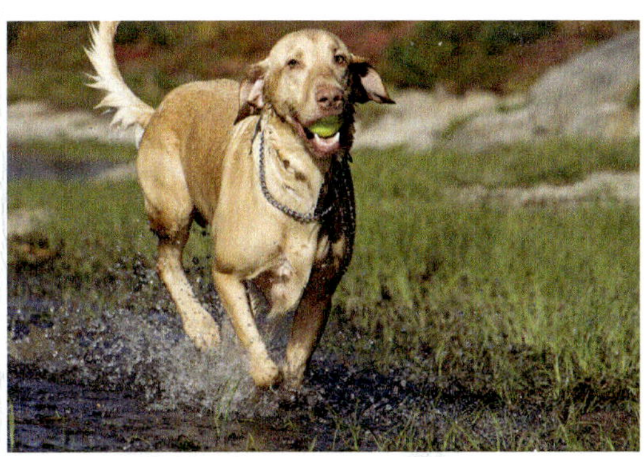
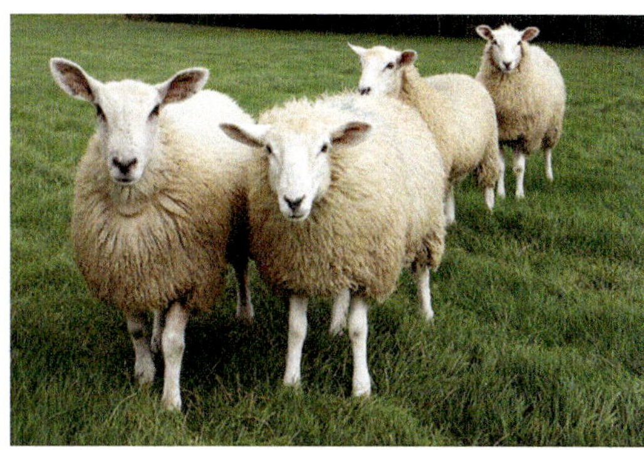
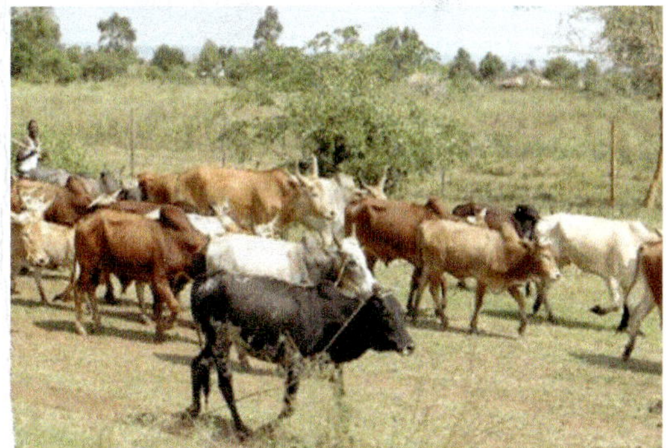
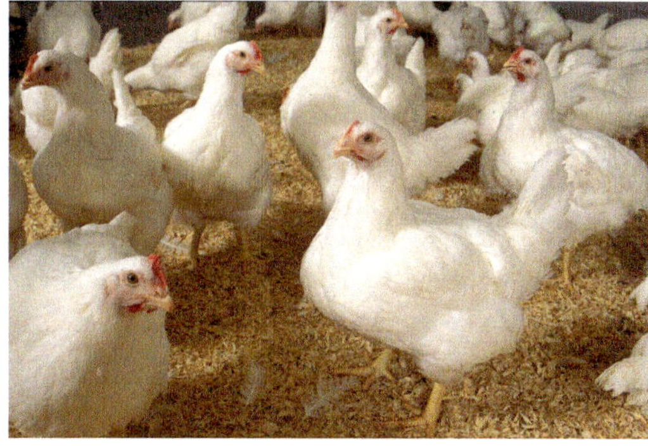

THE AUTHORS

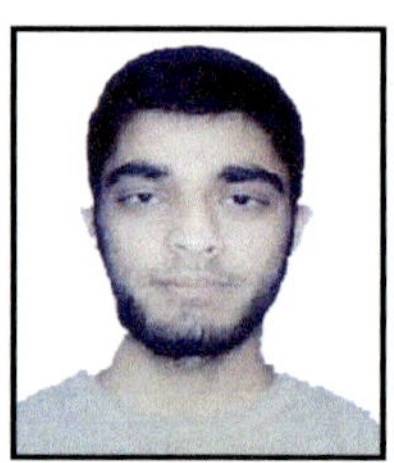

Dr. Omer Mohi-u-din Sofi, obtained his B.V.Sc and AH from SK University of Agricultural Sciences and Technology, Shuhama, Aluestang Srinagar. He done his B.V. Sc in Parasitology from G.B. Pant University of Agriculture & Technology, Pantnagar, Uttarakhand. Presently he is doing his Doctorate from SK University of Agricultural Sciences and Technology, RS Pura, Jammu. He published more than 10 research papers in various International and National journals in addition to attended various International, National and State conferences.

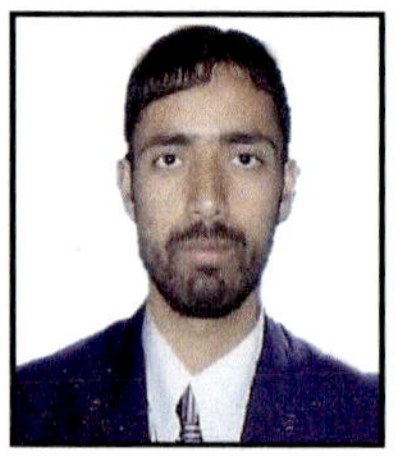

Dr. Tanveer Ahmad Sofi, obtained his M. Sc. Zoology in 2010 from University of Kashmir, Srinagar, completed his M. Phil. in 2012 with "Outstanding" Grades and his Ph.D in 2016 from University of Kashmir, Srinagar. He has edited two Souvenir and Abstracts and published more than 30 research papers in various International Journals, in addition to having attended 05 International conferences, 06 National and 04 State Conferences. Presently, Dr. Tanveer worked as Contractual in Govt. Degree College Sumbal, Sonawari as Assistant Professor in the Department of Zoology. Dr. Tanveer is presently working in JK Sainik School, Manasbal as TGT Biology.

Handbook of Veterinary Preventive Medicine

for

B.V. Sc. & A.H.

Omer Mohi-u-din Sofi
(B.V. Sc and AH; M.VSc)
S.K. University of Agricultural Sciences & Technology
R.S. Pura, Jammu, J&K

Tanveer Ahmad Sofi
(M.Sc. B.Ed. M.Phil; Ph.D)
JK Sainik School, Manasbal
Tullamula Ganderbal, J&K

2021

Daya Publishing House®
A Division of
Astral International Pvt. Ltd.
New Delhi – 110 002

Publisher's Note:

Every possible effort has been made to ensure that the information contained in this book is accurate at the time of going to press, and the publisher and author cannot accept responsibility for any errors or omissions, however caused. No responsibility for loss or damage occasioned to any person acting, or refraining from action, as a result of the material in this publication can be accepted by the editor, the publisher or the author. The Publisher is not associated with any product or vendor mentioned in the book. The contents of this work are intended to further general scientific research, understanding and discussion only. Readers should consult with a specialist where appropriate.

Every effort has been made to trace the owners of copyright material used in this book, if any. The author and the publisher will be grateful for any omission brought to their notice for acknowledgement in the future editions of the book.

Cataloging in Publication Data--DK
Courtesy: D.K. Agencies (P) Ltd. <docinfo@dkagencies.com>

Sofi, Omer Mohi-u-din, author.
Handbook of veterinary preventive medicine : for B.V. Sc. & A.H. / Omer Mohi-u-din Sofi, Tanveer Ahmad Sofi.
pages cm
Includes bibliographical references and index.
ISBN 9789389719635 (HB)

1. Veterinary public health. 2. Veterinary medicine. I. Sofi, Tanveer Ahmad, author. II. Title.

LCC SF740.S64 2021 | DDC 636.0832 23

Published by : **Daya Publishing House®**
A Division of
Astral International Pvt. Ltd.
– ISO 9001:2015 Certified Company –
4736/23, Ansari Road, Darya Ganj
New Delhi-110 002
Ph. 011-43549197, 23278134
E-mail: info@astralint.com
Website: www.astralint.com

Printed at : **Replika Press Pvt. Ltd.**

Foreword

"They say that prevention is better than cure" and that is the very principle of preventive veterinary medicine. Usually, we bring our pets or livestock animals to the veterinarian during instances when they show symptoms of sickness or ill health. Most of the times, the veterinarian can be able to treat the disease and improve the animal's living condition. However, there are certain diseases that may be too difficult to cure and may lead to the death of the animal. In these instances, prevention of the disease is necessary to limit complications to the animal's health. Preventive medicine veterinarians focus on the deterrence; regulation and cure for diseases, promotion of agricultural productivity, and improvement of the health of both animal and human populations. They are the go-to-experts to ask for advice on the precautions to take to avoid an animal from getting sick. They also have extensive knowledge in epidemiology, vaccination, and disease intervention that provide a large impact on society. Veterinarians who work in the field of veterinary preventive medicine also do research, provide diagnosis, and develop methods in order to contain the outbreak of infectious diseases. They are vital to society as their work can extend into the public health, nutrition, agricultural, and economy sectors.

The increase in human and animal lifespan is mainly attributed to proper preventive medicine. Thus, preventive medicine veterinarians may also use their knowledge to help design rural projects and programs that cater to the sustainability needs of livestock, while preventing the spread of zoonotic diseases (diseases of animal origin that affect humans) among the general public. Their contribution to the healthcare sector has freed us from the devastation of epidemic diseases over the years.

It is often said that the history of mankind has been dominated by death from plagues, outbreaks, and pestilence rather than from great wars. Fortunately, veterinary preventive medicine has helped decrease the frequency and severity of epidemic diseases worldwide. Without the continued research and development from preventive medicine veterinarians, our society will crumble due to the damage of infectious diseases. Preventive veterinary medicine is a great career that offers great job variety, plenty of intellectual stimuli, and a huge sense of fulfillment from doing something important for society. As a veterinarian specializing in this field, you will have the opportunity to partake in the battle against the ever evolving infectious agents that affect the world as a whole. Furthermore, the feeling of contributing something beneficial to help improve both animal and human welfare may prove to be worthwhile in considering preventive veterinary medicine as your career of choice.

In the above backdrop the "**Handbook of Veterinary Preventive Medicine**" written by Dr. Omer Mohi-ud-din Sofi and Dr. Tanveer Ahmad Sofi is a valuable contribution. Authors have presented detailed information on the Etiology and Epidemiology, Clinical Manifestations, Diagnosis and Prevention and Control with respect to veterinary diseases. The authors have put in sincere efforts in bringing together information on a wide array of issues related to various diseases of animals of the world. The book contains significant information about the treatment as well as prevention and control of various diseases of animals. I take this opportunity to compliment Dr. Omer Mohi-ud-din Sofi and Dr. Tanveer Ahmad Sofi for doing a good job in bringing out this important Hand book. Simple and interesting to read, I am sure, the book will serve as a valuable source of information to general public, especially the students and teacher community and will help the society a long way in combating many of the animal diseases.

Prof. Bashir Ahmad

Higher Education Department

Preface

This book is designed to be concise information which the users may quickly retrieve in preventive medicine in veterinary sciences. The intent of the book is to provide the readers with an easily used source of information like essential criteria for development of Medicine in livestock sector – basic requirements for Preventive Medicine in livestock and allied sectors (*i.e.* Viral, Bacterial, Fungal, Rickettesial, Parasitic Diseases, *etc.*). The language of the book is simple, lucid, and easy to understand. All the chapters are presented in a systematic manner. In the preparation of this book large number of literature has been consulted. Textbook cannot be written without the support and professional contributions of many people. This book is no exception. There can be no claim to originality except in the manner of presentation. We are grateful to those teachers and colleagues whose stimulating discussions have clarified certain vague points. Although great care has been taken in writing this book, yet the possibility of any error or mistake which may have found its way into this book can not be completely ruled out. We hope this book will not serve the purpose of undergraduates only for whom it is intended but also will be used by allied and higher classes. Although great care has been taken in writing this book, yet the possibility of any error or mistake which may have found its way into this book can not be completely ruled out. Constructive comments and good suggestions from readers will therefore be highly appreciated and incorporated for further improvement in next edition of the book. We are highly thankful to **Prof. M. Z. Chishti** and **Prof. Fayaz Ahmad** for their suggestions and constant encouragement for bringing this book in present form.

Dr. Omer Mohi-u-din Sofi

Dr. Tanveer Ahmad Sofi

Contents

Introduction

Complementary and Alternative Veterinary Medicine (CAVM) as defined in 2001 by the American Veterinary Medical Association, is "a heterogeneous group of preventive, diagnostic and therapeutic philosophies and practices. The theoretical bases and techniques of CAVM may diverge from veterinary medicine routinely taught in North American veterinary medical schools or may differ from current scientific knowledge, or both." Although some of the myriad approaches have been used to treat animals for centuries, many have not. Instead, they have been extrapolated from human approaches without first undergoing assessment for safety and effectiveness in non-human animals.

Despite the popularity of CAVM among some segments of the public, along with intensive promotion by certain groups, much remains unknown regarding the true therapeutic utility of many aspects of CAVM. Thus, to gain a legitimate foothold in modern medicine, CAVM must demonstrate a rational mechanism of action and withstand scientific scrutiny.

The responsibility for protecting and benefiting veterinary patients remains with the scientifically educated clinician. Veterinarians who consider referring patients for CAVM or practice modalities have a responsibility to distinguish tried-and-true from too-good-to-be-true. This is accomplished by conducting well-designed scientific trials to investigate relevant clinical questions and by regularly reviewing the medical literature to reassess which modalities have accumulated independently confirmed data. Even if a certain clinical application has not yet received research scrutiny, studies showing a plausible and unique mechanism of action, as well as a safety record, can help support a rational decision about whether to recommend it.

Parasites

A parasite is an organism that lives on or in another organism (usually referred to as the host), causing harm to the host. Parasites enter the body most often through the mouth or skin. Parasites that enter through the mouth are swallowed and can either remain in the intestine or burrow through the intestinal wall and invade other organs. Parasites that enter through the skin either bore directly through the skin or are introduced through the bites of infected insects. Some parasites enter through the skin or paws when an animal swims or bathes in water contaminated with the parasites.

Diagnosis of a parasitic infection usually requires samples of blood, feces, or urine for laboratory analysis. Repeated sample collections and examinations may be necessary to find the parasite. Less often, a tissue sample, or biopsy, is needed to find the parasite.

Some parasites, particularly those that are single-celled organisms, reproduce inside the host. Other parasites have complex life cycles, producing eggs or larvae that spend time in the environment or in an insect vector before becoming infective. If egg-laying parasites live in the digestive tract, their eggs may be found in the animal's feces when a sample is examined under a microscope.

Infection

Microorganisms are tiny living creatures, such as bacteria and viruses. Microorganisms are present everywhere. Despite their overwhelming abundance, relatively few of the thousands of species of microorganisms invade, multiply, and cause illness in animals and people.

Many microorganisms live on the skin and in the mouth, upper airways, and intestines without causing disease. Whether a microorganism lives harmlessly in or on a pet, or invades and causes disease depends on both the nature of the microorganism and the state of the pet's natural defenses.

Infections in Animals

Many diseases, drugs, and other treatments can cause the body's natural defenses to break down. Such a breakdown can lead to infections, even by microorganisms that normally live harmlessly on or in the body. For example, the risk of infection is greatly increased in animals with extensive burns because damaged skin cannot prevent invasion by harmful microorganisms. Drugs such as the anticancer drugs used in chemotherapy can suppress the immune system. Radiation treatments can also suppress the immune system.

The ability to fight certain infections decreases dramatically in animals with immune disorders. Such animals are at particular risk of opportunistic infections (infections by microorganisms that generally do not cause infection in animals with a healthy immune system). They also become more severely ill from many common infections. Infections are more likely and usually more severe in older animals than in younger ones, probably because aging reduces the immune system's effectiveness.

The practice of veterinary medicine is based primarily on methods designed to prevent or control disease in various animal population groups. Prevention refers to steps taken to preclude the disease's introduction to a group of animals where the disease causing organism (pathogen) is not present. Control programs are designed to lower the occurrence of disease where the pathogen is known to exist in a population. The various groups can include livestock, companion animals, wildlife, and the human population. A common example of prevention, and usually more so control, is vaccination programs aimed at specific disease problems. However, vaccinations are not the only, or sometimes even the best means of keeping our animal populations healthy. Many times animals must live in environments that are contaminated with disease-causing organisms, and many other steps for control of disease occurrence must be instituted. Other examples of prevention and control include cleaning and disinfection, quarantine, test and slaughter, sick animal isolation, closed herds, all-in all-out (AIAO) operations, and probably most important and most overlooked, education.

Preventive Medicine Concepts

The introduction of a disease-causing organism to a naive group of animals could have devastating effects. The idea of prevention is stopping that introduction. Quarantining or sequestering new animals for 30 to 45 days is often the best means to stop inadvertent introduction of pathogens. Animals that have left the farm and have been around other animals should be quarantined when they return. Animal-transport vehicles should be cleaned and sanitise before hauling livestock or coming onto a farm. Visitors to the farm should have clean clothing and boots before working with animals. Large populations of wildlife, birds and feral cats can increase risks for introduction of new pathogens to a farm animal population. Vaccinations are recommended for diseases that are known to be in the state or county but not occurring on the farm. A disease such as rabies poses a threat and would have devastating consequences if introduced to a infected population of expensive animals. A closedherd concept where all replacement animals come from on-farm breeding programs is a good preventive medicine concept because it prevents the introduction of new diseases through infected animals.

Disease Control Concepts

Any method devised to reduce or remove the risk of an animal acquiring a disease that has a history of being on a farm is considered control of disease. Good sanitation and vaccination programs are often the best means to lower the risk of disease. Good sanitation will remove or destroy pathogens and reduce exposure of susceptible animals to these pathogens. Vaccination programs increase resistance to infection by pathogens and also provide protection to the newborn through their mother's milk. Identification and removal of animals harboring pathogens is another method utilized in control of disease. Treatment of infected animals to destroy pathogens is an indirect method of control because the risk to other animals is removed when the diseased and infected animals are free of the pathogen. However, for most diseases only a small portion of infected animals may actually show signs of disease. Because of this fact, isolation of sick animals does little to stop the spread of infection as there may be more infected normal-appearing animals than sick animals. All-in allout operations are a good control strategy because pathogens are theoretically kept confined to groups of animals on the farm.

Disease Eradication

Disease eradication is an extreme disease prevention and control strategy. Eradication usually involves the destruction of infected animals and/or animals exposed to infected animals. Historically in USA such programs had been utilized for removal of diseases that would have far reaching effects when introduced to our animal populations. We have had eradication programs, which successfully eliminated foot and month disease, vesicular exanthema of swine, hog cholera, exotic Newcastle disease and certain avian influenzas. These eradication programs are very costly and in today's market the introduction of certain diseases could seriously affect the cost of meat produced in USA.

OIE-Listed Diseases, Infections and Infestations in Force in 2017

Resolutions passed by the International Committee and recommendations issued by the Regional Commissions instructed the OIE Headquarters to establish a single OIE list of notifiable terrestrial and aquatic animal diseases to replace the former **Lists A and B.**

The aim in drawing up a single list was to be in line with the terminology of the Sanitary and Phytosanitary Agreement of the World Trade Organization, by classifying diseases as specific hazards and giving all listed diseases the same degree of importance in international trade.

In order to create a single list of notifiable diseases, the OIE defined criteria to examine the inclusion or not of a given disease in the OIE single list that were approved in **May 2004**.

In **2005**, the first single list composed of former lists A and B was used, and in the same year, an Ad Hoc Group on disease and pathogenic agents notification was organized to examine diseases according to the adopted criteria for listing diseases, and proposed a new list of diseases meeting the criteria that came into force in **2006**.

The list is reviewed on a regular basis and in case of modifications adopted by the World Assembly of Delegates at its annual General Session, the new list comes into force on 1 January of the following year.

Multiple Species Diseases, Infections and Infestations	*Cattle Diseases and Infections*
☆ Anthrax ☆ Bluetongue ☆ Crimean Congo haemorrhagic fever ☆ Epizootic haemorrhagic disease ☆ Equine encephalomyelitis (Eastern) ☆ Heartwater ☆ Infection with Aujeszky's disease virus ☆ Infection with *Brucella abortus, Brucella melitensis* and *Brucella suis* ☆ Infection with *Echinococcus granulosus* ☆ Infection with *Echinococcus multilocularis* ☆ Infection with foot and mouth disease virus ☆ Infection with rabies virus ☆ Infection with Rift Valley fever virus ☆ Infection with rinderpest virus ☆ Infection with *Trichinella* spp. ☆ Japanese encephalitis ☆ New world screwworm (*Cochliomyia hominivorax*) ☆ Old world screwworm (*Chrysomya bezziana*) ☆ Paratuberculosis ☆ Q fever ☆ Surra (*Trypanosoma evansi*) ☆ Tularemia ☆ West Nile fever	☆ Bovine anaplasmosis ☆ Bovine babesiosis ☆ Bovine genital campylobacteriosis ☆ Bovine spongiform encephalopathy ☆ Bovine tuberculosis ☆ Bovine viral diarrhoea ☆ Enzootic bovine leukosis ☆ Haemorrhagic septicaemia ☆ Infectious bovine rhinotracheitis/ infectious pustular vulvovaginitis ☆ Infection with *Mycoplasma mycoides* subsp. *mycoides* SC (Contagious bovine pleuropneumonia) ☆ Lumpy skin disease ☆ Theileriosis ☆ Trichomonosis ☆ Trypanosomosis (tsetse-transmitted)
Sheep and Goat Diseases and Infections	*Equine Diseases and Infections*
☆ Caprine arthritis/encephalitis ☆ Contagious agalactia ☆ Contagious caprine pleuropneumonia ☆ Infection with *Chlamydophila abortus*(Enzootic abortion of ewes, ovine chlamydiosis) ☆ Infection with peste des petits ruminants virus ☆ Maedi-visna ☆ Nairobi sheep disease ☆ Ovine epididymitis (*Brucella ovis*) ☆ Salmonellosis (*S. abortusovis*) ☆ Scrapie ☆ Sheep pox and goat pox	☆ Contagious equine metritis ☆ Dourine ☆ Equine encephalomyelitis (Western) ☆ Equine infectious anaemia ☆ Equine influenza ☆ Equine piroplasmosis ☆ Glanders ☆ Infection with African horse sickness virus ☆ Infection with equid herpesvirus-1 (EHV-1) ☆ Infection with equine arteritis virus ☆ Venezuelan equine encephalomyelitis

Swine Diseases and Infections	*Avian Diseases and Infections*
✰ African swine fever ✰ Infection with classical swine fever virus ✰ Infection *withTaenia solium* (Porcine cysticercosis) ✰ Nipah virus encephalitis ✰ Porcine reproductive and respiratory syndrome ✰ Transmissible gastroenteritis	✰ Avian chlamydiosis ✰ Avian infectious bronchitis ✰ Avian infectious laryngotracheitis ✰ Avian mycoplasmosis (*Mycoplasma gallisepticum*) ✰ Avian mycoplasmosis (*Mycoplasma synoviae*) ✰ Duck virus hepatitis ✰ Fowl typhoid ✰ Infection with avian influenza viruses ✰ infection with influenza A viruses of high pathogenicity in birds other than poultry including wild birds ✰ Infection with Newcastle disease virus ✰ Infectious bursal disease (Gumboro disease) ✰ Pullorum disease ✰ Turkey rhinotracheitis
Lagomorph Diseases and Infections	*Other Diseases and Infections*
✰ Myxomatosis ✰ Rabbit haemorrhagic disease	✰ Camelpox ✰ Leishmaniosis

OIE-Listed Diseases and Wildlife

Member Countries are obliged to report all detected occurrences of OIE-Listed diseases regardless of the animals affected (whether domestic, wild, captive wild or feral). According to the OIE Terrestrial Animal Health Code (2015), 'wildlife' refers to wild animals, captive wild animals and feral animals. The differentiations are based on whether the animal or group of animals is primarily dependent on care by humans and whether the animal's phenotype has been selected by humans. These classifications can help to delineate approaches to disease prevention and control and identify potential epidemiological roles of each type of animals in disease epidemiology and dynamics.

Surveillance and reporting of OIE-Listed diseases in wildlife are often opportunistic in many countries. Systematic and comprehensive wildlife pathogen surveillance is challenging for several reasons including large geographical host ranges and challenges with access to wildlife, wide diversity of species present in regions, limited resources (especially as many developing countries host the most biodiversity) and lack of infrastructure for wild animal pathogen surveillance (*e.g.*, professional training, best practices, diagnostic facilities, *etc.*). While many countries may conduct livestock disease surveillance through the Ministry of Agriculture or other governmental Veterinary Services, which work closely with the OIE through a delegate generally from the Ministry of Agriculture or Livestock, wild animal health often falls separately under a Ministry of Environment or Forestry, which may or may not have the capacity for running adequate disease surveillance programmes.

The OIE has put in place the concept of wildlife focal points that could be from other national ministries to improve coordination and information sharing on wild animal diseases. The paucity of validated diagnostic tests available for use in most wild animals presents an additional challenge to determining current or previous pathogen infection and significance (Cousins and Florisson 2005).

While the OIE has traditionally focused on livestock, the growing intersection of wild and domestic animals and increasing global wildlife trade warrant a closer look at wildlife pathogen susceptibility. The OIE has demonstrated a strong commitment to integrating wildlife considerations into its disease reporting, prevention and animal health capacity-building efforts. To further this goal, EcoHealth Alliance collaborated with the OIE World Animal Health Information and Analysis Department to generate a database of host wildlife families with species proven to be susceptible to OIE-Listed diseases. The intention of the database was to provide information to better assist OIE Member Countries in their consideration of wildlife surveillance and trade activities, and to provide the OIE with a reference list of potential wildlife hosts based on peer-reviewed scientific literature to be considered for inclusion in the WAHIS reporting system. In general, the database serves to identify a broad scope of known families with host species of OIE-Listed diseases.

Number of Host Species of OIE-Listed Diseases and their Corresponding Families

OIE-Listed Disease		*Wildlife Host Families*		*Number Wildlife Host Species*
African horse sickness	Canidae Elephantidae Equidae	Felidae Hyaenidae	Rhinocerotidae Viverridae	11
Audjeszky's disease	Cricetidae Felidae	Leporidae Muridae	Procyonidae	6
African swine fever	Suidae			2
Anthrax	Bovidae Canidae Elephantidae Equidae Eupleridae Felidae	Giraffidae Hippopotamidae Hominidae Hyaenidae Lorisidae	Mustelidae Myocastoridae Rhinocerotidae Suidae Viverridae	58
Bluetongue	Antilocapridae Bovidae Canidae Cervidae	Elephantidae Felidae Giraffidae Hyaenidae	Muridae Rhinocerotidae Ursidae Viverridae	57
Bovine anaplasmosis	Antilocapridae Bovidae Cervidae	Equidae Giraffidae Nesomyidae	Rhinocerotidae Sciuridae	39
Bovine babesiosis	Bovidae	Cervidae		8

OIE-Listed Disease		*Wildlife Host Families*		*Number Wildlife Host Species*
Bovine genital campylobacteriosis				0
Bovine spongiform encephalopathy				0
Bovine viral diarrhea	Antilocapridae Bovidae	Camelidae Cervidae	Rhinocerotidae Tragulidae	39
Brucella abortus	Bovidae Camelidae Canidae Cervidae Cricetidae	Didelphidae Equidae Giraffidae Heteromyidae Hippopotamidae	Leporidae Muridae Procyonidae Suidae Ursidae	30
Brucella melitensis	Bovidae Camelidae	Cervidae Equidae	Suidae	6
Brucella ovis	Cervidae			2
Brucella suis	Bovidae Canidae	Equidae Leporidae	Suidae Ursidae	6
Camelpox				0
Caprine arthritis/ encephalitis				0
Chlamydophila abortus	Bovidae Phocidae	Ranidae		6
Classical swine fever				0
Contagious agalactia	Bovidae			1
Contageous bovine pleuropneumonia				0
Contagious caprine pleuropneumonia	Bovidae			3
Contagious equine metritis				0
Crimian congo hemorrhagic fever	Bovidae Elephantidae Equidae Erinaceidae Giraffidae	Hystricidae Leporidae Muridae Nesomyidae	Pedetidae Rhinocerotidae Sciuridae Suidae	35
Dourine				0
Echinococcus granulosus	Bovidae Canidae Cervidae	Equidae Felidae Giraffidae	Hippopotamidae Suidae	14

OIE-Listed Disease		*Wildlife Host Families*		*Number Wildlife Host Species*
Echinococcus multilocularis	Cervidae Cricetidae	Felidae Muridae		14
EEEV	Cercopithecidae Cricetidae Dasypodidae	Emballonuridae Molossidae Muridae	Phyllostomidae Sciuridae Vespertilionidaae	23
Enzootic bovine leukosis	Caviidae			1
Epizootic hemorrhagic disease	Antilocapridae Bovidae	Cervidae		12
Equine arteritis	Equidae			1
Equine piroplasmosis	Equidae			1
Equine herpesvirus-1	Equidae	Rhinolophidae	Ursidae	6
Equine infectious anemia				0
Foot and Mouth disease	Bovidae Camelidae Cervidae Elephantidae	Erinaceidae Giraffidae Macropodidae Suidae	Tapiridae Tayassuidae Ursidae	60
Glanders	Felidae	Leporidae		2
Goat pox and sheep pox				0
H3N8 and H7N7				0
Heartwater	Bovidae	Cervidae		8
Hemorrhagic septicemia	Bovidae Cebidae Cervidae	Felidae Hominidae Leporidae	Phocidae	15
Infectious bovine rhinotracheitis	Bovidae	Cervidae		16
Japanese encephalitis	Cercopithecidae Emballonuridae Hipposideridae	Hominidae Pteropodidae	Rhinolophidae Vespertilionidae	25
Leishmania	Bradypodidae Canidae Cebidae Cricetidae Ctenodactylidae Cuniculidae Dasypodidae Dasyproctidae	Didelphidae Echimyidae Felidae Herpestidae Hystricidae Megalonychidae Muridae Mustelidae	Myrmecophagidae Phocidae Phyllostomidae Pitheciidae Procaviidae Procyonidae Rodentia Viverridae	48

OIE-Listed Disease		*Wildlife Host Families*		*Number Wildlife Host Species*
Lumpy skin disease	Bovidae	Giraffidae		10
Maedi-visna				0
Mycobacterium bovis	Bovidae Canidae Cercopithecidae Cervidae Elephantidae Erinaceidae Felidae	Herpestidae Hyaenidae Lemuridae Leporidae Muridae Mustelidae Otariidae	Phalangeridae Procyonidae Rhinocerotidae Suidae Talpidae Ursidae	45
Myxoma virus	Leporidae			5
New world screw worm	Atelidae Bovidae Canidae	Cervidae Didelphidae Leporidae	Mustelidae Pitheciidae	10
Nairobi sheep disease	Antilocapridae Cercopithecidae	Muridae Nesomyidae		3
Nipah virus	Hipposideridae Muridae	Pteropodidae Rhinolophidae	Vespertilionidae	21
Old world screw worm	Aepycerotinae Bovidae Elephantidae	Felidae Giraffidae	Rhinocerotidae Ursidae	8
Paratuberculosis	Bovidae Canidae Cervidae	Corvidae Leporidae	Muridae Mustelidae	15
Peste des petits ruminants	Bovidae			5
Porcine cystocircosis	Hylobatidae Otariidae	Ursidae		3
Porcine reproductive and respiratory syndrome				0
Q fever	Canidae Cricetidae Cricetidae Didelphidae Leporidae	Muridae Otariidae Phocidae Phocoenidae Procyonidae	Sciuridae Suidae Ursidae	15
Rabbit haemorrhagic disease	Leporidae	Muridae		3

OIE-Listed Disease		*Wildlife Host Families*		*Number Wildlife Host Species*
Rabies	Bovidae	Felidae	Myocastoridae	137
	Canidae	Herpestidae	Phyllostomidae	
	Caviidae	Hyaenidae	Procyonidae	
	Cervidae	Mephitidae	Pteropodidae	
	Cricetidae	Molossidae	Rhinolophidae	
	Elephantidae	Mormoopidae	Sciuridae	
	Emballonuridae	Muridae	Vespertilionidae	
	Erethizontidae	Mustelidae	Viverridae	
Rift Valley fever	Bovidae	Muridae	Rhinocerotidae	18
	Hipposideridae	Pteropodidae	Vespertilionidae	
Rinderpest	Bovidae	Giraffidae	Suidae	25
	Cervidae	Hippotamidae	Tayassuidae	
Salmonellosis	Bovidae			1
Scrapie				0
Surra	Caviidae	Cricetidae	Phyllostomidae	9
	Cervidae	Echimyidae	Tayassuidae	
Swine vesicular disease				0
Theileriosis	Bovidae	Cervidae		2
Transmissable gastroenteritis				0
Trichinella	Canidae	Felidae	Mustelidae	59
	Castoridae	Herpestidae	Nandiniidae	
	Cricetidae	Hyaenidae	Odobenidae	
	Crocodylidae	Mephitidae	Procyonidae	
	Dasypodidae	Monodontidae	Sciuridae	
	Dasyuridae	Muridae	Ursidae	
	Didelphidae			
Tritrichomonas foetus	Leporidae	Muridae		2
Trypanosomosis	Bovidae	Felidae	Rhinocerotidae	25
	Camelidae	Hippopotamidae	Suidae	
	Cercopithecidae	Lorisidae		
Tularemia	Cambaridae	Felidae	Muridae	65
	Canidae	Gadidae	Mustelidae	
	Castoridae	Haemulidae	Procyonidae	
	Cervidae	Haliotidae	Salmonidae	
	Cichlidae	Heteromyidae	Sciuridae	
	Cricetidae	Leporidae	Soricidae	

OIE-Listed Disease		*Wildlife Host Families*		*Number Wildlife Host Species*
	Equidae Erinaceidae Falconidae	Mephitidae Moronidae	Talpidae Ursidae	
Venezuelan equine encephalomyelitis	Cricetidae Cuniculidae Didelphidae	Echimyidae Heteromyidae Muridae	Phyllostomidae Sciuridae Vespertilionidae	33
Vesicular stomatitis	Antilocapridae Aotidae Atelidae Bovidae Bradypodidae Camelidae Canidae Cebidae Cervidae	Cricetidae Dasypodidae Dasyproctidae Didelphidae Echimyidae Echimyidae Equidae Erethizontidae Heteromyidae	Leporidae Megalonychidae Mephitidae Muridae Myocastoridae Myrmecophagidae Phyllostomidae Procyonidae Sciuridae	58
West Nile virus	Cercopithecidae Cervidae Cricetidae Didelphidae	Molossidae Muridae Procyonidae	Pteropodidae Sciuridae Vespertilionidae	23
Western equine encephalomyelitis	Colubridae Cricetidae Didelphidae	Leporidae Mephitidae Phyllostomidae	Procyonidae Ranidae Sciuridae	16
Total wildlife host-pathogen relationships				**1146**

Old Classification of Diseases Notifiable to the OIE

List A

Transmissible diseases that have the potential for very serious and rapid spread, irrespective of national borders, that are of serious socio-economic or public health consequence and that are of major importance in the international trade of animals and animal products.

☆ Foot and mouth disease	☆ Vesicular stomatitis
☆ Swine vesicular disease	☆ Rinderpest
☆ Peste des petits ruminants	☆ Contagious bovine pleuropneumonia
☆ Lumpy skin disease	☆ Rift Valley fever
☆ Bluetongue	☆ Sheep pox and goat pox

☆ African horse sickness ☆ Classical swine fever ☆ Newcastle disease	☆ African swine fever ☆ Highly pathogenic avian influenza

List B

Transmissible diseases that are considered to be of socio-economic and/or public health importance within countries and that are significant in the international trade of animals and animal products.

Multiple species diseases	**Cattle diseases**
☆ Anthrax ☆ Aujeszky's disease ☆ Echinococcosis/hydatidosis ☆ Heartwater ☆ Leptospirosis ☆ New world screwworm (*Cochliomyia hominivorax*) ☆ Old world screwworm (*Chrysomya bezziana*) ☆ Paratuberculosis ☆ Q fever ☆ Rabies ☆ Trichinellosis	☆ Bovine anaplasmosis ☆ Bovine babesiosis ☆ Bovine brucellosis ☆ Bovine cysticercosis ☆ Bovine genital campylobacteriosis ☆ Bovine spongiform encephalopathy ☆ Bovine tuberculosis ☆ Dermatophilosis ☆ Enzootic bovine leukosis ☆ Haemorrhagic septicaemia ☆ Infectious bovine rhinotracheitis/infectious pustular vulvovaginitis ☆ Malignant catarrhal fever ☆ Theileriosis ☆ Trichomonosis ☆ Trypanosomosis (tsetse-transmitted)
Sheep and goat diseases	**Equine diseases**
☆ Caprine and ovine brucellosis (excluding *B. ovis*) ☆ Caprine arthritis/encephalitis ☆ Contagious agalactia ☆ Contagious caprine pleuropneumonia ☆ Enzootic abortion of ewes (ovine chlamydiosis) ☆ Maedi-visna ☆ Nairobi sheep disease ☆ Ovine epididymitis (*Brucella ovis*) ☆ Ovine pulmonary adenomatosis ☆ Salmonellosis (S. abortusovis) ☆ Scrapie	☆ Contagious equine metritis ☆ Dourine ☆ Epizootic lymphangitis ☆ Equine encephalomyelitis (Eastern and Western) ☆ Equine infectious anaemia ☆ Equine influenza ☆ Equine piroplasmosis ☆ Equine rhinopneumonitis ☆ Equine viral arteritis ☆ Glanders ☆ Horse mange

	☆ Horse pox ☆ Japanese encephalitis ☆ Surra (*Trypanosoma evansi*) ☆ Venezuelan equine encephalomyelitis
Swine diseases ☆ Atrophic rhinitis of swine ☆ Enterovirus encephalomyelitis ☆ Porcine brucellosis ☆ Porcine cysticercosis ☆ Porcine reproductive and respiratory syndrome ☆ Transmissible gastroenteritis	**Avian diseases** ☆ Avian chlamydiosis ☆ Avian infectious bronchitis ☆ Avian infectious laryngotracheitis ☆ Avian mycoplasmosis (*M. galliseplicum*) ☆ Avian tuberculosis ☆ Duck virus enteritis ☆ Duck virus hepatitis ☆ Fowl cholera ☆ Fowl pox ☆ Fowl typhoid ☆ Infectious bursal disease (Gumboro disease) ☆ Marek's disease ☆ Pullorum disease
Lagomorph diseases ☆ Myxomatosis ☆ Rabbit haemorrhagic disease ☆ Tularemia	

Chapter 1

Viral Diseases

Viral diseases are extremely widespread infections caused by viruses, a type of microorganism. Viruses are the smallest of all infectious agents, averaging about 100 nanometer. There are many types of viruses that cause a wide variety of viral diseases. Viral diseases are contagious and spread from animal to animal when the virus enters the body and begins to multiply. Common ways for infections are: eating food or drinking water contaminated with a virus, contaminated feces, by copulation, by body fluids. Viral diseases result in a wide variety of symptoms that vary in character and severity depending on the type of viral infection and other factors, including the age and overall health. Viral diseases are not treatable with antibiotics, which can only cure bacterial diseases and infections. Many cases of viral diseases can lead dehydration, bacterial pneumonia and other secondary bacterial infections. Cleanless and a good immun system of the animal are the best prerequisites for avoidance viral diseases. There are many viruses which infect animals, some of which cause overt clinical disease while others are asymptomatic. Here we discuss some of the viral diseases which have a veterinary importance.

1.1. African Horse Sickness (AHS)

Synonyms

Perdesiekte, Pestis Equorum, Peste Equina, Peste Equina Africana.

African Horse Sickness (AHS) is an acute or sub acute, febrile, arthropod borne disease of horses characterized by oedema of subcutaneous tissues, lungs, hemorrhage of internal organs and accumulation of serous fluids in the body cavities. This disease is caused by orbi virus belonging to the family Reo viridae, which is a double stranded RNA virus. Horses of all breeds are highly susceptible to natural infection. Mules and zebras are less affected and donkeys are generally resistant. The disease occurs principally in Southern, Eastern and Central Africa.

From there it spreads to Syria, Lebanon, Israel and other parts of Middle East. It has been recorded in Afghanistan, West Pakistan, Turkey and Iraq. It is a seasonal disease, common in late summer in warm, humid, low lying marshy districts. This disease is not directly contagious. Various nocturnal biting insects including mosquitoes are the most important vectors of infection in Africa. Culicoides species of mosquito and insects belonging to Tabanidae family and genus *Stomoxys* have been incriminated in outbreaks in Turkey. Many serotypes have been described. In Africa 9 distinct serotypes are recognized and considerable variation in virulence amongst individual strains within each immunological type occurs. On the other hand only a single antigenic type involved in the Asian outbreak in 1961. Almost all strains grow in the yolk sac of fertile eggs. Virus can be propagated in cell cultures of many different types. Monkey cell lines are most susceptible.

Clinical Manifestations

Incubation period is 6-9 days. There are 4 different clinical forms of illness.

(a) **Very mild form**: only rise in temperature to 41°C.

(b) **Acute or pulmonary form (DUNKOP):** In this, there is severe dyspnoea, pyrexia and coughing with abundant frothy discharge from the nostrils. This form is common in virulent outbreaks and mostly the affected horses die.

(c) **Sub acute form (DIKKOP)**: It is characterized by remarkable swelling of head, neck and supraorbital fossa associated with cardiac dyspnoea. This form usually occurs when the immunity has been broken down by a natural infection or in animals inoculated with mild strains of virus. This form is much milder than the acute form and the affected animals recover.

(d) **Mixed form**: Combination of pulmonary form and cardiac form. Heart is affected.

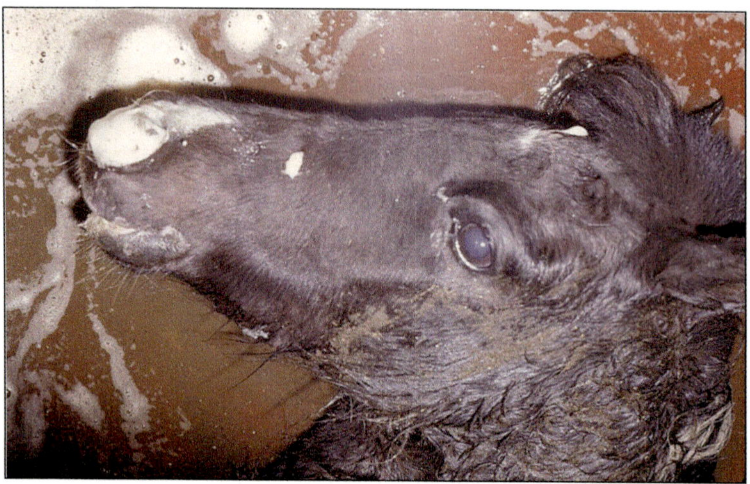

Figure 1.1. Horse, abundant froth draining from the nostrils reflects severe pulmonary edema.

Mortality

In virulent form it is as high as 90 per cent in horses and lower in mules. In milder outbreaks mortality is 25 per cent.

Lesions

It varies depending upon the severity of the case. In acute pulmonary form - extensive oedema of lungs and thorax may contain several litres of fluid. In more chronic cardiac form there is oedematous infiltration of subcutaneous tissue, sub-serosal tissue and other tissues together with gross accumulation of fluid in the pericardial sac.

Diagnosis

In endemic areas, clinical signs and lesions may lead to a presumptive diagnosis. However, laboratory confirmation is essential for definitive diagnosis and determination of the serotype, the latter is important for control measures. Anticoagulated blood should be obtained at the peak of fever and transported (at 4°C) to the laboratory. Spleen samples collected from freshly dead animals should be kept on ice. Presence of virus is best detected by group-specific reverse-transcriptase polymerase chain reaction (RT-PCR). AHSV also can be isolated by intracerebral inoculation of suckling mice or in mammalian or insect cell cultures. Although not widely available, indirect sandwich ELISA is also useful for rapid identification of AHSV antigen in tissues from animals that have died from acute infection. Serotyping of AHSV previously relied on virus neutralization tests using type-specific antisera, which take dikhuaaa 5 days. The recent development of type-specific RT-PCR can now confirm the serotype of an AHSV within 24 hr.

For virus isolation, the tissues of choice for diagnosis are spleen, lung, and lymph nodes, collected at necropsy. Sample preparations can be inoculated in cell cultures, such as Baby Hamster Kidney-21 (BHK-21), Monkey Stable (MS) or African green monkey kidney (Vero), intravenously in embryonated eggs and intracerebrally in newborn mice. Several enzyme-linked immunosorbent assays (ELISAs) for the rapid detection of African Horse Sickness Virus (AHSV) antigen in spleen tissues and supernatant from infected cells have been developed. Identification of AHSV RNA has also been achieved using a reverse-transcription polymerase chain reaction method. Virus isolates can be serotyped by a type-specific serological test such as Virus Neutralisation (VN) and by reverse-transcription polymerase chain reaction and sequencing. Serological tests include complement fixation test, ELISA, immunoblotting and VN.

Prevention and Control

There is no specific treatment for animals with AHS apart from rest and good husbandry. Complicating and secondary infections should be treated appropriately during recovery. AHSV is typically noncontagious and spread exclusively via the bites of infected *Culicoides* spp. or by the direct inoculation of infectious material (*via* blood-feeding insects, needles, *etc.*). Various methods of control may be attempted, such as introducing animal movement restrictions to prevent infected animals initiating new foci of infection and husbandry modification to deny or reduce vector access to susceptible or infected animals (*e.g.*, stabling in vector-proof housing). It is rarely possible to completely eliminate populations of vector *Culicoides*, especially in extensive pasture systems.

Live-attenuated virus vaccines are available for immunization of equids against AHS. These are typically based on cell culture–attenuated viruses and generally provide good, but not absolute protection. Annual revaccination is recommended in regions where these vaccines are used. However, there are increasing concerns regarding use of live-attenuated AHSV vaccines because of their potential reversion to virulence, capacity for transmission by vector *Culicoides* midges and reassortment of their gene segments with other vaccine and field strains of virus, leading to the creation of novel virus progeny. Inactivated and subunit vaccines avoid these potential drawbacks and assuming they are commercially available, would likely be used after incursion of AHSV into previously unaffected regions. Transport of equids from countries where AHSV occurs to virus-free areas is subject to strict regimens of testing and quarantine, although the precise requirements may vary from country to country. The presence of antibodies alone should not preclude such movements as long as AHSV is not present.

1.2. African Swine Fever (ASF)

Synonyms

African pig disease, Wart hog disease.

African swine fever (ASF) highly contagious, mostly acute, febrile disease of domestic swine with cyanosis of the skin hemorrhages of the lymph nodes, kidney, and gastrointestinal mucosa. African swine fever virus (ASFV) belonging to Iridovirus group. The ASFV is immunologically different from swine fever virus. The pigs immunized against swine fever are susceptible to ASF. Domestic pigs, Wart hogs, forest hogs and bush pigs are reservoirs. The virus can be cultivated in developing chicken embryo and tissue culture. Domestic pigs get the infection when they have close contact with the wild pigs. Virus is transmitted via aerosol. The virus is abundantly present in all the secretions and excretions of the affected pigs. The virus is also transmitted through ticks and lice. Mortality is usually 100 per cent in infected pigs. Recovered pigs are the carriers of disease. African Swine Fever (ASF) is a highly contagious hemorrhagic disease of pigs that produces a wide range of clinical signs and lesions that closely resemble those of Classical Swine Fever (CSF). It is an economically important disease that is enzootic in many African countries and the Mediterranean island, Sardinia. In June 2007, ASF was confirmed for the first time in Georgia in the Caucasus region. Since its introduction into Georgia, African Swine Fever Virus (ASFV) has spread rapidly into vast areas of western and southern Russia, where it is currently (2013) circulating out of control in domestic and wild pig populations. The virus has spread to the edges of Europe, with outbreaks reported in both the Ukraine and Belarus in 2013, putting at risk the very large pig populations present in Eastern Europe.

Etiology and Epidemiology

ASFV is a large, enveloped, double-stranded DNA virus that replicates primarily in cells of the mononuclear phagocytic system. It is currently classified as the only member of a family called African swine fever–like viruses (Asfarviridae). The prolonged period during which ASF has been an enzootic disease in Africa is likely to have led to the selection of viruses of varying virulence. Distinct genotypes of ASFV have been differentiated by sequence analysis of the genomes of viruses obtained from different geographic areas over a long time. The virus is highly resistant to a wide pH range and to a freeze/thaw cycle and can remain infectious for many months at room temperature or when stored at 4°C. Virus in body fluids and serum is inactivated in 30 min at 60°C, but virus in unprocessed pig meat, in which it can remain viable for several weeks, can be inactivated only by heating to 70°C for 30 min. Although ASFV can be adapted to grow in cells from different species, it does not replicate readily in any species other than swine.

The disease is limited to all breeds and types of domestic pigs and European wild boar. All age groups are equally susceptible. In Africa, the virus produces inapparent infection in two species of wild swine—warthog (*Phacochoerus aethiopicus*) and bush pig (*Potamochoerus porcus*)—and in the soft tick *Ornithodoros moubata*. When the disease was endemic in southern Spain and Portugal, a different species of soft tick, *O. erraticus*, became infected with the virus. Several other *Ornithodoros* spp. that are not usually associated with pigs or wild swine have been infected experimentally. ASF has been reported in a large number of countries in Africa south of the Sahara, either as an enzootic disease or as sporadic epidemics in domestic pigs. The first spread of the disease outside Africa was into Europe (Portugal) in 1957 as a result of waste from airline flights being fed to pigs near Lisbon airport. Although this incursion of disease was almost certainly eradicated, a further outbreak occurred in 1960 in Lisbon, and ASF then remained endemic in the Iberian Peninsula until the mid-1990s. Outbreaks of ASF were reported in a number of other European countries during the 20th century, including Malta (1978), Italy (1967, 1980), France (1964, 1967, 1977), Belgium (1985), and the Netherlands (1986). The disease was eradicated from each of these countries but has remained endemic in Sardinia since its introduction in 1978. During the 1970s, ASFV spread to the Caribbean and South America. An outbreak in south Brazil in 1978–1979 was eradicated by stamping out, and Brazil regained its ASF-free status in December 1984.

The spread of ASF out of Africa has been a relatively rare event, but in June 2007 ASF was confirmed in pigs in the former Soviet republic of Georgia in the Caucasus region. Genetic analysis revealed the genotype of the Georgia isolate to be closely related to isolates in circulation in Mozambique, Madagascar, and Zambia. It is therefore likely that pigs were fed ASFV-contaminated pig meat transported by ship from the southeastern part of Africa. By July 2007, the outbreak had spread to 56 of 61 districts in Georgia; soon after, outbreaks of ASF were reported in neighboring regions, including the autonomous republic of Abkhazia, Armenia, and Nagorno-Karabakh. Later in the year, infection of wild boar was confirmed in the Russian republic of Chechnya. In 2008, the spread of ASF continued into North Ossetia; it then jumped over 1,000 km into Orenburg, illustrating its potential for rapid spread over long distances. By October 2008, a total of 21 outbreaks of ASF had been officially reported in five Russian administrative divisions. From 2009–2013, the virus has continued to spread within the Russian Federation, and there are currently (Oct. 2013) two main expanding hotbeds of infection in Russia, one in the southern part of the center of the Rostov region (Oblast) and the other in the Tver region (Oblast) and the adjoining areas. In 2013, outbreaks of ASF were reported in both the Ukraine and Belarus, putting at risk large pig populations in Eastern Europe.

Clinical Signs

Incubation period is 5 to 15 days. Common signs are fever, depression, ocular discharge, cough, diarrhea and dehydration. Lesions resemble hog cholera but are more severe. Hemorrhages are present frequently on the epicardium and endocardium, and in lymph nodes, less frequently on the kidneys and bladder. The spleen is enlarged, but there are much less infarcts than in Hog cholera.

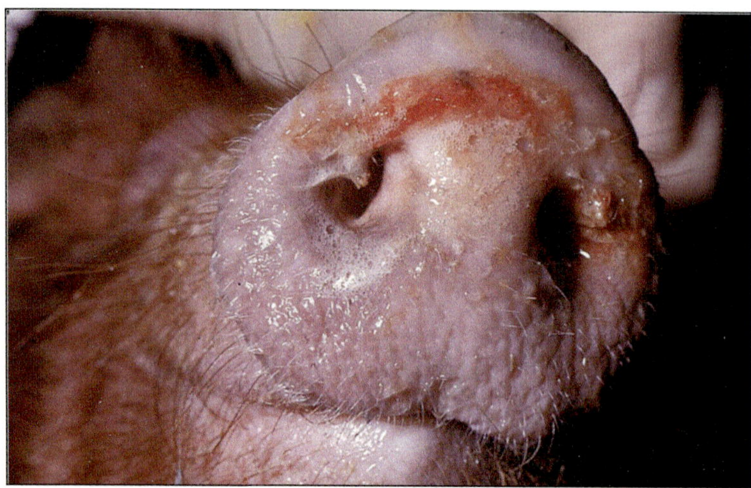

Figure 1.2. Bloody, mucoid, foamy nasal discharge of Pig.

Diagnosis

Samples of blood, spleen, lungs and lymph nodes to be collected; by characteristic clinical signs; isolation of virus in cell culture – bone marrow leucocytes cells; serological tests *viz.*, AGID, ELISA, Radio mmune assay.

Differential Diagnosis

Must be differentiated from, Hog cholera, Erysipelas and Salmonellosis.

Control

There is no treatment for ASF, and all attempts to develop a vaccine have so far been unsuccessful. Prevention depends on ensuring that neither infected live pigs nor pig meat products are introduced into areas free of ASF. All successful eradication programs have involved the rapid diagnosis, slaughter, and disposal of all animals on infected premises. Sanitary measures must also be applied and include control of movement and treatment of waste food. Subsequently, a serologic survey of all pig farms within a specific control zone must be conducted to ensure that all infected pigs have been identified.

1.3. Classical Swine Fever (CSF)

Synonyms

Hog Cholera, Swine Fever, Peste du Porc, Colera Porcina, Virusschweinepest.

Classical swine fever is a contagious, often fatal, disease of pigs clinically characterized by high body temperature, lethargy, yellowish diarrhea, vomiting, and a purple skin discoloration of the ears, lower abdomen, and legs. It was first described in the early 19th century in the USA. Later, a condition in Europe termed "swine fever" was recognized to be the same disease. Both names continue to be used, although in most of the world the disease is now called classical swine fever (CSF) to distinguish it from African swine fever, which is a clinically indistinguishable disease but caused by an unrelated DNA virus. Because of the severe economic impact of CSF, outbreaks are notifiable to the OIE. CSF has the potential to cause devastating epidemics, particularly in countries free of the disease. In these countries, vaccination is allowed only under emergency circumstances. In case of a new outbreak, strict measures are enforced to control spread, *e.g.*, culling of infected and disease suspect herds and strict movement restrictions. This can have severe consequences for the swine industry, especially in densely populated livestock areas. Awareness and vigilance are essential, so that outbreaks are detected early and control measures instituted rapidly to prevent further spread of CSF. The "high risk period," *i.e.*, the time between introduction of the virus and detection of the outbreak, must be kept as short as possible.

Highly contagious viral disease of pigs of all ages, characterized by rapid and sudden onset, high mortality and morbidity with generalized hemorrhages of internal organs. This disease is caused by pantropic RNA virus belonging to the genus Pesti virus, family Flaviviridae. The virus is closely related to Bovine viral diarrhea virus. The disease was widespread in South African countries, Europe, China and Japan and prevalent in moderate to severe proportion in India, Myanmar, Nepal, Pakistan, Bangladesh and Philippines. In India this disease was first reported in West Bengal in the year 1961. Swine are the natural host of the virus. All breeds, sex and ages of pigs are susceptible to this infection. Wild pigs often remain as inapparent carrier of the virus. Young pigs are more susceptible than the adult pigs. Infection is transmitted readily by direct and indirect contact. The virus is usually acquired by ingestion of food and water contaminated with discharges and secretions from infected pig. Urine and nasal and ocular discharges are generally regarded as most infective. The isolation of CSFV should be attempted in the pig kidney (PK-15) cell line, or other suitable cell lines.

Etiology and Epidemiology

CSF is caused by a small, enveloped RNA virus in the genus *Pestivirus* of the family Flaviviridae. Classical swine fever virus (CSFV) is antigenically related to the other pestiviruses, mainly to bovine viral diarrhea virus (BVDV) of cattle and to border disease virus (BDV) of sheep. These viruses are highly prevalent in bovine and ovine populations and can infect pigs. Although infections of pigs with ruminant pestiviruses in most cases do not lead to clinical disease and are rapidly cleared, infections with both BVDV and BVD induce an antibody response in swine. Therefore, antibody discrimination tests must be applied to differentiate CSF infections from infections caused by ruminant pestiviruses. Transmission of ruminant pestiviruses to pigs usually requires direct contact with cattle, sheep, or goats. CSFV naturally infects members of the Suidae family, *i.e*, domestic and wild pigs.

In the laboratory, CSFV is cultured in cells of porcine origin, notably in the PK-15 cell line (porcine kidney), but does not generally cause a visible cytopathic effect. The virus has only one serotype, although some minor antigenic variability between strains is seen. Strains can be typed for epidemiologic mapping purposes by sequencing the entire viral genome or specific regions of the viral genome (*i.e.*, 52UTR, E2, and NS5B regions) combined with phylogenetic analysis.

CSFV is moderately fragile and does not persist in the environment or spread long distances by the airborne route. However, it can survive for prolonged periods in a moist, protein-rich environment such as pork tissues or body fluids, particularly if kept cold or frozen. Virus survival times up to several years have been observed in frozen pork meat. CSFV may also survive months in chilled or cured cuts.

CSF has a worldwide distribution. It is considered endemic in certain countries of Central and South America, in the Caribbean basin, and in many pork-producing countries in Asia. Australia, New Zealand, Canada, and the USA are free of the disease, as well as most countries of western and central Europe, although sporadic outbreaks occur in Europe. CSF is considered endemic in several countries in Eastern Europe. The main source of CSFV infection is the pig, either via infected live animals or via uncooked pork products. In areas where CSF is endemic, the major concern relates to the spread of disease through movement of infected animals, which may lead to widespread outbreaks, particularly in areas where there is large-scale transport of pigs among farms or to slaughter houses. In Europe, CSFV is considered endemic in wild boar populations, and infected wild boars are a source for CSF outbreaks among domestic pigs. However, the most probable source of CSFV infection for wild boars is contaminated garbage or even "spillover" from infected domestic pigs. The outcome of such infections mainly depends on the size and density of the wild boar populations affected. Outbreaks in small populations of wild boars living within natural confines, such as valleys, tend to be self-limiting, and the disease fades away over time. In contrast, infections leading to outbreaks in large areas densely populated with wild boars often become endemic.

Another major risk for CSF outbreaks is the accidental introduction of CSFV into herds through illegally imported pork meat or pork products that often find their way into the porcine food chain via swill feeding. However, CSFV is readily inactivated by heat (*i.e*, cooking), which emphasizes the importance of enforcing regulations for heat treatment of swill feed. In addition, many countries have completely banned swill feeding practices.

Mechanical transmission by vehicles and equipment, as well as by personnel (notably veterinarians) travelling between pig farms, are also significant means of spread of CSF within infected areas. The persistence of CSFV within herds for long periods has been observed. Infections of sows during pregnancy with low to moderately virulent strains of CSFV may lead to in utero infections of eroxidi. These infections lead to litters born persistently infected with CSFV that are carriers of the virus and source for new infections. Persistently infected carrier pigs usually do not show clinical signs but constantly shed CSFV into the environment. Therefore, it is particularly important to consider CSFV infections while investigating herds presenting with unexplained reproductive failures that include clinical manifestations in piglets such as congenital tremor or congenital abnormalities.

Clinical Manifestations

Incubation period is 3-8 days; the disease may appear in three clinical forms;

(a) **Per acute form**: Most commonly noticed in young pigs, disease terminates fatally within about 24 hours of developing disease, no appreciable clinical manifestations except high raise of temperature and erythematous patches in the non-hairy parts of the skin.

(b) **Acute form:** Sharp rise of body temperature, temperature reaction may persist up to 8th day or till death, dullness, depression, anorexia, vomition, constipation, severe foul smelling eroxidi, dehydration and loss of body weight. Hyperemia of the skin with purplish discoloration of snout, ears, abdomen, inner side of the legs, a peculiar blotching effect on the ears, small areas vesicular lesions followed by necrotic lesions on the edges of the ears, tail, lips and vulva. Mucopurulent to purulent discharges from eyes with signs of conjunctivitis, severely affected pigs may suck urine and water due to obvious temperature reaction and dehydration. Central nervous system may be affected; the signs are wobbling gait, ataxia, tremor, convulsion, paralysis, circling, tremor and coma. Reproductive disorders in sows due to low virulent strain with signs of fever and birth of mummified, still birth, abnormal piglets.

(c) **Chronic form:** Chronic diarrhea, chronic pneumonia, gross lesions, degeneration of small blood vessels leading to hemorrhages in kidney, bladder, skin and lymph nodes. Circular or oval raised button ulcers are most prevalent in caecum and proximal portion of the colon. Turkey egg appearance of kidney is the pathognomonic lesion of the disease.

Diagnosis

CSF is first detected by veterinarians in the field. Because clinical signs manifested by CSFV-infected pigs are also seen with other diseases of swine, laboratory confirmation is always required. Clinically, the differential diagnosis varies according to the course of the disease, and primarily includes African swine fever. Hemorrhagic lesions must also be distinguished from those seen in porcine dermatitis and nephropathy syndrome and postweaning multisystemic wasting syndrome. Hemolytic disease of the newborn, porcine reproductive and respiratory syndrome, Aujeszky disease, parvovirus, thrombocytopenic purpura, anticoagulant poisoning (*e.g.*, warfarin), and salt poisoning should also be considered as possible differential diagnoses. Septicemic diseases, including salmonellosis, erysipelas, pasteurellosis, actinobacillosis, *Haemophilus suis* infections, and eperythrozoonosis may resemble CSF. Congenital infections with ruminant pestiviruses can resemble CSF reproductive failures caused by low virulence strains of CSFV. Poor reproductive performance in sows can also be associated with pseudorabies, parvovirus, and other eroxidiseous causes.

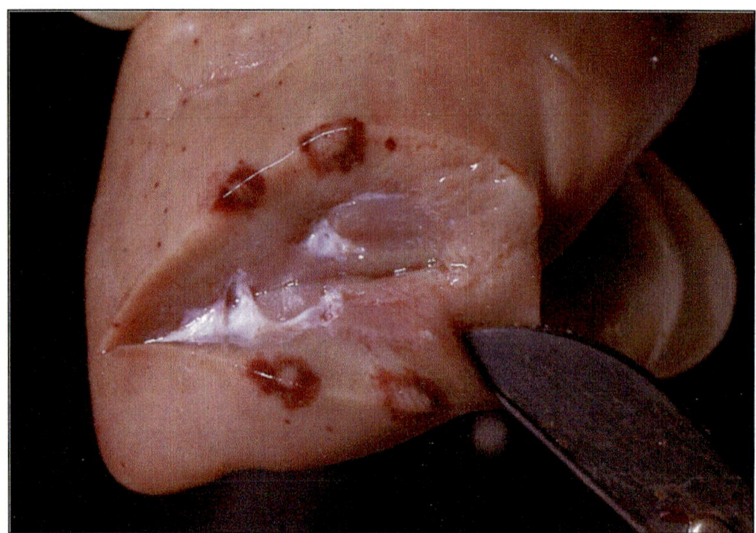

Figure 1.3. Pig. Kidney, the cortex contains multiple petechiae and pale infarcts surrounded by hemorrhage.

Virologic tests are essential to confirm the diagnosis of CSF. Advice on sample submission should be sought from the laboratory. Suitable tissues to detect the presence of the virus are tonsils, lymph nodes (mandibular, retropharyngeal, gastrohepatic, and mesenteric), spleen, kidney, and ileum. Whole blood collected with EDTA as anticoagulant can be used for virus isolation or virus detection, particularly during the viremic phase of the infection. Clotted blood samples (serum) are taken when serologic tests for detection of CSFV antibodies are pursued. Nasal swabs and/or tonsil scrapings are commonly collected clinical samples used to detect the virus (*i.e.*, viral RNA).

Significant amounts of CSFV are shed from infected animals into the environment via the oronasal route, particularly early during infection. Detection of CSFV antigen can be performed using direct immunofluorescence on frozen tissue sections, particularly in tonsil samples using specific antibodies. Antigen detection can also be done using ELISA; however, this assay has low sensitivity and is only useful for screening for the presence of CSFV at the herd level. More commonly, viral nucleic acid detection is done using reverse transcriptase (RT)-PCR. The assay is highly specific and can differentiate CSFV from BVDV and BDV. Standardized methods such as RT-PCR can be scaled up to screen large numbers of samples, giving rapid results while retaining high sensitivity. This is particularly useful to screen herds during an outbreak of CSF.

For virus isolation, cell cultures are inoculated with tissue suspensions or WBCs, fixed after 2–3 days, and the virus is detected using specific antibodies directed against CSFV (*e.g.*, fluorescent or enzymatic methods). Final results may not be available for 4–7 days. This method is labor intensive and time consuming. Virus characterization using virus-specific monoclonal antibodies or RT-PCR is performed to differentiate CSFV from the other pestiviruses. Positive results of antigen detection or virus isolation are not confirmed until virus identification is completed. Virus neutralization tests and ELISA tests are available to detect antibodies against CSFV. Because the virus is noncytopathogenic in culture, the neutralization test requires an additional immunostaining step to reveal the presence of neutralizing antibodies. ELISA tests are suitable for large-scale serology when large number of samples is processed, *i.e*, for surveillance purposes. Cross-reactions between pestivirus antibodies are seen in diagnostic tests. The presence of antibodies against ruminant pestiviruses in pigs may hamper the serologic diagnosis of CSF. BVDV or BDV-specific antibodies are sporadically detected in pig populations. Risk factors related with ruminant pestivirus antibodies in pigs are associated with the presence of cattle on the same farm and high density of sheep and/or goats in the area. Some commercial ELISAs can distinguish CSF from BVDV or BDV antibodies, although confirmatory testing is advised usually via neutralizing eroxidise-linked assays.

New generations of CSFV marker vaccines have been developed to make emergency vaccination compatible with control of CSF. The application of a marker vaccine is possible if tests such as ELISA can distinguish between antibodies produced in response to a natural infection and those produced by vaccination. This is the DIVA principle (differentiation of infected from vaccinated animals) that is based on detection of CSFV-specific antibodies that develop in the host only with CSFV infection but not on vaccination with a marker vaccine. These assays have been developed as necessary companion tests for CSF marker vaccines.

Control

CSF is a notifiable disease. Control is usually strictly regulated by local laws that establish strict sanitary measures. No treatment is available. Outbreaks in countries free of CSF are controlled rapidly via culling of infected animals and preemptive slaughter of susceptible animals within determined distances from the focus. Restriction of movement within a well-defined radius from the outbreak is applied to contain spread of the infection. Eventually, emergency vaccination can be authorized to control the further spread of CSFV. Countries will regain their CSF-free status (no antibodies or virus detected) after establishing that CSFV is no longer present in the national pig herd. Countries free of CSF usually implement preventive measures to avoid outbreaks of CSF by controlling movement of live animals and pork products at borders. Countries free of CSF forbid the use of prophylactic vaccination. In countries where CSF is endemic, prophylactic vaccination is regularly practiced and is mandatory in some cases. Prophylactic vaccination has been used worldwide as a tool to control and eradicate CSF. In these countries, herds affected by an outbreak are quarantined and if possible eliminated. Emergency ring vaccination around the outbreak is done to prevent further spread of CSFV. CSF live attenuated vaccines are safe and highly efficient, being able to induce protection shortly after vaccination (within 3 days after vaccination). Several live attenuated vaccines, such as the Chinese lapinized vaccine (C-strain), the Japanese GPE-strain, and the French Thiverval strain, have been developed and used in different countries. More recently, subunit CSFV vaccines containing only the major viral surface glycoprotein of the virus have been licensed. Although these vaccines have DIVA capabilities, they lack the efficiency of live attenuated vaccines. Oral vaccination of wild boars has been used successfully within the European Union using a live attenuated vaccine delivered via baits. Oral vaccination has been a key strategy to control CSF, particularly where parenteral vaccine delivery is not feasible.

1.4. Aujeskey Disease

Synonyms

Aujeszky's disease, Mad itch, Infectious bulbar paralysis

Pseudorabies is an acute, frequently fatal disease with a worldwide distribution that affects swine primarily and other domestic and wild animals incidentally. The pseudorabies virus has emerged as a significant pathogen in the USA since the 1960s, probably because of the increase in confinement swine housing or perhaps because of the emergence of more virulent strains. Clinical signs in nonporcine animals are similar to those of rabies, hence the name "mad itch" (pigs do not display this sign). Pseudorabies is a reportable disease and has been successfully eradicated from the vast majority of the USA.

This disease is caused by the DNA virus belongs to the alpha-herpesvirinae subfamily, family Herpes viridae and is distributed worldwide. It infects a wide range of natural hosts including mammals and birds. Rodents and pigs are the primary hosts of the virus. This disease is reported world-wide except in few countries including Australia, Canada and Norway. The disease is prevalent in cattle, sheep, goat, pig, horses, dog, cat and mink. Pigs are considered as reservoir host for this virus. The disease is prevalent in pigs all round the year. Pigs may remain as asymptomatic immune carrier and thus may act as a source of infection to other species of animals. The natural way of entry of virus is through a breach in the continuity of skin or integument due to injury, bite or abrasions. Virus may enter through inhalation as aerosol way of transmission. The virus can be grown in susceptible cell line such as porcine kidney (PK-15) or SK6, or primary or secondary kidney cells.

Clinical Manifestations

- ☆ **Cattle:** Incubation period- 3-6 days. Pyrexia along with pruritus starts at the site of entry of virus. Pruritus mostly observed in the nose, eyes, ears, lower jaw, chest or in the udder, limbs, flanks and anal region. Involvement of central nervous system- tremor, continuous or intermittent chewing movements of jaws, profuse salivation and sweating, excitement, bellowing, roll up and down, stumping on the ground, aimless staggering, aggressiveness and circling.

- ☆ **Pigs:** All ages may be affected but very young pigs are more susceptible than older ones. Changes in the respiratory, nervous and reproductive systems. High rise of temperature, with development of nervous signs. Incoordination develops in the posterior limbs which force the animal to move sideways. Muscle tremors and paddling movements, tilting of head, froth at the commissure of mouth, nystagmus, ocular discharge and convulsion, Vomition, diarrhea, signs of blindnesslu.
- ☆ **Sheep, dog, goat, cat and horses:** Similar to that of cattle.
- ☆ **Dogs and cats**: fatal disease where death is eminent within 2 days following manifestation of clinical signs.

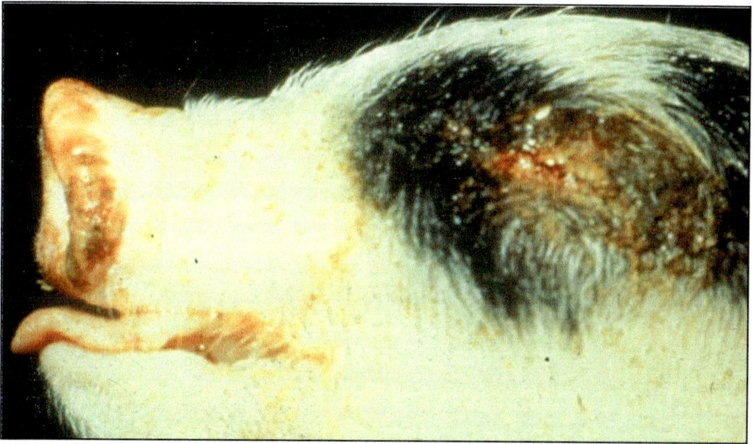

Figure 1.4. Pig head. The mucosal membranes around the eye and nares are crusted and the eye has periorbital serous eexudates.

Lesions

Congestion of meninges, brain, haemorrhage, odema and necrosis of lungs, focal necrosis of liver.

Diagnosis

In addition to the gross and microscopic lesions, other diagnostic aids include virus isolation, fluorescent antibody testing, and serologic testing. Brain, spleen, and lung are the organs of choice for virus isolation. Nasal swabs can be used for isolation of virus from acutely infected animals. The nasal specimens must be stored and transported in cold, sterile saline with antibiotics to suppress bacterial growth. The fluorescent antibody test can be performed using tonsil or brain.

Many serologic tests are now available, including serum neutralization, ELISA, and latex agglutination. Serum neutralization, which is the standard test, requires 48 hr to complete. An ELISA has been developed as a screening assay for large volumes of sera; however, specificity may be poor. False-positive results are typically reassessed using the serum neutralization test. The latex agglutination test, although highly sensitive and rapid, may also have poor specificity. After infection, antibodies can be detected within 6–7 days using the latex agglutination test, within 7–8 days using the ELISA, and within 8–10 days using the serum neutralization test. A differential ELISA has been used to differentiate antibodies produced as a result of vaccination from those produced as a result of natural infection. The vaccines used in swine are based on the deletion of certain genes (gI, gIII, or gX) from the vaccine virus. Swine vaccinated with a gene-deleted vaccine do not mount an antibody response to the protein coded for by the deleted gene. In contrast, infection with field virus results in antibodies against these proteins. Colostral antibodies to pseudorabies virus may be present until pigs are 4 month old (similar to porcine parvovirus). Therefore, paired samples or serologic profiles may be necessary in grower and finisher pigs to assess decreasing levels of maternal antibody and to ensure that pigs are vaccinated at the appropriate time.

Differential Diagnosis

Rabies - no pruritus, biting tendency, dropped jaw, ascending paralysis, demonstration of negri bodies in the neurons of hippocampus and purkinje cells of the cerebellum. Listeriosis - history of intake of silage, facial paralysis. Polyencephalomalacia- history of carbohydrate engorgement, no pyrexia. Poisoning- specific signs depending on the source of poison. Gastric content analysis to pin-point the toxin.

Treatment and Control

Although there is no specific treatment for acute infection with pseudorabies virus, vaccination can alleviate clinical signs in pigs of certain ages. Typically, mass vaccination of all pigs on the farm with a modified-live virus vaccine is recommended. Intranasal vaccination of sows and neonatal piglets 1–7 days old, followed by IM vaccination of all other swine on the premises, helps reduce viral shedding and improve survival. The modified-live virus replicates at the site of injection and in regional lymph nodes. Vaccine virus is shed in such low levels that mucus transmission to other animals is minimal. In gene-deleted vaccines, the thymidine kinase gene has also been deleted; thus, the virus cannot infect and replicate in neurons. It is recommended that breeding herds be vaccinated quarterly and that finisher pigs be vaccinated after levels of maternal antibody decrease. Regular vaccination results in excellent control of the disease. Concurrent antibiotic therapy via feed and IM injection is recommended to control secondary bacterial pathogens.

Numerous programs have been developed for eradication of pseudorabies virus. As of 2014, all 50 states in the USA were considered free of the disease in commercial pigs; however, the virus appeared to be endemic in feral pig populations and had been identified on game ranches. Effective strategies for eradication of pseudorabies include whole-herd depopulation, a test and removal strategy, and offspring segregation. Although effective, whole-herd depopulation is costly and time consuming. Usually, problems other than pseudorabies virus (*e.g.*, genetic improvement) need to be resolved before whole-herd depopulation can be cost effective.

The test and removal strategy consists of blood testing all breeding swine, culling all positive animals, and repeating this procedure until the population tests negative. Naturally infected animals can be culled when such a strategy is used in conjunction with a differential vaccination program. A test and removal strategy can be effective, but it is laborious, and latently infected animals that do not exhibit an antibody response on serologic testing may potentially resume shedding the virus at a later time.

In an offspring segregation program, young piglets (18–21 days old) are removed from vaccinated sows and raised to adulthood at another site. If enough gilts and boars are raised in this manner, the original breeding herd may be depopulated and subsequently repopulated with seronegative replacements. This method also allows seedstock producers to sell animals, even though the breeding herd is infected. In this case, however, all offspring must be individually tested using the serum neutralization test and have negative results before being sold.

1.5. Avian Encephalomyelitis (AE)

Synonym

Epidemic Tremor.

Avian encephalomyelitis (AE) is a viral disease of young chickens, turkeys, Japanese quail, pheasants, and pigeons. Turkeys are less susceptible to natural infection and generally develop a milder clinical disease than chickens. Ducklings and guinea fowl are susceptible to experimental infection. AE is characterized by neurologic signs that result from infection of the CNS with an RNA virus in the family Picornaviridae. Infection occurs via vertical and horizontal transmission. If a breeder flock becomes infected during egg production, the virus is vertically transmitted to the offspring and a major outbreak occurs. The disease often appears in a series of flocks hatched from the infected breeder flock. Field strains of the virus are enterotropic and multiply in the intestine. Infected birds shed the virus in their feces for a few days to a few weeks, which serve to spread the infection to hatchmates. There is no convincing evidence that the virus persists in infected birds. AE virus is resistant to environmental conditions and may remain infectious for long periods.

Avian encephalomyelitis is an acute viral disease of very young chickens (1-21 days) characterized by nervous signs of ataxia, paralysis, tremors in head and neck. Avian encephalomyelitis virus (AEV) is not pathogenic to older chicken even though affected most flocks show no clinical signs of the disease other than a drop in egg production, which is transitory and passed unnoticed. This disease was first described in the New England states of the U.S.A. in 1932 and is now recognized worldwide. In addition to chicken this disease has also been recorded in pheasants, quail and turkeys. Avian encephalomyelitis caused by avian entero virus belongs to the family Picornaviridae. This virus is resistant to lipid solvent, acid pH, trypsin and pepsin. The virus is able to survive very well at ambient temperature. Formaldehyde fumigation is effectively inactivating AEV with an 18 hrs exposure period. Only a single antigenic type but strains vary in virulence. This virus grows very well in yolk sac route of embryonated chicken eggs, chicken embryo fibroblast and chicken embryo kidney cell culture. This disease is an enteric infection and affected chicks shed the virus in the faeces for about 2 weeks. The virus is live in litter material for longer time. Horizontal spread by fomites occurs. Vertical transmission is a very important mode of transmission. Breeder hens get infected. A proportion of the eggs of infected hens are infected. Chicks infected *in ovo* hatch normally but shed virus in their droppings and infect other chicks in the incubator shortly after hatching.

Clinical Manifestations

Incubation period is 1-7 days. Affected chicks exhibit dullness, depression, progressive ataxia, tremors in head and neck and weight loss. They fall on one side or sit back on their hocks or refuse to move. Blindness, paralysis, prostration and coma also occur. Death is mainly due to affected chicks not able to take feed and get trampling by pen mates.

Lesions

No gross lesions are seen in the brain of infected birds. Gray to white foci may be visible on cut surfaces of the muscle of the gizzard. Weeks after infection, opacity of eye lenses (cataracts) may occur in a small percentage of chickens that survive the infection. Microscopic lesions in the CNS are found in the brain (cerebral peduncle, cerebellum, brain stem) and spinal cord and consist of degeneration and necrosis of neurons, perivascular lymphocytic cuffing, and gliosis with formation of glial nodules. In the cerebellum, there are areas of necrosis or loss of Purkinje cells and replacement by glial nodules that extend into the molecular layer of the gray matter. Neuronal lesions of central chromatolysis, shrinkage and increased basophilia, satellitosis, and neuronophagia are best found in neuron clusters (nuclei) in the brain stem, rbour vitae of the cerebellum, and lateral horn (gray matter) of the spinal cord. Central chromatolysis of neurons is characterized by rounding of the cell contour and displacement of Nissl granules to the periphery. Dorsal root ganglia have multifocal nodular collections of lymphocytes. A common microscopic lesion outside the CNS is diffuse or nodular lymphocytic infiltrates in the gizzard muscle, muscular layer of the esophagus and proventriculus, myocardium, and pancreas. Except for cataracts, microscopic lesions generally are not found in infected adults unless they are showing nervous signs, in which case they will have CNS lesions similar to those in young birds.

Diagnosis

Diagnosis is based on history, clinical signs, and characteristic histopathologic lesions in the brain and spinal cord. The diagnosis is best confirmed by isolation and identification of the virus. Tissues collected for virus isolation must include the brain and duodenum with the pancreas. Demonstration of AE virus antigen in the brain, spinal cord, and other tissues by immunofluorescent and immunohistochemical staining is a reliable method of diagnosis. The major differential diagnosis for

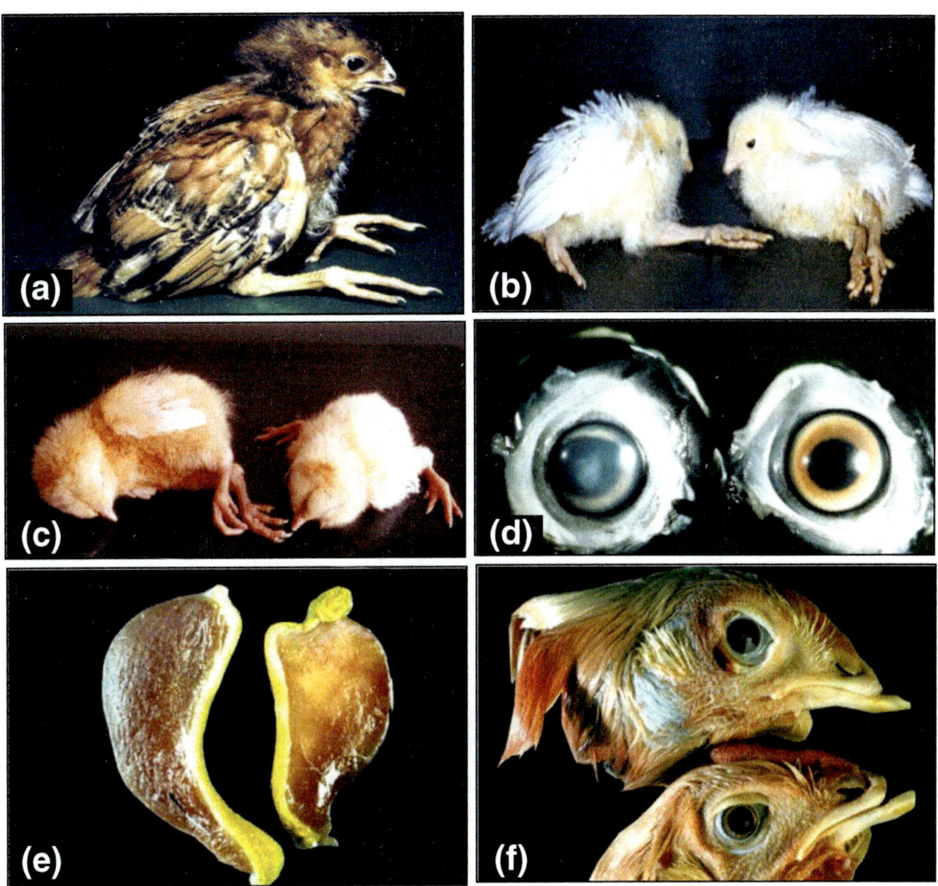

Figure 1.5

(a) Hock slitting posture- Avian encephalomyelitis; (b) Neurological signs-Avian encephalomyelitis; (c) Paralysis and prostration- Avian encephalomyelitis; (d) Extensive cataract- Avian encephalomyelitis; (e) Extensive ventriculitis- Avian encephalomyelitis; (f) Cataract- Avian encephalomyelitis.

neurologic signs in very young chicks is bacterial or mycotic encephalitis. Rickets and nutritional encephalomalacia are next in the list of differential diagnoses, although the clinical manifestations of these diseases differ from those in AE. In adults, serologic testing of acute and convalescent sera to demonstrate an increase in antibody titers helps establish a diagnosis.

Serological Tests

Some of them are FAT, AGID, ELISA, IPT and virus neutralization test. At the age of 18dayold, all the (100 per cent) embryos exhibit paralysis and severe muscular dystrophy. Differential diagnosis should be made with New Castle disease.

Control

Depopulation, attenuated live-virus vaccine administered in the drinking water to be administered after chickens reaches 10 wks of age or 4 weeks before laying-Passive immunization. High levels of maternal antibodies protect the chicks up to 21 days. Inactivated vaccine may also be used.

1.6. Avian Leukosis

Synonyms

Avian sarcoma, Big liver disease, visceral lymphoid leukosis, lymphomatosis.

Under natural conditions, lymphoid leukosis has been the most common form of the leukosis/sarcoma group of diseases seen in chicken flocks, although in the 1990s myeloid leukosis become prevalent in meat-type chickens. The International Committee on Taxonomy of Viruses placed viruses of the avian leukosis/sarcoma group in the *Alpharetrovirus* genus of the family Retroviridae. Members of this RNA group of viruses have similar physical and molecular characteristics and share a common group-specific antigen. Detection of the major antigen present in the core of leukosis/sarcoma viruses forms the basis of several diagnostic tests. Lymphoid leukosis occurs naturally only in chickens. Experimentally, some of the viruses of the leukosis/sarcoma group can infect and produce tumors in other species of birds or even mammals. The infection is known to exist in virtually all chicken flocks except for some SPF flocks from which it has been eradicated. Tumor mortality commonly accounts for ~1 per cent –2 per cent of birds, with occasional losses of dikhuaaa 20 per cent. Subclinical infection, to which most flocks are subject, decreases several important performance traits, including egg production and quality. The frequency of infection has been reduced substantially in the primary breeding stocks of several commercial poultry breeding companies, particularly egg-type breeders. In recent years this control program has expanded, and infection has become infrequent or absent in certain commercial flocks. The frequency of lymphoid leukosis tumors even in heavily infected flocks is typically low (<4 per cent), and disease is often inapparent. As much as 1.5 per cent excess mortality per wk has been reported in commercial broiler-breeder flocks naturally infected with subgroup Javian leukosis virus.

Avian leukosis is an infectious cancerous condition of the mature birds involving the haemopoietic and lymphoid tissues like liver, bursa, spleen, gonads, kidneys bones, *etc.* The avian leukosis group of viruses (ALGV) is comprised of 10 subgroups, A to J, based on differences in envelope glycoproteins. Subgroups A to E, and J viruses infect chickens. The other subgroup viruses occur in quail, partridges and pheasants. Subgroup 'A' viruses cause most outbreaks of avian leukosis that manifest as a lymphoid leukosis, a B cell lymphoma. This is the most important and common neoplasm associated with the disease. Viruses of subgroup J have been associated with myeloid leukosis in broilers. Most of the viruses causing avian leukosis are exogenous. Endogenous ALGVs, which mostly belong to subgroup E and occur commonly in chickens and other avian species, are of little or no pathogenicity. These proviral DNA sequences are integrated into germ line cells and are thus transmitted vertically. Avian leukosis viruses occur commonly in chickens, quail, partridges and pheasants worldwide and the disease is of great economic importance. Although transmission may occur by contact, as virus is present in feces and saliva, the principle means of transmission is via the egg. Blood-sucking parasites are potential vectors. Endogenous viruses, which are common in the chicken but not important as causes of leukosis, are also transmitted genetically in the germ line from parent to offspring.

Diagnosis

Plasma, serum, tumours, whole bird with extremities, visceral organs (liver, kidney, spleen), oral washings, faeces. Based on clinical signs and gross and histopathologic lesions, but lymphoid leukosis may be confused with the acute form in older birds. Differential features, nodular tumors in the bursa of fabricius as opposed to diffuse enlargement with Marek's disease; intrafollicular cell proliferation in the bursa of fabricius as opposed to interfollicular cell proliferation with Marek's disease; and the cytologic appearance of lymphoid cells that are uniformly "blast" cells with lymphoid leukosis but a mixture of mature and immature pleomorphic cells with Marek's disease. Isolation of the virus or the demonstration of antibody is not considered to be of value in diagnosis because avian leukosis group viruses are ubiquitous in chickens.

Prevention

There is no vaccine available and eradication is the preferred method of control. Since the viruses are primarily transmitted via the egg, virus infected breeders are detected by testing the egg albumin for viral antigen by an ELISA method. Positive birds are eliminated. ELISA and Immunofluorescence assays are used to detect antibodies in serum and egg yolk. Most commercial flocks of chickens are now free of exogenous ALG viruses. Some birds are genetically more resistant to fowl leukosis; they have decreased numbers of specific cell surface viral receptors. Incubators should be clean and adequately disinfected. Control blood-sucking parasites.

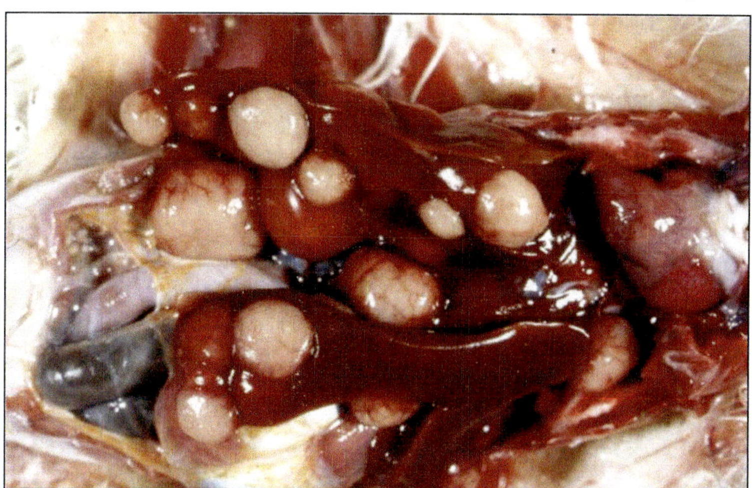

Figure 1.6. Avian Leukosis.

Clinical Manifestations

All avian leukemia group viruses are oncogenic, except those belonging to subgroup E. The mechanisms involved in the development of neoplasia by viruses, that is, oncogenesis. Such factors as genetics (autosomally transmitted susceptibility or resistant avian cells) and the age and sex of the host can also be important in the development of tumors. The incubation period is variable and may be as long as months or years. Viruses of subgroups A through D are associated with a variety of neoplastic conditions in chickens, including lymphoid leukosis, erythroblastosis, myeloblastosis, myleocytoblastosis, osteopetrosis and nephroblast

1.7. Blue Tongue (BT)

Synonyms

Sore mouth or sore muzzle, ovine catarrhal fever. Malignant head catarrh, Snotsiekte, Catarrhal fever, Gangrenous coryza.

Bluetongue (BT) is an orbiviral disease of wild and domestic ruminants, mainly sheep. In Sicily, the first Bluetongue outbreak occurred in October 2000; there have been 76 recorded outbreaks so far. The National Surveillance Plan, based on European Union Commission Decision 138/2001/CE, establishes serological and entomological surveys. This plan consists of controls of seronegative cattle, called 'sentry' as indicators for the presence and circulation of virus in defined areas. Malignant catarrhal fever (MCF) is an infectious systemic disease that presents as a variable complex of lesions affecting mainly ruminants and rarely swine. It is principally a disease of domestic cattle, water buffalo, Bali cattle (banteng), American bison, and deer. In addition to these farmed animals, MCF has been described in a variety of captive ruminants in mixed zoologic collections. In some species, such as bison and some deer, MCF is acute and highly lethal, capable of affecting large numbers of animals. With occasional exceptions, the disease in cattle normally is seen sporadically and affects single animals. MCF is typically fatal; however, there are outbreaks in which several animals are affected, with evidence of recovery and mild or inapparent infections in some cases. It also occasionally presents as chronic alopecia and weight loss. Its distribution is essentially worldwide, mirroring that of the principal carriers, domestic sheep and wildebeest. MCF has long been a major problem in farmed deer operations and in recent years has emerged as a severe threat to the commercial bison industry.

Blue tongue (BT) is an infectious, non-contagious acute arthropod borne virus, primarily affecting sheep characterized by catarrhal inflammation of the mucous membrane of buccal mucosa and gastrointestinal tract. This disease frequently involves the udder, coronary band of the foot and sensitive laminae of the hoof. There is epithelial desquamation but no vesicle formation occurs. Blue tongue virus (BTV) is the double stranded RNA virus, species of the *Orbi* virus genus, family Reoviridae. The disease first recognized in Africa and reported from Canada, Japan, Australia, Brazil, West Indies, USA, Egypt, Israel, Cyprus, and in some other countries. This disease first reported in India in 1964. The distribution of the disease is dependent on the presences of reservoir and amplifying host such as cattle and on suitable species of *Culicoides* being present in large numbers to effect transmission to sheep. It is basically a disease of sheep but amongst sheep susceptibility varies in different age groups.Young sheep within the age group of one year are more prone to infection. Goats, cattle and wild ruminants exhibit milder symptoms and may act as non-clinical carriers. Horses, dogs, cats, ferrets, rabbits and guinea pigs are not susceptible to natural infection. The disease spread through blood sucking midges of the genus *Culicoides*. Besides mosquitoes and other ectoparasites like sheep ked, *Melophagus ovinus*, may transmit the disease mechanically. Wild animal reservoirs play an important role in maintaining the infection during the interepizootic period. Stress factors like lower plane of nutrition, worm burden, inclement weather, and fatigue due to transportation are predisposing factors for the disease. Blue tongue virus can most readily be identified isolated by inoculating into a 10-12 days old embryonated chicken eggs. Primary isolation can only achieved by inoculating the suspected materials into intracerebral inoculation of new-born mice or in monolayer cell cultures such as BHK-21, mouse L cells, vero cells.

Clinical Manifestations

Incubation period one week. The disease has been arbitrarily divided into three forms.

(a) **Acute form**: High rise of temperature, nasal discharge, salivation and lacrymation. Hyperemia, Petechiation and swelling of the buccal mucosa, dental pads and tongue. Later hyperaemic regions become "cyanotic" or "purplish blue." Extensive necrosis of the dental pad, Muzzle turns dry show burnt appearance, Cyanotic and bluish appearance of tongue. Blood stained diarrhoea occurs when the intestinal mucosa is involved which is always fatal. There may be involvement of sensitive laminae and breaking of wool fibres. Heavy mortality occurs in early stages and chronically affected animals become thin and emaciated. Morbidity is 50 per cent.

(b) **Subacute form or subclinical form:** Common in cattle and generally passed unnoticed.

(c) **Abortive form**: Abortion of pregnant ewes, which results in the loss of entire breeding season. Young animals and Merino sheep are particularly susceptible.

Lesions

Blue Tongue and gangrenous, Legs shows coronary band show congestion and hemorrhage, Lungs show pneumonic changes.

Diagnosis

Based on history, clinical findings, and seasonal occurrence. Samples to be collected -unclotted blood from febrile animals or fresh spleen and lymph node collected at post mortem. Virus isolation in unweaned mice or growing in susceptible cell cultures or in embryonated eggs (i/v or yolk sac routes). The virus propagated in primary cultures of calf kidney, adrenal and testis, HeLa cell cultures and also

BHK21. CPE within 24-72 hours, which consists of foci of enlarged and retractile cells. Other tests – CFT, SNT, Plaque inhibition test, Microgel diffusion test, FAT, AGID, ELISA.

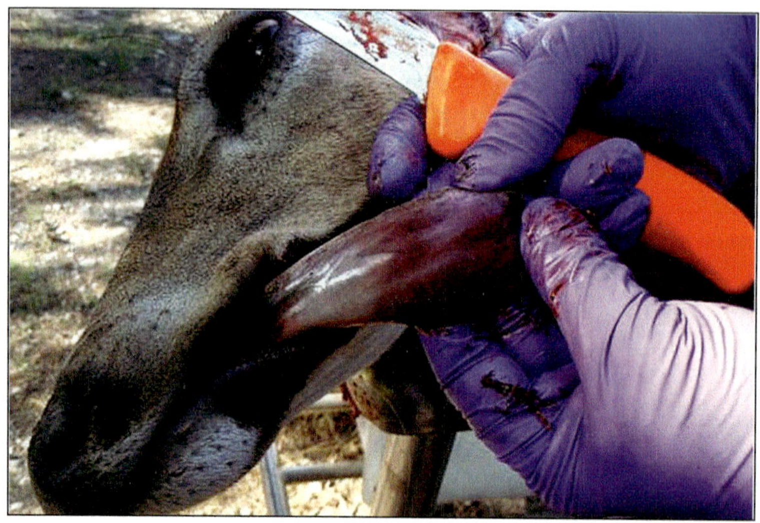

Figure 1.7. Blue tongue.

Differential Diagnosis

Foot and mouth disease, malignant catarrhal fever, Photosensitization.

Prevention and Control

The recovered sheep are immune for 6 months. Grazing of the animals should be avoided in areas where there is lot of vectors. Vector control by applying insecticides and good water management. Quarantine of the newly purchased animals.

Vaccination: Live, attenuated, avianated vaccines are used as monovalent strain or quadrivalent vaccine. Live vaccines should not be used in pregnant sheep. Sheep are vaccinated annually, and several weeks before service and before the start of rainy season. Lambs vaccinated at 6 months of age and booster vaccination at once in a year.

1.8. Bovine Viral Diarrhoea (BVD)

Bovine Viral Diarrhea (BVD) or Bovine Viral Diarrhoea (UK English), and previously referred to as Bovine Virus Diarrhoea (BVD), is a significant economic disease of cattle which is endemic in the majority of countries throughout the world. The causative agent, bovine viral diarrhea virus (BVDV) is a member of the Pestivirus genus of the family Flaviviridae. BVD infection results in a wide variety of clinical signs, due to its immunosuppressive effects, as well as having a direct effect on respiratory disease and fertility. In addition, BVD infection of a susceptible dam during a certain period of gestation can result in the production of a Persistently Infected (PI) fetus.

Bovine viral opular (BVD) and Mucosal Disease (MD) are clinically dissimilar disease syndromes, and were originally described as separate diseases, but they are now known to have a common viral etiology. The virus can cause both acute disease, bovine viral opular and a protracted form of illness, mucosal disease, arising from persistent infection. BVD may occur at any age. MD is a persistent infection acquired *in utero* and characterized by high mortality and low morbidity. The BVD virus can be either non cytopathogenic or cytopathogenic. Isolation and demonstration from both BVD and MD were serologically similar and gave the same experimental disease. The clinical evidence that abortions were constant finding of field outbreaks of BVD and also the demonstration of transplacental transfer of the virus to the fetus. Early fetal infection with BVD virus may lead to persistent viraemia and a failure to develop antibodies. Persistently viraemic animals could subsequently develop MD. Persistently viraemic animals are infected with only non-cytopathogenic virus, whereas those developing MD are infected with both non-cytopathogenic and cytopathogenic forms. Mucosal disease is almost invariably fatal disease with low morbidity. It occurs in cattle, which have a persistent BVD infection acquired as fetuses characterized by a specific immune tolerance to the infecting virus strains and consequent lack of antibody to it. In MD, if the fetus infected at 110-120 days of gestation, *i.e.*, before the age of immunocompetence, the virus become accepted as self and persist through out the life of the animal. This explains the lack of antibody to persisting virus and the continued state of opula tolerance. Sometimes after birth, when the animal is about 6-18 months of age, super infection of these persistently viraemic animals with the cytopathogenic bio-type may occur causing MD. Bovine viral opular virus (BVDV) is a SS-RNA virus, genus Pestivirus in the family Flaviviridae and is closely related to classical swine fever and Ovine Border disease viruses. This virus affects domestic and wild ruminants and pigs. There are two genotypes of the BVDV recognized. Both viral genotypes have been co-circulating in cattle throughout the world. This disease reported from most regions of the world. Natural infections and disease occur not only in cattle but also in sheep, pigs, goats and a wide range of captive, free-living ruminants. BVDV also classified into two biotypes-Non cytopathogenic and cytopathogenic biotypes. The most important sources of BVDV in nature are opula-tolerant, persistently infected animals. High virus levels are usually present in their nasal secretions, saliva, tears, semen, milk, urine and faeces. Animals in contact with a persistently infected animal rapidly become infected. Vertical and horizontal transmission may occur. Disease transmits by direct or indirect contact. The virus may be isolated in a number of bovine monolayer cell cultures (*e.g.*, kidney, lung, testis or turbinate). Growth of both biotypes is usually satisfactory.

Clinical Manifestations

The clinical and pathologic manifestation of infection in individual cattle varies with age and pregnancy status. Postnatal infection of susceptible non-pregnant cattle. Three situations are considered; (i) Postnatal infection in non pregnant cattle (ii) Infection in pregnant cattle and (iii) persistent infection in calves and mucosal disease.

Acute Infection

Infection is most common in animals 8-24 months of age. Although calves may receive antibodies in opulars, antibody levels decline by 3-8 months of age and animals can then become infected. Incubation period 5-7 days followed by pyrexia (40-41°C), leucopenia, viraemia. In majority it is sub clinical infection. There may be opular of explosive nature with very high morbidity but no mortality. Drop in milk yield in dairy cows, oculo-nasal discharge and mouth ulcers is referred to as BVD. Animals develop serum neutralizing antibodies which persists life long.

Immuno Suppression

Virus induces transient but profound opula suppression. The virus suppresses the interferon production, affects lymphocyte function, humoral antibody production and phagocytosis which paves way for many respiratory and other diseases in calves.

Venereal Infection

Semen from persistently infected bulls by AI or natural service infects cows which results in early embryonic mortality and repeat breeding. Infection of susceptible pregnant cattle.

Transplacental Infection

The infection to the fetus causes abortion, weak calves, under sized calves and congenitally deformed calves. The virus replicates in almost all the fetal tissues and the extent of damage is more in actively dividing cells. Regarding the nervous system it causes cerebellar hypoplasia, dysplasia, cavitation of the cerebrum and retinal displacement.

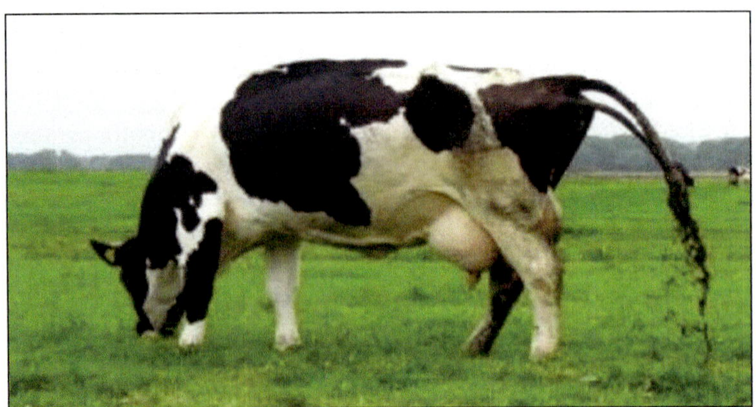

Figure 1.8. Bovine viral opular.

Immunological Competence of the Fetus

Infection in early fetal life becomes persistent viral infection in many tissues and organs. After birth, the calf remains infected for life. These calves excrete the virus in large quantity and transmit to all susceptible healthy animals. Therefore, high probability of development of MD is possible.

Persistently Infected Cattle

In susceptible healthy herds in which virus was recently introduced, high proportion of calves in the next calving season become persistently infected. Mortality rate exceeds 50 per cent in the preslaughter age, *i.e.*, 6-18 months age and the most classical clinical manifestations are that of MD. This disease is characterized by pyrexia, anorexia, profuse watery opular, nasal discharge, buccal ulceration and sometimes lameness. Death is within a few days to 3 weeks.

Diagnosis

Clinical diagnosis is a complex problem. Signs of the different syndromes may appear alone or in combination. Although many of the signs are similar to RP, the mortality in that disease is much higher. The oral lesions are very important, but their absence does not exclude BVD. This disease must be differentiated from conditions in cattle causing opular, erosions/ulcerations of the gastrointestinal tract, reproductive failure, teratology, skin disease, laminitis, poor growth and respiratory tract disease such as vesicular diseases, ingestion of caustic substances, mucosal disease complex: Rinderpest, bluetongue, opular stomatitis, malignant catarrhal fever.

Laboratory Diagnosis

Samples to be collected- nasal, ocular discharges, blood, spleen, lymph nodes, lungs, and liver. Identification of the agent- Persistently viraemic healthy animals resulting from congenital infection can be readily identified by isolation of noncytopathogenic virus in cell cultures from blood or serum. It is necessary to use an immune-labelling method to detect the growth of virus in the cultures. Alternative methods based on direct detection of viral antigen or viral RNA in leukocytes is also available. Persistence of virus should be confirmed by resampling after an interval of at least 3 weeks. These animals will usually have no or low levels of antibodies to BVDV.

Serological Tests

Acute infection with BVDV is best confirmed by demonstrating seroconversion using sequential paired samples from several animals in the group. The testing of paired sera (acute and convalescent samples) should be done a minimum of 21 days apart and samples should be tested side by side. The enzyme-linked immunosorbent assay (ELISA) for antibody and the virus neutralization test are the most widely used. Demonstration of the BVDV by CPE (but many BVDV strains do not produce CPE), FAT, PCR a much more productive method, are necessary for definitive diagnosis.

Prevention and Control

Primary goal of a control strategy is removal of persistently infected animals from a herd. All cattle should be screened for the virus including calves born in the herd for nine months after initiation the programme. Newly introduced animals should be tested for the disease before their introduction. Quarantine period for newly purchased animals is 30 days. Strict managemental practices. Replacement animals especially breeding bulls. Cattle should not be allowed to mix with sheep and goats.

Vaccination

Modified Live BVD vaccine – not recommended for pregnant cattle or in stressed populations. Killed BVD vaccine, which is safer for administration even to pregnant cattle. A booster dose after 3 to 4 weeks of initial vaccination. Calves should be vaccinated at 4-6 months of age and again when they are 8-12 months old. Calves less than three months of age generally not vaccinated because of potential vaccination failure associated with the presence of colostral immunity. Heifers and cows should be revaccinated 30-60 days before breeding and booster dose one month before calving or in the last trimester.

1.9. Canine Distemper

Synonyms

Carre's disease, Hard-pad disease, Canine influenza.

Canine distemper is a highly contagious, systemic, viral disease of dogs seen worldwide. Clinically, it is characterized by a diphasic fever, eucopenia, GI and respiratory catarrh, and frequently pneumonic and neurologic complications. Its epidemiology is complicated by the large number of species susceptible to infection. The disease is seen in Canidae (dog, fox, wolf, raccoon dog), Mustelidae (ferret, mink, skunk, wolverine, marten, badger, otter), most Procyonidae (raccoon, coatimundi), some Viveridae (binturong, palm civet), Ailuridae (red panda), Ursidae (bear), Elephantidae (Asian elephant), primates (Japanese monkey), and large Felidae. Domestic dogs (including feral populations) are considered to be the reservoir species in most, if not all, locations. Antigenic drift and strain diversity is increasingly documented in association with outbreaks in wild species, domestic dogs, and exotic animals held in zoos and parks. This is an acute febrile systemic, infectious and contagious disease of dogs caused by morbili virus and the disease is characterized by biphasic fever, acute catarrhal inflammation of various mucous membranes, pneumonia and in some cases skin lesions and involvement of nervous system. This disease is caused by canine distemper virus (CDV) is an enveloped single stranded RNA virus. This virus is the member of genus morbili virus sub-family Paramyxo virinae, family Paramyxoviridae. This virus is antigenically related to Rinderpest, Peste des petits ruminants and measles viruses. There is only one serotype causing this disease in canines. There are three strains of this virus namely A, B and C. The strains A and B were more virulent than C strain. All these strains vary in their pathogenicity and tissue trophism. This disease has a worldwide distribution except in hot and arid regions such as parts of Africa. All members of canidae (dogs, wolves, dingo, fox, coyote, jackal), Mustelidae (ferret, skunk, mink, otter, weasel), Viveridae (Binturong) and Procyonidae (Raccoon, panda, coati) are susceptible to distemper. Canine distemper virus causes higher morbidity and mortality than any other virus that infects dogs. Incidence is more in foreign breeds than Indigenous breeds. The disease is more common in dogs at the age group of

3-6 months. The rate of incidence gradually declines with the attainment of age. More the age, lesser the rate of infection.

Clinical Manifestation

The disease is most important among dogs. The disease may be noted in all age groups, but the young ones between age group of 3-6 months are more susceptible and case fatality rate in this age group are maximum. There is high rise of temperature. This temperature reaction is characteristic and is known as biphasic reaction. The body temperature of the animal raises up to 103° to104°F. In this stage the nose of the animal will turn dry and hot and eyes will turn congested. The animal is markedly depressed and refuses to take food. Within few days yellowish green discharge is voided from the eyes and nose. The temperature is usually for 3-4 days and then drops. The temperature is normal till 11th or 12th day which again shows a rise which remains continuous during the course of the systemic infection. The second rise of temperature is accompanied by rhinitis, conjunctivitis, gastroenteritis and bronchopneumonia. The clinical manifestations vary in respect to severity and involvement of the system concerned.

There are five different forms of manifestation of clinical signs.

(a) **Pulmonary form:** A coryza like syndrome is characterized by oculonasal discharge, pharyngitis, bronchitis , *etc*. Bronchopneumonia is the common feature. The pulmonary form is more prevalent than digestive form. The pneumonic condition may persist for a long period.

(b) **Gastrointestinal form:** This form is characterized by loss of appetite, vomition and abdominal pain. The faeces are semisolid or loose; foul smelling. The diarrheic faeces may contain blood. The hemorrhagic enteritis is commonly seen in young pup.

(c) **Ocular form:** This is manifested as swollen eye lids, conjunctivitis and purulent discharge from the eyes. Ulceration of the cornea and transient keratitis may also be located.

(d) **Nervous form:** The affection of the nerve cells lead to neurological disorders. These are characterized by restlessness, excitement, chewing movements, excessive salivation and convulsion. The nervous manifestations are noted when the animal can resist the primary infection and suffer from secondary complication. Lymphopaenia is the distinct feature of distemper but this may not occur in dogs with delayed encephalitis. A condition known as "old dog encephalitis" characterized by mental disorders, motor deterioration and death as clinical features. The nervous form may be characterized by jerky movements of group of muscles. The muscular spasms may be observed in the lips, cheeks, jaws, head, neck or limb muscles.

(e) **Cutaneous form:** There is appearance of rash, vesicles and pustules on the body of the affected dog especially on the ventral aspect of the abdomen and on the inner parts of the thigh. In some cases the skin of the foot pads and nose may become hard due to hyperkeratitis and the condition is ascribed as hardpad disease.

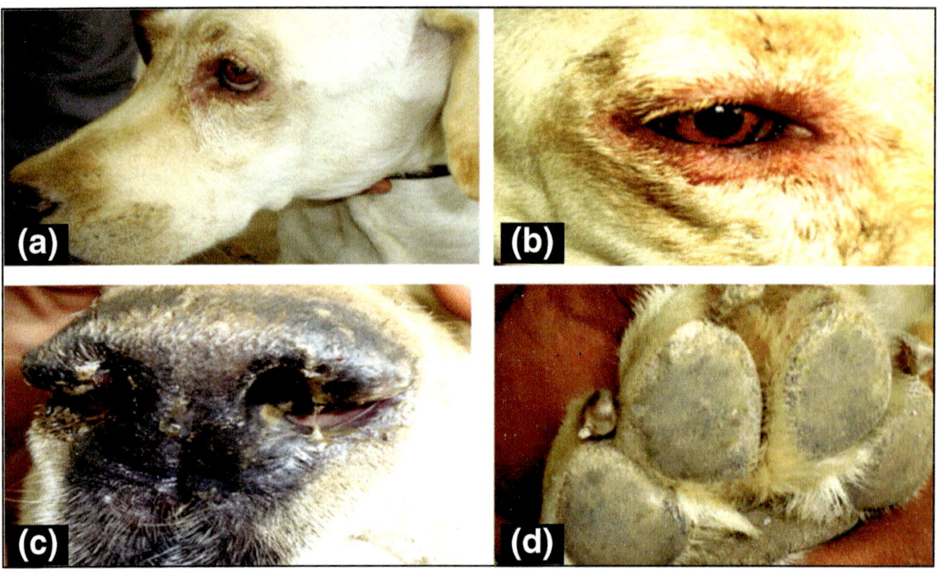

Figure 1.9

(a) Serous ocular discharge, (b) Blepharitis along with cloudiness of eyes, (c) Scanty nasal discharge (d) Hyper keratinization of pads in dog suffering from nervous form of canine distemper.

Diagnosis

Distemper should be considered in the diagnosis of any febrile condition in dogs with multisystemic manifestations. Characteristic signs sometimes do not appear until late in the disease, and the clinical picture may be modified by concurrent parasitism and numerous viral or bacterial infections. Distemper is sometimes confused with other systemic infections such as leptospirosis, infectious canine hepatitis, or Rocky Mountain spotted fever. Intoxicants such as lead or organophosphates can cause simultaneous GI and neurologic signs. A febrile catarrhal illness with neurologic sequelae justifies a clinical diagnosis of distemper.

In dogs with multisystemic signs, the following can be examined by immunofluorescent assay or reverse transcriptase (RT) PCR: smears of conjunctival, tracheal, vaginal, or other epithelium; the buffy coat of the blood; urine sediment; or bone marrow aspirates. Commercially available quantitative RT-PCR can usually distinguish natural infection from vaccinal virus. A combined two-step RT-PCR to distinguish vaccinal strains from emerging wild-type strains has also been described; this assay would be of particular value in epidemiologic investigations or in outbreaks in non-canine species. Antibody titers or ELISA can be performed on CSF and compared with peripheral blood; a relatively higher level in the CSF is typical of natural infection versus vaccination. Viral antigen immunofluorescent assay (IFA) or fluorescent in situ hybridization for viral DNA can be performed on biopsies from the footpads or from the haired skin of the dorsal neck.

At necropsy, diagnosis is usually confirmed by histologic lesions, IFA, or both. These samples are often negative when the dog is showing only neurologic manifestations or when circulating antibody is present (or both), requiring that the diagnosis be made by CSF evaluation or RT-PCR as described above.

Animal Inoculation

Dogs or ferrets are to be inoculated with the suspected materials and observations are to be recorded about clinical signs, lesions and inclusion bodies.

Detection of Inclusion Bodies

In living clinically affected dogs, intracytoplasmic eosinophilic inclusion bodies are noted in the conjunctival or vaginal epithelial impressions. These inclusions are reliable aid in diagnosis of canine distemper.

Fluorescent Antibody Technique (FAT)

The direct or indirect FAT is employed to detect the presence of viral antigen. This test offers reliable clue for the demonstration of the virus in tissue smears and sections. Impressions of mucous membrane and tissues from foot pad are the samples for this disease diagnosis by FAT. The virus used to persist in foot pad for a longer period of time.

Isolation of the Virus

Isolation of the virus from nasal or conjunctival swabs and inoculation in the cell cultures and embryonated chicken eggs.

Prevention and Control

Canine distemper vaccine alone or in combination with other diseases may be used with the first dose of vaccine at 6-8 weeks of age with additional doses at 3-4 weeks intervals until puppies are 14 weeks of age. Annual revaccination may be required at enzootic areas. Besides immunization, isolation of CD diseased dogs appears to be the most important measure in controlling the disease. As the virus is shed in all body secretions and excretions during the acute systemic disease and direct dog-to-dog contact appears to be the main route of viral spread. Disinfection of a CDV contaminated environment can be accomplished with commonly used disinfectants because the enveloped virus destroyed outside the host.

1.10. Canine Parvo Viral Infection (CPV)

Canine parvovirus is a highly contagious virus that can affect all dogs, but unvaccinated dogs and puppies younger than four months old are the most at risk. Dogs that are ill from canine parvovirus infection are often said to have "parvo." The virus affects dogs' gastrointestinal tracts and is spread by direct dog-to-dog contact and contact with contaminated feces (stool), environments, or people. The virus can also contaminate kennel surfaces, food and water bowls, collars and leashes, and the hands and clothing of people who handle infected dogs. It is resistant to heat, cold, humidity, and drying, and can survive in the environment for long periods of time. Even trace amounts of feces from an infected dog may harbor the virus and infect other dogs that come into the infected environment. The virus is readily transmitted from place to place on the hair or feet of dogs or via contaminated cages, shoes, or other objects. Canine parvo viral infection is caused by canine parvo virus 1 (CPV), smallest DNA virus belonging to the family Parvo viridae. Wide varieties of hosts are affected with Parvo virus including cattle, pigs, dogs, cats. Breeds of dogs like Dobermann and Labrador are highly susceptible than other breeds of dogs. The virus is transmitted through direct contact with the infected animal or its excretions. Virus excreted in large quantities in the faeces of the affected dogs. Infection spreads when the dogs are placed in close aggregation in large breeding establishments, pet shops, clinics.

Clinical Manifestations

Two forms of manifestations are observed in parvo virus infection.

(a) **Parvoviral enteritis:** Hemorrhagic gastroenteritis occurs in dogs of any age but serious proportions in pups, slight to high rise of temperature in initial stage of disease but gradually turn to subnormal level with advancement of vomition and iarrhea, inappetance, polydipsia, frothy yellow coloured vomitus, retching, dehydration and exhaustion, death due to dehydration leading to peripheral circulatory failure.

(b) **Parvo virus myocarditis:** Common in pups under 10 weeks of age, heart muscles damaged, affected animals show the signs of circulatory failure, pulmonary oedema, death due to cardiogenic shock, death in dogs of 4-8 weeks of age.

Signs of Parvovirus

Some of the signs of parvovirus include lethargy; loss of appetite; abdominal pain and bloating; fever or low body temperature (hypothermia); vomiting; and severe, often bloody, diarrhea. Persistent vomiting and diarrhea can cause rapid dehydration, and damage to the intestines and immune system can cause septic shock. Most deaths from parvovirus occur within 48 to 72 hours following the onset of clinical signs. If your puppy or dog shows any of these signs, you should contact your veterinarian immediately.

Diagnosis and Treatment

Parvovirus infection is often suspected based on the dog's history, physical examination, and laboratory tests. Fecal testing can confirm the diagnosis. No specific drug is available that will kill the virus in infected dogs, and treatment is intended to support the dog's body systems until the dog's immune system can fight off the viral infection. Treatment should be started immediately and consists primarily of intensive care efforts to combat dehydration by replacing electrolyte, protein and fluid losses, controlling vomiting and diarrhea, and preventing secondary infections. Sick dogs should be kept warm and receive good nursing care. When a dog develops parvo, treatment can be very expensive, and the dog may die despite aggressive treatment. Early recognition and aggressive treatment are very important in successful outcomes. With proper treatment, survival rates can approach 90 per cent. Since parvovirus is highly contagious, isolation of infected dogs is necessary to minimize spread of infection. Proper cleaning and disinfection of contaminated kennels and other areas where infected dogs are (or have been) housed is essential to control the spread of parvovirus. The virus is not easily killed, so consult your veterinarian for specific guidance on cleaning and disinfecting agents.

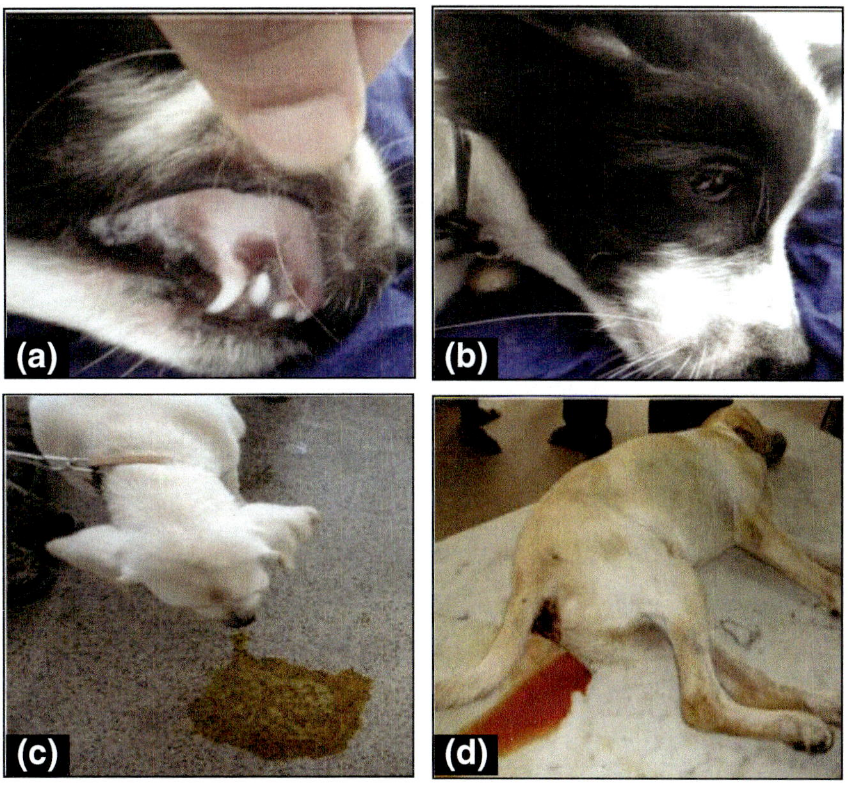

Figure 1.10

(a) Canine parvo viral infection- pale buccal mucous membrane, (b) Canine parvo viral infection- shunken eyeball, (c) Vomiltion in Canine parvo viral infection (d) Canine parvo viral infection- Haemorrhagic enteritis.

Preventing Parvovirus

Vaccination and good hygiene are critical components of prevention. Young puppies are very susceptible to infection, particularly because the natural immunity provided in their mothers' milk may wear off before the puppies' own immune systems are mature enough to fight off infection. If a puppy is exposed to canine parvovirus during this gap in protection, it may become ill. An additional concern is that immunity provided by a mother's milk may interfere with an effective response to vaccination. This means even vaccinated puppies may occasionally be infected by parvovirus and develop disease. To reduce gaps in protection and provide the best protection against parvovirus during the first few months of life, a series of puppy vaccinations are administered. Puppies should receive a dose of canine parvovirus vaccine between 14 and 16 weeks of age, regardless of how many doses they received earlier, to develop adequate protection. To protect their adult dogs, pet owners should be sure that their dog's parvovirus vaccination is up-to-date. There are titers available that measure the dog's level of antibodies against the canine parvovirus, but the antibody level may not directly translate to protection if the dog is exposed to the virus. Ask your veterinarian about a recommended prevention program for your dog.

Until a puppy has received its complete series of vaccinations, pet owners should use caution when bringing their pet to places where young puppies congregate (*e.g.* pet shops, parks, puppy classes, obedience classes, doggy daycare, kennels, and grooming establishments). Reputable establishments and training programs reduce exposure risk by requiring vaccinations, health examinations, good hygiene, and isolation of ill puppies and dogs. Contact with known infected dogs and their premises should always be avoided. In spite of proper vaccination, a small percentage of dogs do not develop protective immunity and remain susceptible to infection. Finally, do not let your puppy or adult dog to come into contact with the fecal waste of other dogs while walking or playing outdoors. Prompt and proper disposal of waste material is always advisable as a way to limit spread of canine parvovirus infection as well as other diseases that can infect humans and animals. Dogs with vomiting or diarrhea or other dogs which have been exposed to ill dogs should not be taken to kennels, show grounds, dog parks, or other areas where they will come into contact with other dogs. Similarly, unvaccinated dogs should not be exposed to ill dogs or those with unknown vaccination histories. People who are in contact with sick or exposed dogs should avoid handling of other dogs or at least wash their hands and change their clothes before doing so.

1.11. Bovine Epihemeral Fever (BEF)

Synonyms

Bovine Epizootic Fever, Ephemeral Fever, Three-Day Sickness, Three-Day Stiffsickness, Dragon Boat Disease, Lazy Man's Disease, Dengue of Cattle.

Bovine ephemeral fever (BEF) also known as Three Day Sickness is an arthropod vector-borne disease of cattle and is caused by bovine ephemeral fever virus (BEFV), a member of the genus *Ephemerovirus* in the family Rhabdoviridae. Bovine ephemeral fever (or 3-day sickness) is an acute febrile illness of cattle and water buffaloes. Caused by an arthropod-borne rhabdovirus, bovine ephemeral fever virus (BEFV), the disease occurs seasonally over a vast expanse of the globe encompassing much of Africa, the Middle East, Asia and Australia. Although mortality rates are typically low, infection prevalence and morbidity rates during outbreaks are often very high, causing serious economic impacts through loss of milk production, poor cattle condition at sale and loss of traction power at harvest. There are also significant impacts on trade to regions in which the disease does not occur, including the Americas and most of Europe. In recent years, unusually severe outbreaks of bovine ephemeral fever have been reported from several regions in

Asia and the Middle East, with mortality rates through disease or culling in excess of 10–20 per cent. There are also concerns that, like other vector-borne diseases of livestock, the geographic distribution of bovine ephemeral fever could expand into regions that have historically been free of the disease.

Bovine ephemeral fever (BEF) is a benign acute, non-contagious, arthropod-borne viral disease of cattle and water buffalo characterized by sudden onset, lameness and quick recovery with high morbidity and low mortality. This disease occurs in tropical and subtropical regions of Africa, Asia and Australia. The BEF virus belongs to the genus Rhabdovirus. This virus is related to dengue fever virus in human. All breeds of cattle are susceptible. Among the cattle, 6 months to 2 years are more susceptible. This disease is prevalent both in indigenous and exotic breeds of cattle as well as water buffalo. The disease is not reported in goat, sheep, pig and dog. Virus transmitted mainly by sand flies (Ceratopogonidae family). Mosquitoes (*Aedes, Anophles and Culex*), and biting midges are playing a major role in transmission. Strong wind can transport vectors for longer distances. Epizootics associated with recent rainfall. The virus does not spread by any other modes.

Clinical Manifestations

The incubation period is 2 to 10 days, calves are least affected, those less than 6 months of age showing no clinical signs. After an incubation period of 2-10 days, there is sudden onset of fever. A biphasic or triphasic fever and sharp fall in milk yield are commonly observed. There is severe ruminal stasis followed by constipation. Muscular signs become more evident on the second day with severe stiffness. Swellings in shoulders neck and back may be seen. A posture similar to that of acute laminitis, with all four feet bunched under the body is characteristic. On the third day the animal begins eating and ruminating and the febrile reaction disappear. Some animal's remains standing in acute stage and exhibit terna recumbency associated with hypocalcaemia (Milk fever posture). Most recovered animals develop a solid immunity. The morbidity rate may reach 100 per cent and the fatality rate is 1 per cent. Milk yield returns to normal within 2 to 3 weeks.

Post Disease Complications

Fall in milk yield, increased susceptibility to mastitis, delay in next estrus, pneumonia due to prolonged recumbency.

Lesions

Enlargement and edema of the lymph nodes, polysinovitis, tendovaginitis and periarthritis, pulmonary and pleural congestion, edema and haemorrhages of the brain and meninges, necrotic changes in the skeletal muscle.

Diagnosis

Sample of choice – blood (Buffy coat) and serum is the highly suitable specimen. Based on clinical signs – rapid and short course affecting a large number of cattle in an area. Virus isolation by intracerebral inoculation of mice or hamster or isolation in cell culture such as Baby hamster kidney cell lines and monkey kidney cell lines. Other tests are – CFT, AGID, FAT, ELISA. Based on clinical pathology – increased level of plasma fibrinogen and decreased serum calcium level, high level of creatinine kinase and marked leukocytosis.

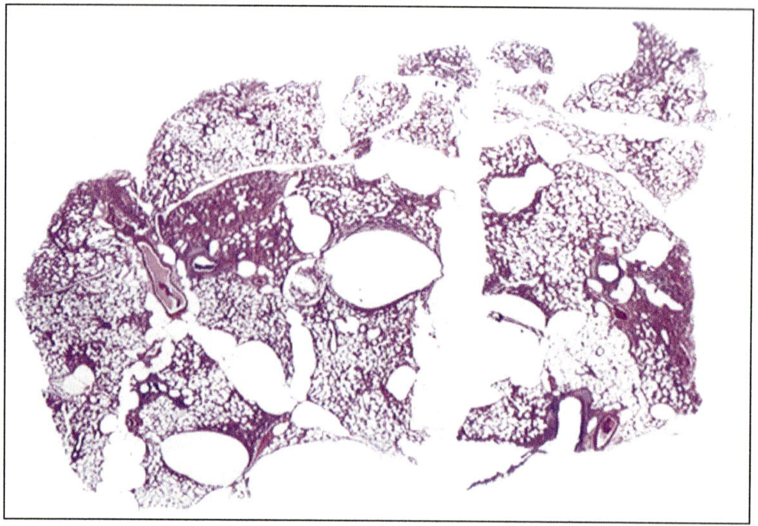

Figure 1.11. Interstitial pneumonia with interlobular emphysema.

Differential Diagnosis

Laminitis, milk fever.

Prevention and Control

Treatment revolves around the generalized inflammation and the depression of serum calcium. The inflammation can be treated with phenylbutazone given intramuscularly for eight hourly periods of up to 3 days depending on response. Treatment with calcium borogluconate is warranted when signs of hypocalcemia are present. Supplementary antibiotic treatments to avoid secondary pneumonia or mastitis are warranted. Vector control is usually impractical in endemic areas. In endemic areas, it is important to immunize cattle; particularly highly valuable animals. Both formalin killed and attenuated vaccines are available. Calves aged more than six months vaccinated. Trials have been carried out using a limited vaccine based on the envelope-glycoprotein has been developed.

1.12. Equine Infectious Anaemia (EIA)

Synonyms

Swamp Fever, Mountain Fever, Slow Fever, Equine Malarial Fever, Coggins Disease.

Equine infectious anemia or equine infectious anaemia (EIA), also known by horsemen as swamp fever, is a horse disease caused by a retrovirus and transmitted by bloodsucking insects. The virus (EIAV) is endemic in the Americas, parts of Europe, the Middle and Far East, Russia, and South Africa. The virus is a lentivirus, like human immunodeficiency virus (HIV). Like HIV, EIA can be transmitted through blood, milk, and body secretions. Transmission is primarily through biting flies, such as the horse-fly and deer-fly. The virus survives up to 4 hours in the vector. Contaminated surgical equipment and recycled needles and syringes, and bits can transmit the disease. Mares can transmit the disease to their foals via the placenta. The risk of transmitting the disease is greatest when an infected horse is ill, as the blood levels of the virus are then highest.

It is a chronic persisting infectious viral disease of equines characterized by emaciation, anaemia, intermittent fever and generalized lymphoproliferative changes and odema. The anaemia may be for few days or may persist for a longer period and this is considered to be immunologically induced problem. The etiological agent for this disease is a RNA virus belonging to Lenti virinae, subfamily Retroviridae family. The virus can be cultivated in tissue culture and the virus can be killed by exposing them to heat and commonly available detergents. The members of the Equidae family are the principle hosts for this disease. This disease is transmitted through blood sucking arthropods such as Tabanus, Stomaxys and mosquitoes. Fly breeding season actually augment the spread of the disease. It is also transmitted by iatrogenic transmission.

There are three stages, which includes;

(a) **Acute:** The acute form is a sudden onset of the disease at full-force. Symptoms include high fever, anemia (due to the breakdown of red blood cells), weakness, swelling of the lower abdomen and legs, weak pulse, and irregular heartbeat. The horse may die suddenly.

(b) **Subacute:** A slower, less severe progression of the disease. Symptoms include recurrent fever, weight loss, an enlarged spleen (felt during a rectal examination), anemia, and swelling of the lower chest, abdominal wall, penile sheath, scrotum, and legs.

(c) **Chronic:** Horse tires easily and is unsuitable for work. May have a recurrent fever and anemia, may relapse to the subacute or acute form even several years after the original attack.

A horse may also not appear to have any symptoms, yet still tests positive for EIA antibodies. This horse can still pass on the disease. According to most veterinarians, horses diagnosed EIA positive are usually not showing any sign of sickness or disease. EIA may cause abortion in pregnant mares. This may occur at any time during the pregnancy if there is a relapse when the virus enters the blood. Most infected mares will abort, however some give birth to healthy foals. Foals are not necessarily infected.

Studies indicate that there are breeds with a tolerance to EIA. Recent studies in Brazil on living wild horses have shown that in the Pantanal, about 30 per cent of domesticated and about 5.5 per cent of the wild horses are chronically infected with EIA.

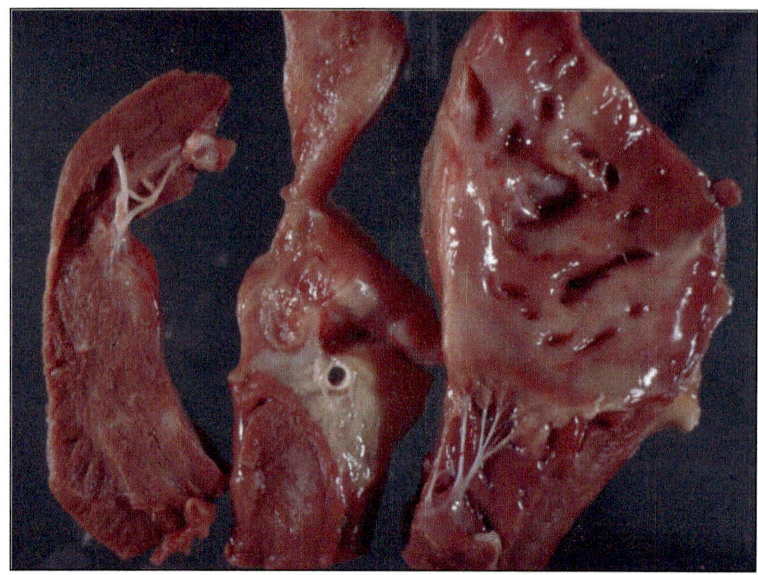

Figure 1.12. Horse, heart. Pale cardiac muscle, focal white areas of myocardial degeneration, and reddened hemorrhagic areas (possible hypoxia during death).

Clinical Manifestations

Long incubation period- 1-4 weeks. Varied clinical manifestation- anorexia, pyrexia, depression, odema of dependent parts, icterus, wasting and anaemia.

Lesions

Entire carcass – subcutaneous odema, submucosal and subserous hemorrhages, generalized lymphadenopathy, Hepatomegaly and spleenomegaly.

Diagnosis

Based on history and clinical signs. Laboratory tests- Coggin's agar gel immunodiffusion test, ELISA-Alternative test for AGID.

Differential Diagnosis

Should be differentiated with other diseases of horses including Babesisois, trypanosomiasis where anaemia is the important clinical picture. The above diseases ruled out with peripheral blood smear examination, AGID and ELISA. Viral arteritis –have clinical resemblance but can be differentiated be looking at the ocular changes characterized by palpebral odema, photophobia and lacrymation.

Prevention and Control

Limit the movements of carrier animals. Suspected animals should be isolated and identified by a serological test. Disease is mostly prevalent in swampy areas where the vectors are abundant, so such areas should be avoided for equine rearing. Strict vector control measures. Vaccination with different subtypes of the virus prevalent in the particular area.

1.13. Equine Influenza

Synonyms

Equine distemper, Typhoid fever, pink eye.

Equine influenza is highly contagious and spreads rapidly among naive horses. Horses 1–5 year old are the most susceptible to infection. Orthomyxovirus A/equine-2 was first recognized in 1963 as a cause of widespread epidemics and has subsequently become endemic in many countries, except for New Zealand and Iceland. China, Japan, and Australia experienced devastating epidemics of equine influenza affecting tens of thousands of horses in 2007. Equine influenza had not been reported in China since 1993, in Japan since 1972, and had never been reported in Australia. Endemicity is maintained by sporadic clinical cases and by inapparent infection in susceptible horses introduced into the population by birth, through waning immunity, or after movement from other areas or countries. A carrier state is not recognized for equine influenza. The clinical outcome after viral exposure largely depends on immune status; clinical disease varies from a mild, inapparent infection to severe disease in susceptible animals. Influenza is rarely fatal except in donkeys, zebras, and debilitated horses. Transmission occurs by inhalation of respiratory secretions. Epidemics arise when one or more acutely infected horses are introduced into a susceptible group. The epidemiologic outcome depends on the antigenic characteristics of the circulating virus and the immune status of a given population of horses at time of exposure. Frequent natural exposure or regular vaccination may contribute to the degree of antigenic drift seen with specific strains of A/equine-2 virus in some parts of the world.

Equine influenza is an acute febrile highly infectious disease of horses characterized by general septicemia, respiratory problem accompanied by severe persistent dry cough. This is an economically important disease occurs worldwide except in Australia, New Zealand and Iceland. Two immunologically distinct subtypes of influenza "A" virus are described in horses. The virus, first isolated from horses in 1956, was designated A/equine/Prague/1/56 (H7N7) or influenza A/equine 1. In 1963, a second subtype was isolated in the USA and designated A/equine/Miami/2/63 (H3N8) or influenza A/equine 2. Infection or vaccination with one subtype does not induce protection against infection with the other subtype. Although the last outbreak of disease attributed to influenza A/equine I occurred in 1979, there is serological evidence that this subtype continues to circulate in the horse population. Antigenic drift accounts for several variants of influenza A/equine 2 with two antigenically and genetically distinct lineages identified in Europe and the Americas. In contrast, the H3N8 subtype isolated from horses in China was more closely related to avian strains than to the H3N8 subtype circulating in horses elsewhere. Outbreaks are associated with movement and assembly of horses for shows, sales, racing or training. The initial source of infection is often a partially immune horse shedding virus without showing clinical signs. Equine influenza is highly contagious disease and spreads rapidly among susceptible horses. Large quantities of virus are shed in aerosols by the frequent coughing of affected animals.

Infection can be acquired at distances up to 30 metres. Indirect transmission through contamination of clothing, equipment and vehicles can also occur.

Clinical Findings and Lesions

The incubation period of influenza is ~1–3 days. Clinical signs begin abruptly and include high fever (up to 106°F [41.1°C]), serous nasal discharge, submandibular lymphadenopathy, and coughing that is dry, harsh, and on-productive. Depression, anorexia, and weakness are frequently seen. Clinical signs usually last <3 days in uncomplicated cases. Influenza virus replicates within respiratory epithelial cells, resulting in destruction of tracheal and bronchial epithelium and cilia. Cough develops early in the course of infection and may persist for several weeks. Nasal discharge, although scant and serous initially, may become mucopurulent due to secondary bacterial infection. Mildly affected horses recover uneventfully in 2–3 wks; severely affected horses may convalesce as long as 6 mo. Recovery may be hastened by complete restriction of strenuous physical activity. Respiratory tract epithelium takes ~21 days to regenerate; during this time, horses are susceptible to development of secondary bacterial complications such as pneumonia, pleuropneumonia, and chronic bronchitis. Complications are minimized by restricting exercise, controlling dust, providing superior ventilation, and practicing good stable hygiene. Primary complications of vasculitis, myositis, and myocarditis are seen infrequently.

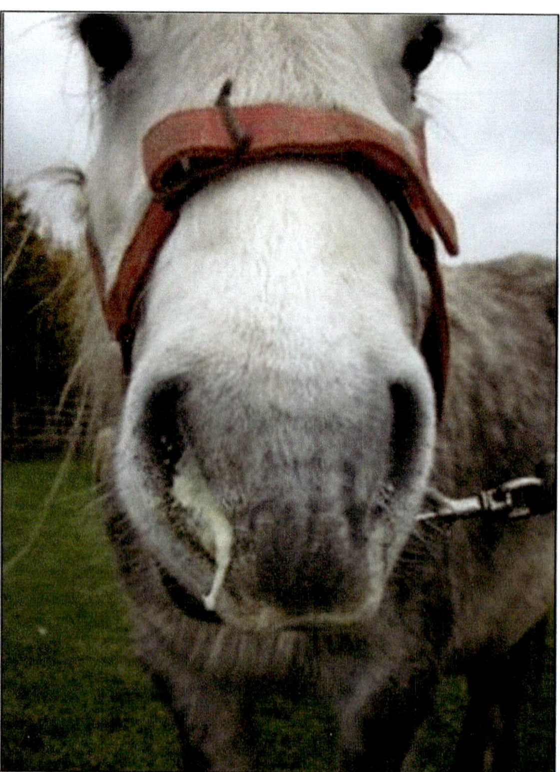

Figure 1.13. Equine influenza.

Diagnosis

The presence of a rapidly spreading respiratory infection in a group of horses characterized by rapid onset, high fever, depression, and cough is presumptive evidence of equine influenza. Definitive diagnosis can be determined by virus isolation, influenza A antigen detection (patient-side kit), or paired serum samples (hemagglutination inhibition). Nasopharyngeal swabs are obtained for virus isolation and antigen detection. These samples should be obtained soon after the onset of illness. Virus isolation in chick embryos is highly specific but less sensitive for detection of influenza because of bacterial contamination of the sample. Antigen detection is performed using a human influenza A kit, which provides immediate results that are not affected by bacterial contamination.

Identification of the Agent

Embryonated hen's eggs and/or cell cultures can be used for virus isolation from nasopharyngeal swabs or nasal and tracheal washes. Viral growth is monitored by haemagglutination (HA) or, in cell cultures, by haemadsorption (HAD) using chicken or guinea-pig red blood cells. Isolates can be characterized by haemagglutination inhibition (HI) using strain specific antisera. Isolates should always be sent immediately to an International Reference Laboratory (OIE or World Health Organization). Samples that yield negative results should be repassaged up to five passages may be necessary to isolate viruses from vaccinated horses. Infection may also be demonstrated by detection of viral antigen in respiratory secretions using an enzyme-linked immunosorbent assay.

Serological Tests

Diagnosis of influenza virus infections is usually only accomplished by tests on paired sera; the first sample should be taken as soon as possible after the onset of clinical signs and the second approximately 2 weeks later. Antibody levels are determined by HI or single radial haemolysis (SRH).

Treatment and Control

Supportive therapy and rest is indicated for affected horses. Several inactivated vaccines are commercially available. However, immunity is usually short-lived and booster injections are required in accordance with manufacturer's instructions. The incorporation of polymer adjuvants or Quil-A based immune-stimulating complexes (ISCOMs) into vaccine preparations extends the duration of protective levels of immunity. Vaccinated horses generally exhibit milder clinical signs and shed virus for shorter periods than unvaccinated animals. Vaccine manufacturers must update vaccinal strains regularly. Vaccines should include antigenic material representative of the influenza "A" virus subtypes prevalent in the horse population. In addition to vaccination, control of equine influenza requires isolation of affected horses and cleaning, disinfection and isolation of infected premises. Animal movement should cease until contaminated premises have been cleaned and disinfected.

1.14. Foot and Mouth Disease (FMD)

Synonyms

Aphthous fever, Epizootic aphthea, Aftosa, Fast Moving Disease.

Foot-and-mouth disease or hoof-and-mouth disease (*Aphthae epizooticae*) is an infectious and sometimes fatal viral disease that affects cloven-hoofed animals, including domestic and wild bovids. The virus causes a high fever for approximately two to six days, followed by blisters inside the mouth and on the feet that may rupture and cause lameness. Foot-and-mouth disease (FMD) has severe implications for animal farming, since it is highly infectious and can be spread by infected animals through aerosols, through contact with contaminated farming equipment, vehicles, clothing, or feed, and by domestic and wild predators. Its containment demands considerable efforts in vaccination, strict monitoring, trade restrictions, and quarantines, and occasionally the killing of animals. Susceptible animals include cattle, water buffalo, sheep, goats, pigs, antelope, deer, and bison. It has also been known to infect hedgehogs and elephants; llamas and alpacas may develop mild symptoms, but are resistant to the disease and do not pass it on to others of the same species. In laboratory experiments, mice, rats, and chickens have been successfully infected by artificial means, but they are not believed to contract the disease under natural conditions. Humans are very rarely infected. The virus responsible for the disease is a picornavirus, the prototypic member of the genus *Aphthovirus*. Infection occurs when the virus particle is taken into a cell of the host. The cell is then forced to manufacture thousands of copies of the virus, and eventually bursts, releasing the new particles in the blood. The virus is genetically highly variable, which limits the effectiveness of vaccination.

Foot and Mouth Disease (FMD) is an acute, febrile, highly contagious disease of almost all cloven hoofed animals characterized by the formation of vesicles (fluid-filled blisters) and erosions in the mouth, nose, teats and feet with high morbidity and low mortality. The causative agent is Apthovirus, is an infectious, positive sense, ss-RNA virus. There are 7 serotypes of the virus: Types O, A, C, South African Territories 1, 2 and 3 (SAT-1,-2,-3) and Asia-1. Large numbers of subtypes were also identified. In our country only four major serotypes, O, A, C and Asia 1 are known to occur. Among which A 22, A 5 and A 10 subtypes are more commonly occur. Infection with one serotype does not confer immunity against another. This disease occurs naturally in cloven-hoofed animals (Both domestic and wild animals). Cattle are most susceptible followed by pigs and the disease is rare in sheep and goats. Several wildlife species including African buffalo, elephants, hedgehogs, deer and antelopes are also susceptible. Man may contact the disease with mild symptoms such as vesicles on the hand. Horse is refractory to Foot and Mouth Disease virus (FMDV) infection. The healthy animals are infected by contact with the secretions and excretions of the FMD affected animals. The main route of transmission is by inhalation and aerosol route. In addition to inhalation, transmission also occurs by direct or indirect contact with infected animals such as through abraded skin, conjunctiva, ingestion of contaminated garbage, inoculation with contaminated vaccines and insemination. Mechanical transmission may also occur with wild animals, birds and other non-susceptible domestic animals. The virus grows very well in cell cultures. The cell cultures that are commonly used are primary bovine tongue epithelium or bovine thyroid cells, primary pig kidney, calf kidney and lamb kidney cells. Cell lines such as Baby Hamster Kidney-21 (BHK-21) and IB-RS-2 cells are highly suitable. Most strains of the virus multiply to produce cytopathic effect within 24-48 hrs. This virus is highly cytolytic. Guinea pigs, suckling mice, hamsters and rabbits are used as experimental animals. Some strains grow in embryonated eggs (14 days old). Route is chorioallantoic membrane or intravenous route.

Clinical Manifestations

Incubation period is 2 days to 3 weeks. In pigs, the incubation period is as short as 1-3 days.

Cattle

The onset is heralded by a precipitate fall in milk yield and a high fever (40-41°C) accompanied by loss of appetite, depression. This is followed by appearance of painful stomatitis and the temperature subsides. There is profuse salivation, the saliva hanging in long, ropy strings, a characteristic smacking of the lips, and the animal chews carefully. Vesicles and bullae (1-2 cm in diameter) appear on the buccal mucosa, dental pad, udder and tongue. The vesicles are thin walled contain a straw coloured fluid. Vesicles rupture within 24 hrs, leaving a raw painful surface, which heals in about 1 week. Vesicles appear on the feet, particularly in the clefts and on the coronet. The lesions on the tongue often heal within a few days but those on the feet and nasal cavities are contaminated with bacteria, maggots, which result in lameness and muco purulent discharge. Vesicles may also develop on the teats, which results in severe mastitis. The virus does not cross the placenta but the abortion mostly during second trimester of pregnancy mainly due to fever. Morbidity is high (reaches 100 per cent) and mortality is very low (less than 2 per cent). Due to myocarditis the mortality in young calves up to 6 months of age, is very high. A sequel to FMD in cattle due to endocrine damage is a chronic syndrome of dyspnea, deleterious effects on testes causing production of poor quality of semen, anaemia, over growth of hair and lack of heat tolerance described as 'panting'.

Sheep and Goats

The pronounced clinical sign is sudden and acute lameness. The vesicles develop in the interdigital space of the feet, which rupture in about 2-3 days. Sometimes, the upper layer of the hoof is lost. Oral lesions are rare or they may develop only on the tongue and upper palate but there is no salivation.

Pigs

Large vesicles and bullae occur in the snout and feet and these may rupture to expose large raw surface. Lameness is the first sign. The foot lesions are very painful. Vesicles in the mouth are very less prominent.

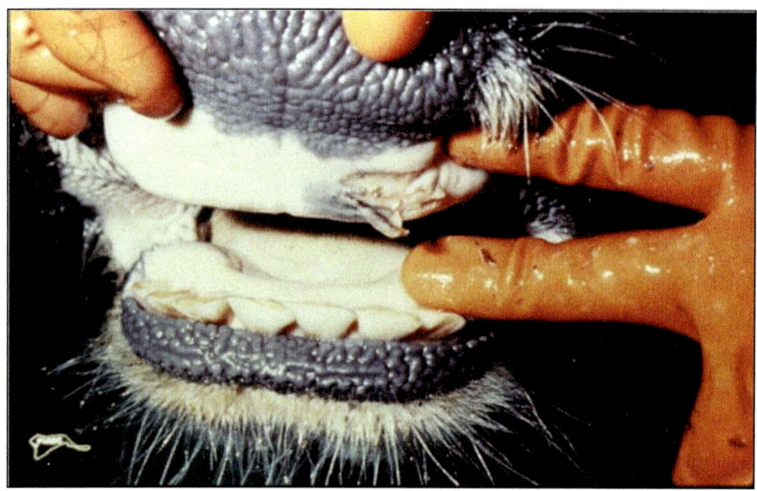

Figure 1.14. Foot and mouth disease.

Diagnosis

The highly contagious nature of the disease, profuse salivation and the presence of typical raised vesicles with blanched covering epithelium filled with a clear straw colour fluid are usually pathognomonic.

Samples to be Collected

Vesicular fluids, epithelial fragments of recent vesicles especially from lesions of tongue, feet, udder or lips of about 1 gm. Pieces of cardiac muscle and pancreas of dead animals. Transport medium – the samples should be kept in a solution of phosphate buffer saline at pH 7.6 which contain equal parts of glycerol and 0.00196 phenol red indicator. The outside of the container should be disinfected with 4 per cent Na_2 CO_3 or 0.2 per cent citric acid. The container is wrapped with cotton wool and kept in a sealed fluid tight container packed in a strong outer box of wood and sent to the lab.

By Serological Tests

Complement fixation test (CFT) is the most commonly used and important test to identify the type of virus. The suspension of the original serum is used as antibody. Virus and serum neutralization tests may be used to detect specific antibodies in the serum of recovered animals or for identifying the causative virus. The test is done with known hyperimmune sera Gel diffusion test, Fluorescent Anitbody Test (FAT), Immunoperoxidase test (IPT) and ISO electric focusing is also useful. Enzyme Linked Immunosorbent Assay (ELISA) and Polymerase Chain Reaction (PCR) are now standard methods for virus detection and typing in reference laboratories.

Cell Culture

Monolayers of bovine thyroid or pig kidney cells are inoculated and CPE develops within 24-48 hours at 37°C.

Mouse Inoculation

The suspected material is inoculated in unweaned mice and the mice die within 1-7 days.

Cross Immunity

For accurate identification inoculation of groups of susceptible and immune cattle are used.

Differential Diagnosis

Animal Species	*Route of Inoculation*	*FMD*	*VS*	*VE*	*SVD*
Natural infection					
Cattle		+	+	-	-
Pig		+	+	+	+
Sheep and goat		+	+	-	-
Horse		-	+	-	-
Experimental infection					
Horse	Intra dermal in tongue	-	+	+	-
Guinea-pig	Intra dermal in foot pad	+	+	-	-
Suckling mice	Intra dermal in foot pad	+	+	-	+
Adult chicken	Intra dermal in tongue	+	+	-	-

Control

Spread by air borne route is very difficult to control. Control of movement of livestock is one of the effective measures. Where the disease is not endemic the policy of quarantine, slaughter and disinfection of infected premises has proved efficient and economical also. Slaughter of infected animal stops the production of virus and slaughter of animals in direct or indirect contact with the source of infection breaks the infective chain. This is an economic method only in countries where disease incidence is low. In other countries, it may not be economically or socially acceptable and there vaccination is carried out. Where the disease is not endemic the policy of quarantine, slaughter and disinfection of infected premises has proved efficient and economical. Inactivated vaccines containing serotypes predominant in the geographical areas are available commercially. Vaccines may be monovalent, bivalent, trivalent or polyvalent. To establish a satisfactory level of immunity it is usual to give a primary course of two inoculations, 2-4 weeks apart, followed by revaccination every 4-12 months. In young animals maternal antibody may last for 3-6 months and can interfere with immunization. To avoid gap in protection, countries recommend first vaccination at ages ranging from 2-6 months. For calves usually first vaccination is given at the age of 4 months, followed by booster at 2-4 weeks interval, revaccination every 6 months or 4-12 months once. Sheep and pigs vaccinated at 6 months of age. The dosage of vaccine in sheep is one-third of that of cattle. The first vaccination leads to immunity in ruminants for about 3-6 months. Subsequent vaccinations may give protection for a year in cattle but only about 6 months in sheep. In the areas where the greatest risk of infection is likely, ruminants are vaccinated three times a year. With a medium risk, animals are vaccinated twice a year. In countries where the infection is low ruminants are vaccinated twice the first year and subsequently annually. The choice of strains of FMDV to use in the vaccine is important.

1.15. Fowl Pox

Fowl pox is the worldwide disease of poultry caused by viruses of the family Poxviridae and the genus *Avipoxvirus*. The viruses causing fowlpox are distinct from one another but antigenically similar, possible hosts including chickens, turkeys, quail, canaries, pigeons, and many other species of birds. There are two forms of the disease. The first is spread by biting insects (especially mosquitoes) and wound contamination and causes lesions on the comb, wattles, and beak. Birds affected by this form usually recover within a few weeks. The second form is spread by inhalation of the virus and causes a diphtheritic membrane to form in the mouth, pharynx, larynx, and sometimes the trachea. The prognosis for this form is poor.

Fowl pox is a slow spreading disease characterized by the development of discrete, nodular proliferative skin lesions on the unfeathered parts of the body (cutaneous form) or fibrino-necrotic and proliferative lesions in the mucous membrane of the upper respiratory tract, mouth and esophagus (diphtheritic form). Fowl pox is a common viral disease of domestic birds and has been reported in more than 60 species of wild birds representing 20 families. It affects chicken of all ages, sexes and breeds. Fowl pox virus (FPV) belongs to the genus Avi pox, sub-family Chordopoxvirinae, family Pox viridae. Pox virus infection occurs through mechanical transmission of the virus to the injured or lacerated skin. Insects mechanically transmit the disease. For isolation and propagation of FPV chicken embryos, and cell culture of chicken origin such as chicken embryo fibroblasts, chicken embryo dermis and kidney cells are used.

Clinical Manifestations

Incubation period varies from 4-10 days. The disease may occur in one of the two forms such as diphtheritic or cutaneous or both. Signs vary depending upon the susceptibility of the host, virulence of the virus, distribution of the lesions and other complicating factors. Cutaneous form- nodular lesions on the comb, wattle, eyelids and other unfeathered areas of the body. Diphtheritic form (wet pox)- cankers or diphtheritic yellowish lesions on the mucous membranes of mouth, esophagus or trachea with accompanying coryza like mild or severe respiratory signs when the lesions involve the trachea. Mortality in severe cases may be as high as 50 per cent.

Lesions

Cutaneous form: Local epithelial hyperplasia involving epidermis and underlying feather follicles with formation of nodules. **Diphtheritic form**: Slightly elevated white opaque nodules on the mucous membrane of the mouth, oesophagus and trachea.

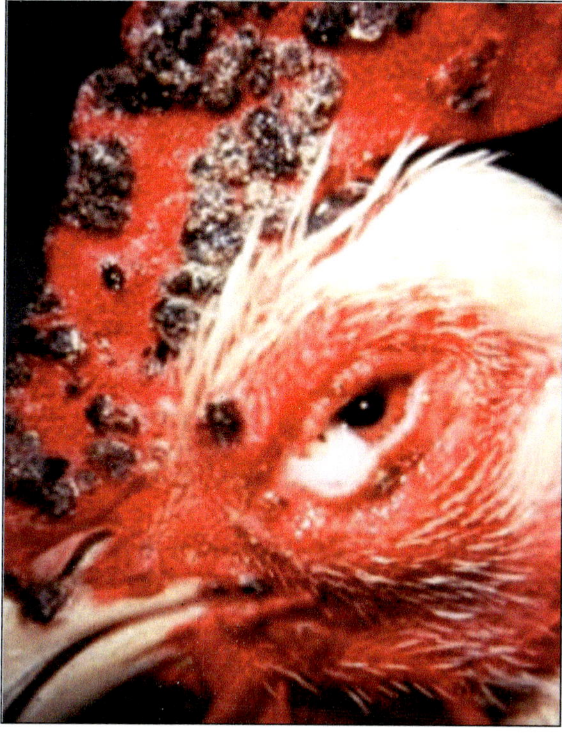

Figure 1.15. Fowl pox.

Diagnosis

Cutaneous infections usually produce characteristic gross and microscopic lesions. When only small cutaneous lesions are present, it is often difficult to distinguish them from abrasions caused by fighting. Microscopic examination of affected tissues stained with H and E reveals eosinophilic cytoplasmic inclusion bodies. Cytoplasmic inclusions are also detectable by fluorescent antibody and immunohistochemical methods (using antibodies against fowlpox virus antigens). The elementary bodies in the inclusion bodies can be detected in smears from lesions stained by the Gimenez method. Viral particles with typical poxvirus morphology can be demonstrated by negative-staining electron microscopy as well as in ultrathin sections of the lesions. The virus can be isolated by inoculating chorioallantoic membrane of developing chicken embryos, susceptible birds, or cell cultures of avian origin. Chicken embryos (9–12 days old) from an SPF flock are the preferred and convenient host for virus isolation. The genomic profiles of field isolates and vaccine strains of fowlpox virus can be compared by restriction fragment length polymorphism. This method is useful to compare closely related DNA genomes. However, because of the large size of the genome, minor differences are difficult to detect by this method. Detailed genetic analysis reveals differences between vaccine strains and field strains responsible for outbreaks of fowlpox in previously vaccinated chicken flocks. Whereas vaccine strains of fowlpox virus contain remnants of long terminal repeats of reticuloendotheliosis virus (REV), most field strains contain full-length REV in their genome.

Nucleic acid probes derived from cloned genomic fragments of fowlpox virus can also be used for diagnosis. This procedure is especially useful for differentiation of the diphtheritic form of fowlpox (involving the trachea) from infectious laryngotracheitis.

PCR can be used to amplify genomic DNA sequences of various sizes using specific primers. This procedure is useful when an extremely small amount of viral DNA is present in the sample. PCR has been used effectively to differentiate field and vaccine strains of the virus, whether full-length REV is present in those strains that are associated with outbreaks in vaccinated birds. DNA isolated from the formalin-fixed tissue sections of birds that are histologically positive for fowlpox can be used for PCR amplification of genomic fragments using specific primers. Because most outbreaks of fowlpox in previously vaccinated chickens are caused by strains with a genome that contains full-length REV, use of REV envelope-specific primers to determine the presence of full-length REV is helpful in such cases. Two monoclonal antibodies that recognize different fowlpox virus antigens have been developed. These monoclonal antibodies are useful for strain differentiation by immunoblotting. The complete nucleotide sequence of the fowlpox virus genome has been determined. It is useful in comparing the sequences of selected genes of other avian poxviruses.

Prevention and Treatment

Where fowlpox is prevalent, chickens and turkeys should be vaccinated with a live-embryo or cell-culture-propagated virus vaccine. The most widely used vaccines are attenuated fowlpox virus and pigeonpox virus isolates of high immunogenicity and low pathogenicity. In high-risk areas, vaccination with an attenuated vaccine of cell-culture origin in the first few weeks of life and revaccination at 12–16 wks is often sufficient. Health of birds, extent of exposure, and type of operation determine the timing of vaccinations. Because the infection spreads slowly, vaccination is often useful in limiting spread in affected flocks if administered when <20 per cent of the birds have lesions. Passive immunity may interfere with multiplication of vaccine virus; progeny from recently vaccinated or recently infected flocks should be vaccinated only after passive immunity has declined. Vaccinated birds should be examined 1 wk later for swelling and scab formation ("take") at the site of vaccination. Absence of "take" indicates lack of potency of vaccine, passive or acquired immunity, or improper vaccination. Revaccination with another serial lot of vaccine may be indicated. Naturally infected or vaccinated birds develop humoral as well as cell-mediated immune responses. Humoral immune responses can be measured by ELISA or virus neutralization tests.

Zoonotic Risk

There is no zoonotic risk associated with fowlpox virus. Avian poxviruses cause a productive infection in avian species but a nonproductive infection in mammalian hosts. Consequently, avianpox viruses have been used as vectors for expression of genes from mammalian pathogens in the development of safe recombinant vaccines.

1.16. Goat Pox

Synonyms

Variola capra.

Variola caprina (Goat Pox) is a contagious viral disease caused by a pox virus that affects goats. The virus usually spreads via the respiratory system, and sometimes spreads through abraded skin. It is most likely to occur in crowded stock. Sources of the virus include cutaneous lesions, saliva, nasal secretions and faeces. There are two types of the disease; the papulo-vesicular form and nodular form (stone pox). The incubation period is usually between 8–13 days, but it may be as short as 4 days. It is thought the same virus spreads sheep pox, to which European sheep breeds are highly susceptible. The virus may be present in dried scabs for up to 6 months. In endemic areas the morbidity rate is 70-90 per cent and the mortality rate is 5-10 per cent. The mortality rate may reach nearly 100 per cent in imported animals. Resistant animals may show only a mild form of the disease, which may be missed as only a few lesions are present, usually around the ears or the tail.

It is a malignant disease of goats characterized by fever and appearance of generalized pock lesions. It is caused by a member of the genus *Capripox* virus, sub-family chorodopox virinae, family Pox viridae. Goat pox virus, sheep pox virus and virus of bovine lumpy skin disease constitute Capri pox genus of pox viruses and they cannot be distinguished serologically. The disease has been reported from various parts of the world. The disease has been reported from different states of India. All breeds of goats are susceptible. The usual mode of transmission of this disease is by contact with the infected animal. The viral entry is through wound and abrasions. The biting insects, dogs are mechanically transmits the disease. Aerosol or droplet infection is quite possible.

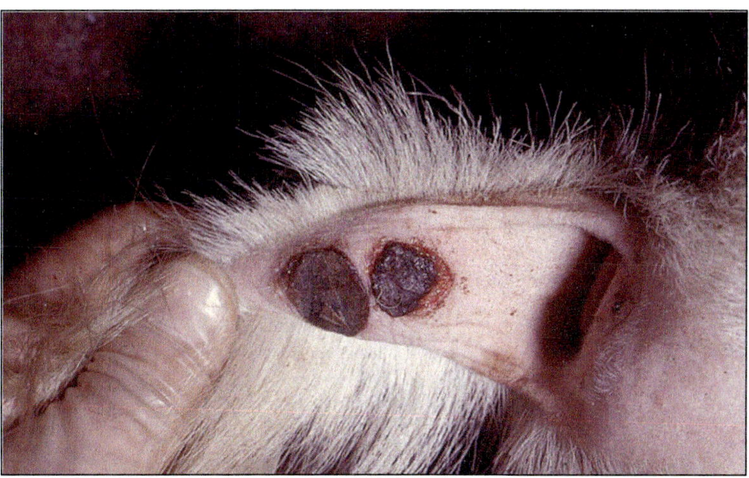

Figure 1.16. Goat. Two pox on the ventral tail have dessicated, dark red, undermined (necrotic and sloughing) centers.

Clinical Manifestations

Incubation period is 4-8 days after natural infection. Fever, formation of skin papules in the hairless regions at 2-5 days following fever. Papule later converted into macules. After papules formation rhinitis and conjunctivitis. Swelling of superficial lymph nodes and eye lids. Mucopurulent discharge from nose and eye. Macules convert into scabs. Death due to labored breathing due to bronchopneumonia.

Diagnosis

Samples of choice – scabs, based on clinical findings, isolation of the virus in cell cultures, SNT, AGID.

Differential Diagnosis

Contagious ecthyma or ORF, FMD.

Prevention and Control

Strict sanitary measures, disinfection of the goat shed with 1-3 per cent formalin, acids, caustic soda and virucidal disinfectants, caprination. The lymph from the vesicles is to be withdrawn and to be inoculated in the underside of tail or inner surface of the ear of young goat. Alternatively, the lymph may be rubbed on scarified surface of the skin. This will produce mild form of the disease and will protect against subsequent virulent attack

1.17. Highly Pathogenic Avian Influenza (HPAI)

Avian influenza (AI) viruses infect domestic poultry as well as pet, zoo, and wild birds. In domestic poultry, AI viruses are typically of low pathogenicity (LP), causing subclinical infections, respiratory disease, or drops in egg production. However, a few AI viruses cause severe systemic infections with high mortality. This highly pathogenic (HP) form of the disease has historically been called fowl plague. In most wild birds, AI viral infections are subclinical except for the recent H5N1 HPAI viruses of Eurasian lineage.

Influenza is an infection or disease syndrome caused by any type "A" influenza virus, a member of the Orthomyxoviridae family. Influenza "A" viruses are responsible for major disease problems in birds, as well as in human and lower mammals. Avian influenza viruses are distributed throughout the world in many domestic birds including turkeys, chickens, guinea fowl, chukars, quails, pheasants, geese and other waterfowls. Domestic turkeys and chickens have experienced the most substantial disease problems due to influenza. The disease caused in chickens and turkeys by HPAI viruses has historically been termed "fowl plague". The highly pathogenic avian influenza viruses should be used to describe viruses causing high mortality upon experimental infections of chickens.

HPAI Infections of Chickens and Turkeys

None of the clinical signs seen in HPAI infections of turkeys and chickens is pathognomonic. Many symptoms and post mortem lesions are similar to avian pasteurellosis. In general, more clinical signs are seen the longer the birds survive

HPAI infections, and in birds surviving >48 hours post infection, the following series of classical clinical signs can be seen, sudden onset of high mortality, cessation of egg laying, respiratory signs, excessive lacrymation, sinusitis, odema of the head, face and neck, cyanosis of unfeathered skin, particularly the comb and wattles and diarrhea, the very virulent viruses cause only sudden death.

HPAI in Ducks

Ducks are refractory to even the most pathogenic influenza viruses for chickens and turkeys, and this may be important in the epizootiology of HPAI.

Clinical Manifestations

The signs of disease are extremely variable and depend on the species affected, age, sex, concurrent infections, virus, environmental factors, *etc.* Signs may reflect abnormalities of the respiratory or enteric or reproductive or nervous systems. The signs most commonly reported include pronounced depression and decreased activity, decreased feed consumption and emaciation, increased broodiness of hens and decreased egg production, mild to severe respiratory signs including coughing, sneezing, rales and excessive lacrymation, huddling, ruffled feathers, odema of head and face, cyanosis of unfeathered skin, nervous disorder and mmunea. Any of these signs may occur singly or in various combinations.

Diagnosis

LP and HP AI viruses can be readily isolated from oropharyngeal and cloacal swabs, and HP AI viruses from many internal organs. AI viruses grow well in the allantoic sac of 9- to 11-day-old embryonating chicken eggs, and they agglutinate RBCs. The hemagglutination is not inhibited by Newcastle disease or other paramyxoviral antiserum. AI viruses are identified by demonstrating the presence of 1) influenza A matrix or nucleoprotein antigens using AGID or other suitable immunoassays, or 2) viral RNA using an influenza A–specific reverse transcriptase-PCR test.

LP AI must be differentiated from other respiratory diseases or causes of decreased egg production, including 1) acute to subacute viral diseases such as infectious bronchitis, infectious laryngotracheitis, low virulent Newcastle disease, and infections by other paramyxoviruses; 2) bacterial diseases such as mycoplasmosis, infectious coryza, ornithobacteriosis, turkey coryza, and the respiratory form of fowl cholera; and 3) fungal diseases such as aspergillosis. HP AI must be differentiated from other causes of high mortality such as virulent Newcastle disease, peracute septicemic fowl cholera, heat exhaustion, and severe water deprivation.

Dead Birds

Intestinal contents (faeces) or cloacal swabs, oropharyngeal swabs, samples from trachea, lungs, air sacs, intestine, spleen, kidney, brain, liver and heart should also collected and processed either separately or as a pool

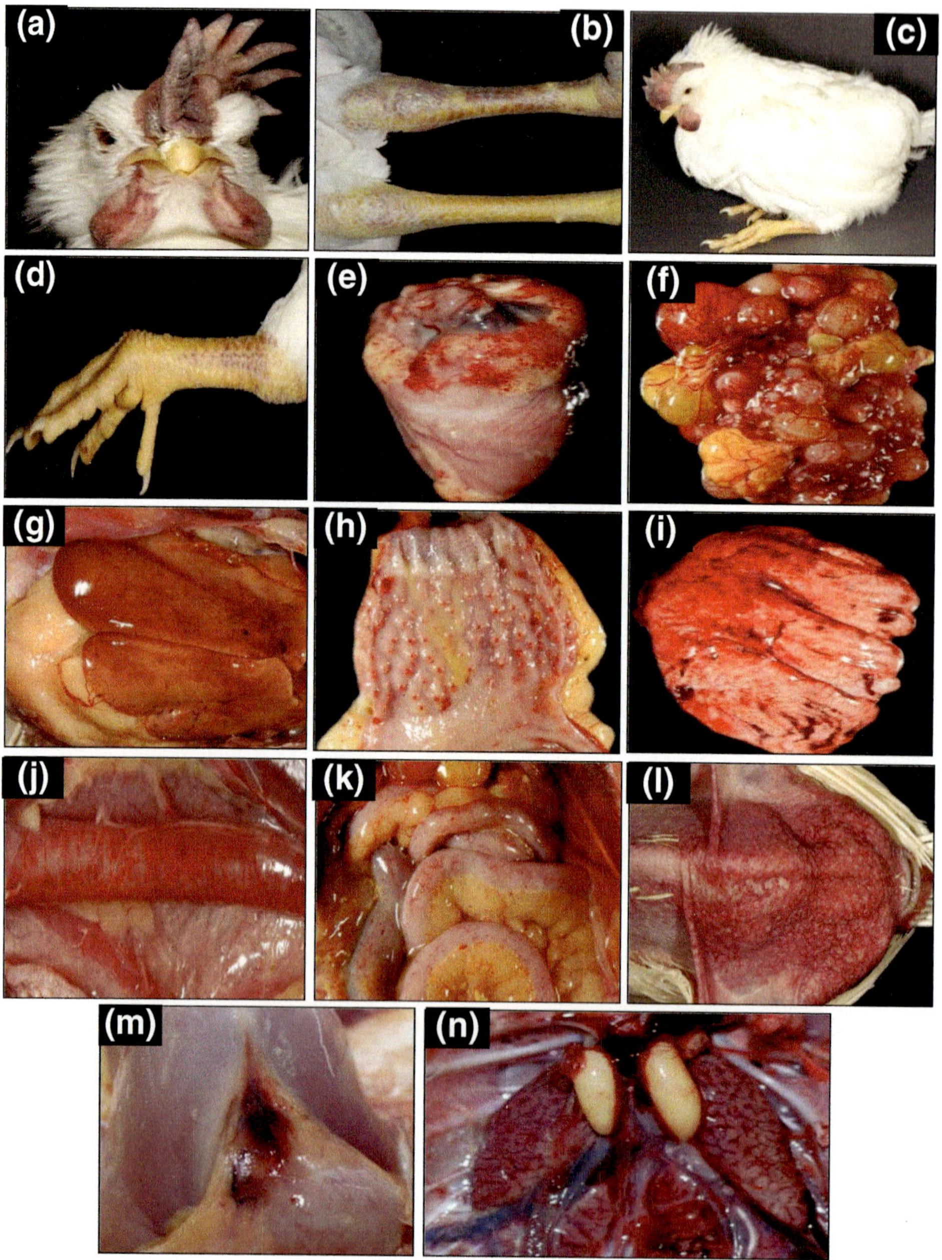

Figure 1.17

(a) Bilateral odema on face, (b) Different degree of haemorrhages on shank, (c) Depression of the bird with echymoses on the comb, (d) Ecchymotic haemorrage in the skin, (e) Petechiae in heart, (f) Congestion and haemorrhage in ovarian follicle, (g) Diffuse haemorrhage on the liver with hepatopathy, (h) Haemorrhage in proventriculus, (i) Haemorrhage in lungs, (j) Haemorrhagic tracheitis, (k) Multifocal haemorrhages in intestine, (l) Subcutaneous haemorrhage in skin, (m) Haemorrhage in fat, (n) Swollen kidneys.

Live Birds

Oropharyngeal and cloacal swabs. Swabbing of small delicate birds should be done with the use of especially small swabs that are usually commercially available and intended for use in humans. Where these are not available, the collection of fresh faeces may serve as an alternative.

Other Specimens

Drinking water or water from the water sources frequented by the birds. All samples should be placed in PBS pH 7.0-7.4 containing antibiotics. Faeces and tissue should be homogenized in PBS to give a suspension of 10-20 per cent w/v. The range and concentration of antibiotics are penicillin 2000 units/ml, streptomycin 2mg/ml, gentamycin 50µg/ml and mycostatin 1000 units/ml. These levels are suitable for tracheal swabs and tissue suspensions. But 5 fold higher concentrations should be used for cloacal swabs and faeces. Samples should be processed as soon as possible, but they may be stored in the antibiotic solution for up to 2 days at 4°C or for longer periods in the freezer at -70°C or on dry ice. Samples should be left in antibiotic solution at room temperature for 1-2 hours before inoculation. Embryonated fowl eggs are the most commonly used growth system for Influenza "A" viruses. Sample volume of 0.2 ml is inoculated into the amnio-allantoic cavity of five 8-10 day old embryonated fowl eggs. Tissue and faeces samples may need centrifugation at 1000 X g for 10 minutes before samples are taken for inoculation. Inoculated eggs are usually incubated at 37°C and their viability is monitored twice a day by candling. Dying or dead embryos as they arise and all eggs at 5 days post inoculation are chilled to 4°C and the harvested amnio-allantoic fluids are tested for HA activity. Negative fluids should be passaged, undiluted once more.

Serological Diagnosis

Haemagglutination inhibition (HI), Agar gel mmune diffusion (AGID) test.

Differential Diagnosis

This disease should be differentiated from the other diseases such as Newcastle disease (ND) and other Paramyxo viral infections, Chlamydia, Mycoplasma infections.

Prevention

Separation of susceptible birds from infected birds and their secretions and excretions, Entry of wild birds and swine into the farm premises should be prevented, following strict insecurity measures

Vaccination

Selection of subtype of the HPAI virus dominant in the particular area and an inactivated vaccine was prepared from the particular strain of the virus and used for vaccination.

Control

All methods for controlling the spread of influenza are based on preventing the contamination of, and controlling the movement of, people and equipment. Persons have direct contact with birds or their manure should not be moved from farm to farm, and it is important to keep the traffic area near the poultry house from becoming not contaminated with manure. In high risk areas such as those on migratory waterfowl routes, all domestic poultry will have to be reared in bird-proofed confinement, if freedom from infection is to be maintained. Prevention of secondary spread is also important. Secondary spread is prevented by Controlled marketing and depopulation of infected flocks after recovery from acute disease. Cleaning and disinfection of buildings after depopulation. A rest period of 3-4 weeks before repopulation, Controlled movement of people and strict sanitary procedures, Prevention of access of wild birds to poultry flocks, Vaccination. In HPAI outbreaks governmental eradication procedures (quarantine, slaughter, disposal and cleanup are employed.

Zoonotic Risk

AI viruses exhibit host adaptation to birds. Human infections have occurred, usually as isolated, rare, individual cases. Most human cases have originated from infection with Eurasian H5N1 HP AI virus and, most recently, Chinese H7N9 LP AI virus. The total accumulated human cases of H5N1 HP AI virus in Asia and Africa from 2003–2013 is 648, of which 384 were fatal. The primary risk factor for human infection has been direct contact with live or dead infected poultry, but a few cases have resulted from consumption of uncooked poultry products, defeathering of infected wild swans, or close contact with human cases. Respiratory infection has been the most frequent presentation of human H5N1 cases. For H7N9 LP AI, total accumulated human cases in China for 2013 are 137, of which 45 were fatal. Most cases had exposure risk to live-poultry markets. Conjunctivitis was the most frequent symptom in human cases of H7N7 HP AI virus infection in the Netherlands during 2003, with 89 confirmed cases and 1 fatality. Other HP AI viruses and all LP AI viruses have produced very rare or no human infections.

1.18. Infectious Bursal Disease (IBD)

Synonyms

Gumboro disease, Avian bursitis, Infectious nephritis.

Infectious bursal disease (IBD) is seen in domestic chickens worldwide. It can present as a clinical or subclinical disease, but immunosuppression and related secondary infections are typically seen. Severity of the immunosuppression depends on the virulence of the infecting virus and age of the host. Infectious bursal disease (IBD) is an acute, highly contagious viral infection of young chickens that has lymphoid tissue as its primary target with a special predilection for the bursa of fabricius. Gumboro disease was recognized as a disease of chicken in 1957, and a virus reported in Gumboro (USA) in 1962 by Coxgrove. In India this disease was first reported by Mohanty *et.al.* (1971) in Uttar Pradesh. Chicken are the only natural hosts for the virus in which natural infection occurs. All breeds were affected, White leghorns more susceptible. Infectious bursal disease is most severe in chicks 3-6 weeks old, when the target organ, the bursa of fabricius, reaches its maximal stage of development. Naturally virus has special affinity for pre-B lymphocytes of the bursa of fabricius, leading to acquired B-lymphocyte deficiency in affected birds. Infectious bursal disease virus (IBDV) is a double stranded RNA virus and is a member of the Birna viridae family, genus Birna virus. It is inhibited by formalin and not by ether, chloroform and phenol *etc.* It is stable at pH-2, but inactivated at pH 12. There are three serotypes of the virus. Infectious bursal disease virus replicates in both chicken and mammalian cells. Chicken embryo kidney cell culture is good for isolation. Cytopathogenic effect is seen in 3-5 days. Chicken embryo fibroblasts are more sensitive than fertile eggs for viral titration.

Clinical Manifestations

Incubation period is very short -2-3 days, earliest sign – birds picking their own vents, soiled vent feathers, whitish or watery peciali, anorexia, depression, ruffled feathers, trembling, severe prostration and death, affected birds became dehydrated, subnormal temperature in terminal stages, morbidity 100 per cent, mortality 20-30 per cent.

Lesions

Dehydration, hemorrhages in the leg and thigh muscles, hepatic infarcts, enlarged kidneys with pronounced tubules. Bursa highly enlarged twice or 2-4 times of its normal size-approximately three days after infection and becomes edematous and hemorrhagic, atrophies by 12 days, post infection. Spleen slightly enlarged and mottled with deep red spots. Hemorrhagic lesions present in the proventriculus and hypertrophy of the liver is noticed.

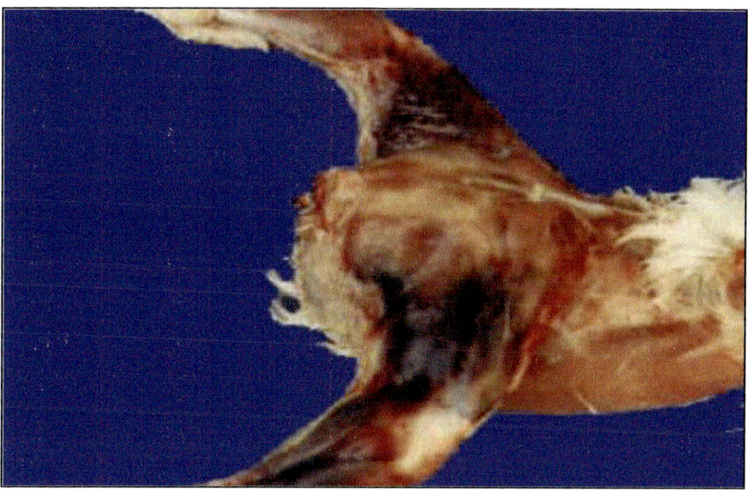

Figure 1.18. Infectious bursal disease.

Immunosuppressive Properties

Infectious bursal disease (IBD) infection reduces the HI antibody titers and lgG levels for Newcastle disease vaccination. Further humoral antibody response to various vaccines was also suppressed. Immunosuppressive property as been recorded in the cases of Infectious bronchitis (IB) and Infectious laryngeotracheitis (ILT) also. Report of suppression of CMI by IBD also has been recorded.

Diagnosis

Specimens

Bursa, spleen, blood, based on history and clinical signs, identification of the agent, isolation of IBDV are not usually carried out as a routine diagnostic procedure. Specific antibody-negative chickens may be used for this purpose, as may cell cultures or embryonating eggs from specific antibody-negative sources. However, some difficulty may be experienced if using the latter two systems as the virus does not readily adapt to them. If successful, the identity of the virus can be confirmed by the virus pecializedon (VN) test. The agar gel immunodiffusion (AGID) test can be used to detect viral antigen in the bursa of fabricius. A portion of the bursa is removed, homogenized, and used as antigen in a test against known positive antiserum. This is particularly useful in the early stages of the infection, before the development of an antibody response. An Immunofluorescence test using IBDV-specific chicken antiserum can also be used to detect antigen in bursal tissue. Antigen-capture enzyme-linked immunosorbent assays (ELISAs) based on plates coated with IBDV-specific antibodies have also been described for the demonstration of IBDV antigens in bursal homogenates. The reverse transcription polymerase chain reaction (RT-PCR) with specific primers may be used to detect viral genomic RNA in the bursa of fabricius.

Strain Characterization

IBDV strains can be further identified by testing their pathogenicity in specific antibody-negative chickens, by investigating their antigenic reactivity in cross VN assays or in tests based on monoclonal antibodies, by determining the nucleotide sequence of RT-PCR amplification products derived from IBDV genome, or by studying the number and size of the restriction fragments obtained following digestion of such RT-PCR products with restriction endonucleases. Tests should be performed by pecialized laboratories and should include a panel of reference strains as controls. Although the molecular basis for antigenic variation is now better understood, no validated virulence marker has been described yet.

Prevention and Control

Maternal antibodies protect day old chicks against death and clinical IBD. **Vaccination**: Ideal age of vaccination –14 to 16 days of age by using IV95/ Intermediate plus/MB strain and this vaccine should be repeated after one week. Vaccination of breeders to produce high maternal antibody level in the offspring to prevent infection during first week of age. Vaccination of the progeny at day old to prevent early infection. Long lasting and more uniform levels of maternal antibody was present in, the chicks which were from breeders receiving two live IBD vaccines and are inactivated oil emulsion IBD vaccine during the growing period.

1.19. Infectious Bovine Rhinotracheitis

Synonyms

Viral bovine rhinotracheitis, Red nose, Necrotic rhinitis.

Infectious Bovine Rhinotracheitis (IBR) is a highly contagious, infectious respiratory disease that is caused by Bovine Herpesvirus-1 (BHV-1). It can affect young and older cattle. In addition to causing respiratory disease, this virus can cause conjunctivitis, abortions, encephalitis, and eutralizat systemic infections. IBR is eutralizatio by acute inflammation of the upper respiratory tract. It is an acute highly contagious viral disease of cattle characterized by high temperature, rhinitis, dyspnoea, abortion, meningoencephalitis, keratoconjunctivitis and pustular vulvovaginitis. Dairy and beef cattle are equally susceptible. Besides cattle, the disease also reported in goat, swine and water buffaloes. The disease is widely prevalent in all parts of the world. In India the disease has been recorded from various states including Uttar Pradesh, Kerala, Gujarat, Tamil Nadu, Odisha, Andhra Pradesh and Karnataka. The disease is caused by a DNA virus called bovine herpes virus-1 belonging to the family herpes viridae, subfamily Alpha herpes virinae and genus *Varicello* virus. Cattle of all ages are affected. Dairy and beef cattle are equally susceptible. Besides cattle the disease also reported in goat, swine and water buffaloes and in wild ruminants. The virus is transmitted through infected feed and water. The virus can spread through ocular, nasal and reproductive secretion and excretion of infected cattle. Droplet infection is the important way of transmission.

Clinical Manifestations

The clinical signs have been grouped as respiratory form, vulvo-vaginal form, ocular form, encephalomyelitic form, abortive form.

(a) **Respiratory form:** This form is characterized by mild to severe rise of temperature, depression of appetite, acceleration of respiration and dyspnoea. The nasal discharges are initially serous which later turn to mucopurulent. Whole of the upper respiratory tract show hyperemia, edema along with mucopurulent exudation causing dyspnoea. Affected cattle may exhibit open mouth breathing in severe cases. Animal may show signs of bronchitis and pneumonitis. The nasal mucosa is severely congested hence the disease is named as "Red nose". The recovered cattle may remain as carrier and thus shed the virus for a considerable period.

(b) **Vulvo-vaginal form:** This form is characterized by sharp fall in milk yield and appearance of erythematous and pustular lesions on the vulvar and vaginal mucosa. There is swelling of vulva and frequent urination. There may be mucopurulent discharge from vulva and vagina. Animal is unable to put its tail in normal position after urination due to pain. The virus produces pustular balanoposthitis in bull. The semen of the affected bull become contaminated and thus pose problem in natural or artificial breeding.

(c) **Ocular form:** This form may appear along with respiratory form. There is inflammation of the conjunctiva in addition to respiratory changes. But in some occasions severe conjunctivitis and ocular discharges may be noted without respiratory involvement. The ocular discharges vary from serous to purulent. Petechial hemorrhages may be noted on the conjunctiva and sometime corneal opacity may appear as main attribute of the disease.

(d) **Encephalomyelitic form:** The virus may produce severe encephalomyelitis syndrome in calf terminating to death. The signs of encephalomyelitis comprise of high rise of temperature, incoordination, tremor, circling, falling, coma and death. Death ensures within 4 days following appearance of neurological signs.

(e) **Abortive form:** The pregnant cattle may abort following infection. The abortion may supervene as "abortion storm". Foetus died at 4 months of gestation and expelled. Foetus is autolysed in most cases.

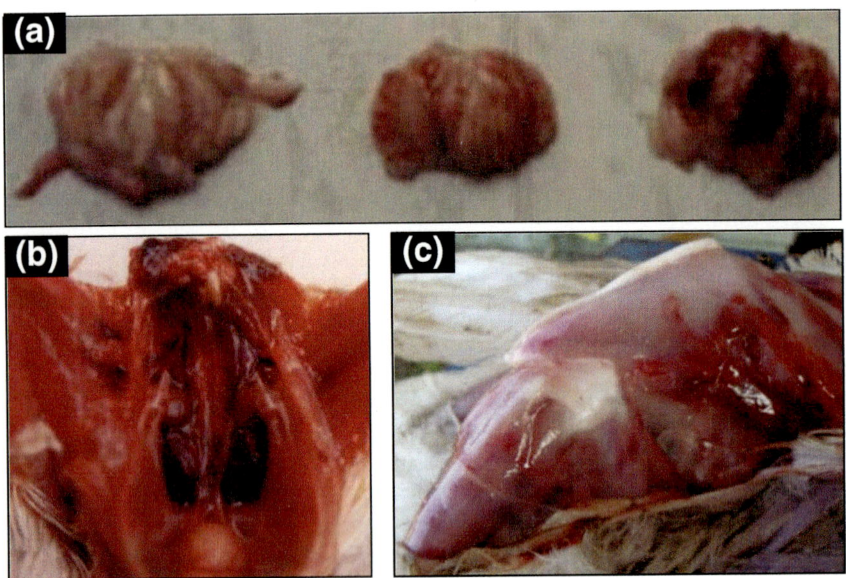

Figure 1.19

(a) IBD-Haemorrhage in bursa, (b) IBD-Enlarged bursa, (c) IBD-Haemorrhage in breast muscles.

Diagnosis

Samples of live animals to be collected from nasal swabs or genital swabs or conjunctival swabs during the acute phase of infection, aborted materials, tissue samples from the fetal liver, brain, and spleen, semen, placenta, uterine mucus and serum. Samples of dead animals to be collected from lymph nodes, liver, lungs, brain, aborted foetal liver, brain and spleen.

Based on Clinical Signs

Identification of the Agent

The virus can be isolated from nasal swabs or genital swabs, from animals with vulvovaginitis or balanoposthitis, taken during the acute phase of the infection, and from various organs collected at post-mortem. For virus isolation, various cell cultures of bovine origin are used, for example, secondary lung or kidney cells or the Madin–Darby bovine kidney cell line. The virus produces a cytopathic effect in 2– 4 days. It is identified by neutralization or antigen detection methods using monospecific antisera or monoclonal antibodies. Viral DNA detection methods have been developed, and the polymerase chain reaction technique is increasingly used in routine diagnosis.

Serological Tests

The virus eutralization test and various enzyme-linked immunosorbent assays (ELISA) are most widely used for antibody detection. ELISA antibodies can be detected in serum and with lower sensitivity in milk. Fluorescent antibody technique (FAT) and electron microscopy can be made for diagnosis of disease.

Differential Diagnosis

This disease should be differentiated from;

Pasteurellosis	Respiratory signs alone present and responds to broad spectrum antibiotic therapy
Parainfluenza	Toxaemia, dyspnea, - Antibiotic treatment for secondary bacterial complications and recovery in 3-5 days
Verminous pneumonia	Respiratory signs, esinophilia, responds to broad spectrum antibiotic therapy
CBPP	Fibrinous pneumonia, pleurisy, deep cough, extension of head, abduction of elbow, pleural rub, differentiated with IBR with serological tests

Prevention and Control

No successful treatment, antibiotics given to avoid or prevent secondary bacterial complications. Best way to control this disease is to prevent contact between infected animals and seronegative animals. Since the virus is latent in seropositive animals, they should be identified and eliminate them from the herd. Good hygiene, management and isolation do not seem control the disease adequately.

Vaccination

The best practice is to vaccinate females kept for breeding once or twice prior to their first breeding with modified live virus vaccines or inactivated vaccine. Age of vaccination in calves after 5 months of age. Immunity develops within 10-14 days. Live vaccines induce a relatively rapid immune response comprising both humoral and cell-mediated responses, including mucosal immunity that resembles a natural infection. Live attenuated vaccine administered through intramuscular or intranasal route, but modified live virus (MLV) vaccines contraindicated in pregnant cows because MLV have the property of abortigenicity. In outbreaks-intranasal route selected. Vaccine may be instilled into one or two nostrils. Killed vaccines are administered by intramuscular route. Primary and secondary inoculation should be given four weeks apart followed by booster inoculations annually.

1.20. Inclusion Body Hepatitis (IBH)/ Hydropericardium Syndrome

Adenoviruses are widespread throughout all avian species. Studies have demonstrated the presence of antibodies in healthy poultry, and viruses have been isolated from normal birds. Despite their widespread distribution, most adenoviruses cause no or only mild disease; however, some are associated with specific clinical conditions. Avian adenoviruses (AAVs) in chickens are the etiologic agents of two important diseases known as inclusion body hepatitis (IBH) and hydropericardium syndrome (HP). Although in some cases each disease is observed separately, the two conditions have been frequently observed as a single entity; therefore, the name hepatitis hydropericardium has been widely used to describe the pathologic condition. The syndrome is an acute disease of young chickens associated with anemia, hemorrhagic disorders, and hydropericardium. It is a common disease in several countries, where broilers are severely affected, resulting in high mortality rates.

Inclusion body hepatitis/hydropericardium syndrome is an acute disease of young chickens associated with anemia, hemorrhagic disorders, and hydropericardium. It is a common disease in several countries, where broilers are severely affected, resulting in high mortality rates. It is caused by avian adenovirus. Although there are 12 different serotypes of AAV, the most common viruses isolated in cases of IBH/HP belong to serotypes 4 and 8. This disease commonly affects the broiler birds of 3-6 weeks age. Sometimes layer and breeder pullets also affected. This disease was first reported in Pakisthan in the year 1987 and first reported in India in the year 1994. Horizontal and vertical transmission plays an important role in IBH/HP. In the breeder flocks the vertical transmission of IBH/HP reported when the progeny from breeder flocks infected with AAV serotypes 4 and 8. Young chicks in contact with infected chicks can die of peracute IBH/HP. Chicks and young chickens are commonly affected. Infection with some strains of AAV may result in minimal hepatic disease; however, the disease becomes more severe when there is combination of infection with immunosuppressive diseases such as infectious bursal disease and chicken infectious anaemia.

Clinical Signs and Lesions

Sudden onset of mortality, dullness, huddling together, ruffled feathers and mucoid/yellowish dropping. Sudden mortality usually is seen in chickens < 6 wkold and as young as 4 days of age. In chickens of < 3 weeks age mortality normally ranges from 2-40 per cent. However, there have been outbreaks in which mortality has reached 80 per cent. Mortality rates also vary depending on the pathogenicity of the virus and infection with other viral or bacterial agents. Signs associated with diseases caused by other pathogens (*e.g.*, bacteria, fungi, or viruses) commonly occur if birds are immunosuppressed. Gross lesions include up to 10 mL of a straw-colored transudate in the pericardial sac, generalized congestion, and an enlarged, pale, friable liver.

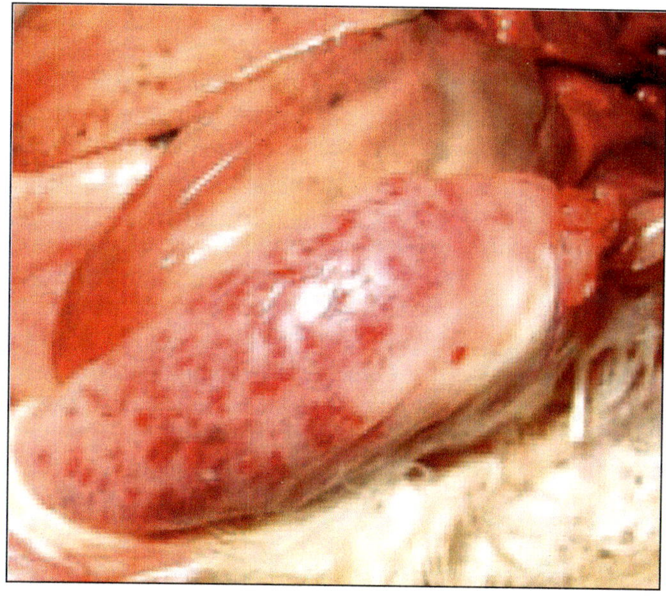

Figure 1.20. Inclusion body hepatitis/hydropericardium syndrome.

Diagnosis

Virus Isolation

Virus isolation by inoculation of 10 per cent suspension of the affected organ and faeces suspension into cell cultures such as chick embryo liver or lung cells or chick kidney cell cultures.

Serology

AGID or double immunodiffusion, IFAT, ELISA, SNT.

Prevention and Control

Both live and inactivated vaccines are used to control the syndrome. The AAV serotypes most frequently used to prepare commercial vaccines are serotypes 4 and 8. Sometimes autogenous inactivated vaccines are also used to ensure the transfer of maternal immunity from breeding flocks to their progeny. When breeders are properly vaccinated, antibodies generated by the vaccine are transmitted to the progeny, providing protection against field infections and clinical disease. Broilers are vaccinated at < 10 days of age when their parents either do not have serotype-specific adenovirus antibodies or maternal antibody transmission is erratic due to improper vaccination procedures that result in a substantial number of unvaccinated birds.

1.21. Infectious Bronchitis

Synonym

Gasping disease.

Infectious bronchitis is an acute, highly contagious disease of major economic importance in commercial chicken flocks throughout the world. It is usually characterized by respiratory signs, although decreased egg production and poor egg quality are sometimes seen in breeders and layers. Some strains of the etiologic agent, infectious bronchitis virus (IBV), are nephropathogenic, causing interstitial nephritis, particularly in chicks. Associations with myopathy and proventriculitis have also been reported. An acute, highly contagious respiratory disease of chickens characterized by respiratory signs such as coughing, sneezing, tracheal rales with accumulation of mucus in the bronchi and depression, heavy mortality in young chickens, stunting growth, nephritis, increased feed convertion ratio, long-term reproductive problem, decreased egg production and affect both internal and external quality of egg. This disease is distributed worldwide. Infectious bronchitis virus (IBV) is a member of the family Coronaviridae, genus Coronavirus positive stranded linear ssRNA virus. Chicken is the only bird that is usually infected by IBV. All ages are susceptible, but the disease is most severe in baby chicks. This virus spreads rapidly among chicks by aerosol transmission.

Clinical Signs

The incubation period of IB is 18-36 hour depending on the route of inoculation. The characteristic respiratory signs of IB in chicks are gasping, coughing, sneezing, tracheal rales and nasal discharges. Wet eyes may be observed and occasional swollen sinuses. The chicks appear depressed, may be seen huddled under a heat source and feed consumption and weight gain are significantly reduced. In chickens over 6 weeks of age and in adult birds the signs are similar to those in chicks, but nasal discharge does not occur as frequently and the disease may go unnoticed unless the flock is examined carefully by handling the birds or listening to them at night when the birds are normally quiet. In laying flocks there is declined egg production and quality are seen in addition to respiratory signs. Internal qualities of eggs also affected. The albumen of the egg maybe thin and watery without definite demarcation between the thick and thin albumen.

Gross Lesions

Infected chickens have serous, catarrhal or caseous eexudates in the trachea, nasal passages and sinuses. Airsacs may appear cloudy or contain yellow caseous eexudates. A caseous plug may be found in the lower trachea or bronchi of the chicks die due to the disease. In affected layer birds fluid yolk material may be found in the abdominal cavity.

Diagnosis

Laboratory confirmation is required for diagnosis of respiratory forms because of similarities to mild forms of disease caused by agents such as Newcastle disease virus, avian metapneumovirus, infectious laryngotracheitis virus, mycoplasmas, *A.*

paragallinarum, and *Ornithobacterium rhinotracheale*. Demonstration of seroconversion or a rise in antibody titer against IBV by ELISA, or hemagglutination inhibition or virus neutralization tests can be used for diagnosis when there is a history of respiratory disease or reduced egg production.

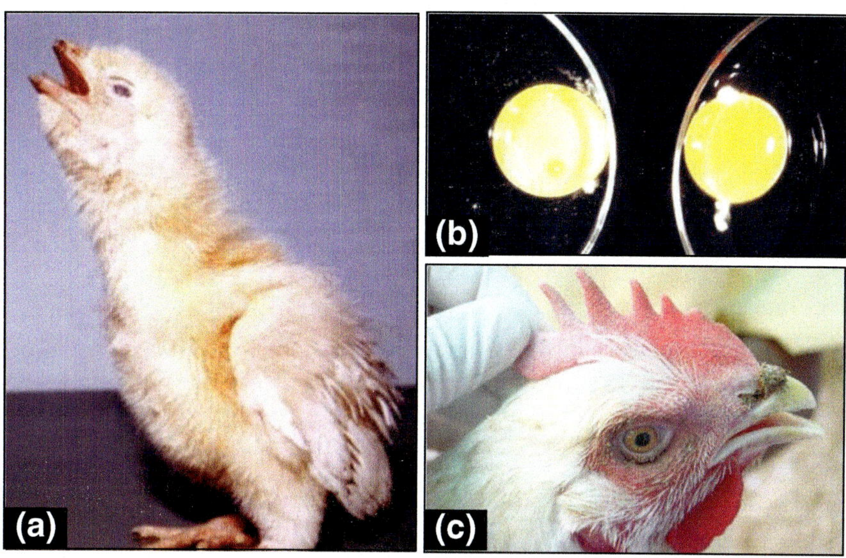

Figure 1.21

(a) IB-Chick with open mouthed breathing, (b) IB- Altered internal quality of egg (left) with normal egg (right), (c) IB-Muccoprulent nasal discharge

Definitive diagnosis is generally based on virus detection and identification. Virus can be isolated by inoculation of homogenates of tracheal, cecal tonsil, and/or kidney tissue into 9- to 11-day-old SPF chicken embryos, with growth of IBV indicated by embryo stunting and curling, and deposition of urates in the mesonephros, with variable mortality. Alternatively, IBV may be isolated in tracheal organ cultures, with growth of virus indicated by cessation of cilial motility. Several blind passages of the virus may be necessary for isolation of some field strains. More rapid diagnosis may be achieved using reverse transcriptase-polymerase chain reaction (RT-PCR) assays to detect viral RNA in nucleic acid extracts of tracheal, cecal tonsil, or kidney tissue.

Typing viruses can help distinguish vaccine and field strains and may help diagnose outbreaks caused by serotypes distinct from those of the vaccines used in a flock. Serotypes have been identified using sera from SPF chickens inoculated with known serotypes in virus neutralization tests. However, because this is expensive and time consuming, it is not readily available. A restricted range of serotype-specific monoclonal antibodies (MAb) have been developed for serotyping, but direct detection viral antigen using these Mabs to immunohistochemically stain tissue sections from diseased birds is of limited value because of the low concentration of antigen in tissues. The Mabs have been best used after propagation in chicken embryos, to detect viral antigen in the chorioallantoic membranes by immunofluorescence or immunoperoxidase staining, or in the allantoic fluid by ELISA. Analyses of the products of RT-PCR assays are now commonly used to identify the virus serotype and to identify individual strains within serotypes. The S1 region of the spike glycoprotein gene determines the serotype, and RT-PCR products derived from this region can be subjected to restriction fragment length polymorphism analysis, analyzed by nucleotide sequencing, or compared with reference strains using high-resolution melting curve analysis. Genotype determination based on the S1 region can be complemented by analyzing other regions of the viral genome, including the nucleocapsid gene and the 5′ untranslated region. These analyses can also aid in rapid detection of novel recombinant IBVs.

Prevention and Control

Management Procedures

Ideal managemental procedures include strict isolation and repopulation with only day old chicks, following the cleaning and disinfection of the poultry house. Ventilating houses with filtered air under positive pressure.

Vaccination

Both live and inactivated virus vaccines used for IB immunization. Live vaccines are used in broilers and for initial vaccination of breeders and layers. Inactivated oil emulsion vaccines are used primarily at point of lay in breeders and layers. Live vaccine administered individually by eye drop, intratracheal or intranasal route. Mass application methods include administration of vaccine as coarse spray, aerosol and drinking water. Inactivated vaccines require injection of individual birds. These vaccines are usually given after priming with live virus and are administered a few weeks before production commences.

Time of Vaccination

Two weeks of age is frequently used as the time for initial immunization. Booster doses administered at 7-12 or 16-18 weeks of age.

1.22. Infectious Canine Hepatitis

Synonyms

Rubarth's disease, contagious hepatitis.

Infectious canine hepatitis (ICH) is a worldwide, contagious disease of dogs with signs that vary from a slight fever and congestion of the mucous membranes to severe depression, marked iarrheaa, and coagulation disorders. It also is seen in foxes, wolves, coyotes, bears, lynx, and some pinnipeds; other carnivores may become infected without developing clinical illness. In recent years, the disease has become uncommon in areas where routine immunization is done, but periodic outbreaks, which may reflect maintenance of the disease in wild and feral hosts, reinforce the need for continued vaccination. It is an acute infectious viral disease of dogs of all ages, characterized by high rise of temperature, vomition, iarrhea and convulsion. This disease is caused by a DNA virus belongs to adenovirus. Among the members of the Canidae family dogs and foxes are more important species to suffer from this disease. Among the dogs younger dogs under one year of age suffer with acute form of the disease after which the dogs are inapparently infected with periodic relapses. Excretions and secretions are the important sources of the virus to healthy animals.

Clinical Manifestation

Signs vary from a slight fever to death. The mortality rate ranges from 10 per cent –30 per cent and is typically highest in very young dogs. Concurrent parvoviral or distemper infection worsens the prognosis. The incubation period is 4–9 days. The first sign is a fever of >104°F (40°C), which lasts 1–6 days and is usually biphasic. If the fever is of short duration, iarrheaa may be the only other sign, but if it persists for >1 day, acute illness develops. Signs are apathy, anorexia, thirst, conjunctivitis, serous discharge from the eyes and nose, and occasionally abdominal pain and vomiting. Intense hyperemia or petechiae of the oral mucosa, as well as enlarged tonsils, may be seen. Tachycardia out of proportion to the fever may occur. There may be subcutaneous edema of the head, neck, and trunk. Despite hepatic involvement, there is a notable absence of icterus in most acute clinical cases. Clotting time is directly correlated with the severity of illness and is the result of disseminated intravascular coagulation induced by vascular endothelial compromise, coupled with failure of the liver to rapidly replace consumed clotting factors. It may be difficult to control hemorrhage, which is manifest by bleeding around deciduous teeth and by spontaneous hematomas. CNS involvement is unusual and is typically the result of vascular injury. Severely infected dogs may develop convulsions from forebrain damage. Paresis may result from brain stem hemorrhages, and ataxia and central blindness have also been described. Foxes more consistently have CNS signs and intermittent convulsions during the course of illness, and paralysis may involve one or more limbs or the entire body. Respiratory signs usually are not seen in dogs with ICH; however, CAV-1 has been recovered from dogs with signs of infectious tracheobronchitis despite high serologic titers against parenteral disease. Clinicopathologic findings reflect the coagulopathy (prolonged prothrombin time, thrombocytopenia, and increased fibrin degradation products). Severely affected dogs show acute hepatocellular injury (increased ALT and AST). Proteinuria is common. Leukopenia typically persists throughout the febrile period. The degree of iarrheaa varies and seems to be correlated with the severity of illness. On recovery, dogs eat well but regain weight slowly. Hepatic transaminase activities peak around day 14 of infection and then decline slowly. In ~25 per cent of recovered dogs, bilateral corneal opacity develops 7–10 days after acute signs disappear and usually resolves spontaneously. In mild cases, transient corneal opacity may be the only sign of disease. It has long been thought that chronic hepatitis may develop in dogs that have low levels of passive antibody when exposed, although a recent PCR-based study did not confirm this theory.

Lesions

Endothelial damage results in "paint-brush" hemorrhages on the gastric serosa, lymph nodes, thymus, pancreas, and subcutaneous tissues. Hepatic cell necrosis produces a variegated color change in the liver, which may be normal in size or swollen. Histologically, there is centrilobular necrosis, with neutrophilic and monocytic infiltration, and hepatocellular intranuclear inclusions. The gallbladder wall is typically edematous and thickened; edema of the thymus may be found. Grayish white foci may be seen in the kidney cortex.

Acute Form

Acute form of the disease starts with apathy, anorexia and high rise of temperature up to 105°F. There is often vomition and iarrhea. The faeces are often blood tinged and abdominal pain also evinced. The first rise of temperature usually falls after 24-48 hours without leveling to normal temperature; it rises again to form a saddle curve which will last for 6 days. Animal shows intense thirst and the buccal mucous membrane turn fiery red or even hemorrhagic. There is swelling of liver capsule which results in pain on palpation of xiphoid region. The dogs may show "tucked up" condition of the abdomen. After 1-3 weeks following disappearance of clinical signs, a transient corneal opacity may develop. This condition is known as "Blue eye". This is due to iridocyclitis and corneal oedema.

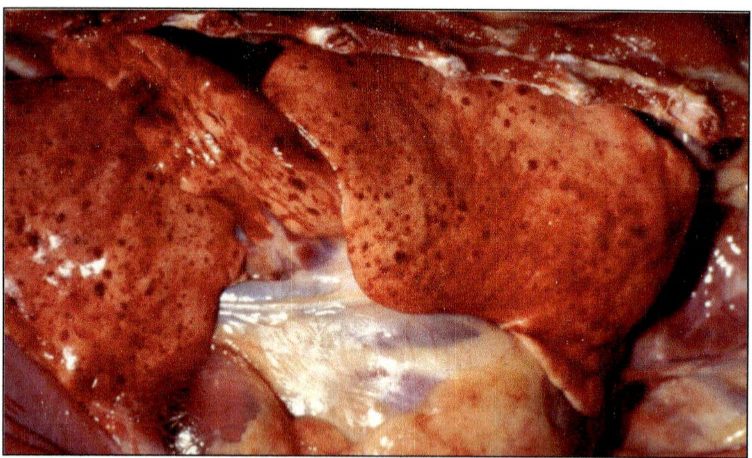

Figure 1.22. Infectious canine hepatitis.

Diagnosis

Usually, the abrupt onset of illness and bleeding suggest ICH, although clinical evidence is not always sufficient to differentiate ICH from distemper. Definitive antemortem diagnosis is not required before institution of supportive care but can be pursued with commercially available ELISA, serologic, and PCR testing. PCR or restriction fragment length polymorphism is required to definitively distinguish CAV-1 from CAV-2, if clinically necessary. Postmortem gross changes in the liver and gallbladder are more conclusive, and diagnosis is confirmed by virus isolation, immunofluorescence, characteristic intranuclear inclusion bodies in the liver, or PCR or fluorescence in situ hybridization studies of infected tissue.

Treatment

Treatment is symptomatic and supportive. The goals of therapy are to limit secondary bacterial invasion, support fluid balance, and control hemorrhagic tendencies. Broad-spectrum antibiotics and intravenously administered balanced electrolyte solutions with 5 per cent dextrose supplementation are indicated. Plasma or whole blood transfusions may be necessary in severely ill dogs. Although the transient corneal opacity (which may be seen during the course of ICH or associated with vaccination with attenuated CAV-1 vaccines) usually requires no treatment, atropine ophthalmic ointment may alleviate the painful ciliary spasm sometimes associated with it. Dogs with corneal clouding should be protected against bright light. Systemic corticosteroids are contraindicated for treatment of corneal opacity associated with ICH.

Prevention

Modified-live virus (MLV) injectable vaccines are available and are often combined with other vaccines. Vaccination against ICH is recommended at the time of canine distemper vaccinations. Maternal antibody from immune bitches interferes with active immunization in puppies until they are 9–12 wk-old. Attenuated CAV-1 vaccines have produced transient unilateral or bilateral opacities of the cornea, and the virus may be shed in urine. For these reasons, CAV-2 attenuated live virus strains, which provide cross-protection against CAV-1, are preferentially used because they have very little tendency to produce corneal opacities or uveitis, and the virus is not shed in urine. Historically, annual revaccination against ICH was standard, and vaccines are labelled for annual use. Increasing evidence suggests that immunity induced by MLV CAV-1 injectable vaccines lasts dikhuaaa 3 year, although this remains an extra-label use of commercially available vaccines.

1.23. Infectious Laryngotracheitis (ILT)

Infectious laryngotracheitis (ILT) is an acute, highly contagious, herpesvirus infection of chickens and pheasants characterized by severe dyspnea, coughing, and rales. It can also be a subacute disease with nasal and ocular discharge, tracheitis, conjunctivitis, and mild rales. The disease is caused by *Gallid herpesvirus I*, commonly known as infectious laryngotracheitis virus (ILTV). It has been reported from most areas of the USA in which poultry are intensively reared, as well as from many other countries. Infectious laryngotracheitis (ILT) is a viral respiratory tract infection of chickens that may result in severe production losses due to mortality result and decreased egg production. This disease is caused by gallid herpes virus 1, belonging to the sub family Alphaherpesvirinae, family Herpesviridae. In areas of intensive production and large concentrations of poultry such as in the United States, Europe, China, Southeast Asia and Australia ILT is usually endemic. The chicken is the primary natural host of this virus. Birds of all age groups are affected but this disease is mostly common in adult birds. Natural portals of entry for infectious laryngotracheitis virus (ILTV) are through the upper respiratory and ocular routes. Ingestion is also a mode of infection. Transmission occurs more readily from acutely infected birds than through contact with clinically recovered carrier birds.

Clinical Manifestations

Incubation period for this disease is 6-12 days. This disease causes an acute respiratory disease in chickens. Characteristic clinical signs include nasal discharge and moist rales followed by coughing and gasping. Marked dyspnea and expectoration of blood stained mucus is characteristic of severe forms of the disease. Clinical signs associated with mild enzootic forms include unthirftiness, reduction in egg production, watery eyes, conjunctivitis, swelling of infraorbital sinuses, persistent nasal discharge.

Gross Lesions

Gross lesions found at conjunctiva and throughout respiratory tract of ILTV infected chickens, but most consistently observed in larynx and trachea. Tissue changes include excess mucus, hemorrhagic and diphtheritic changes.

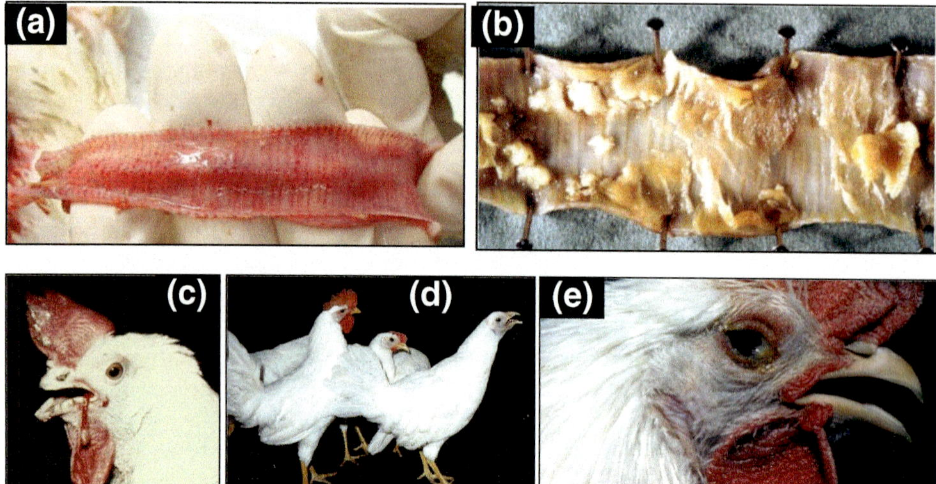

Figure 1.23

(a) ILT- Multifocal haemorrhage in trachea, (b) ILT-diptheritic changes in the trachea, (c) ILT-Expectoration of bloody mucus, (d) ILT- Open mouthed breathing, (e) ILT-Conjunctivitis.

Diagnosis

The acute disease is characterized by the presence of blood, mucus, yellow caseous eexudates, or a hollow caseous cast in the trachea. Microscopically, a desquamative, necrotizing tracheitis is characteristic of acute disease. In the subacute form, punctiform hemorrhagic areas in the trachea and larynx and mild conjunctivitis with lacrimation may be detected. A rapid diagnosis can be achieved by detection of intranuclear inclusion bodies in the tracheal epithelium early in the course of the disease; results of the microscopic examination can be rapidly confirmed by detection of viral DNA using virus-specific PCR assays. Isolation and identification of the virus is done in chicken embryos or tissue culture from embryo liver or kidney cells or from kidney cells from adult chickens. Chicken embryos are preferred for virus isolation. Chorioallantoic membrane of developing chicken embryos (9–12 days old) is inoculated with the specimen. Microscopic examination of the chorioallantoic membrane lesion shows intranuclear inclusions. On microscopic examination of the trachea, intranuclear inclusion lesions produced by ILTV infection must be differentiated from the diphtheritic form of fowlpox infection that produces intracytoplasmic inclusions.

Method of Isolation

Inoculation of suspensions of samples into 9-12 day old embryonated chicken eggs through CAM route or onto susceptible cell cultures. Cell cultures of choice are Chicken embryo liver cells (CEL), and CK cells. A maximum of two passages in CEL and CK cell cultures required.

Other Tests

FAT, ELISA, IPT, DNA hybridization techniques and PCR techniques.

Control

In endemic areas and on farms where a specific diagnosis is made, the disease is controlled by implementation of biosecurity measures and vaccination. Vaccination is done with live attenuated vaccines and viral vector recombinant vaccines. Live vaccines originated from virulent isolates that were attenuated by consecutive passages in embryos or tissue culture. These are applied via eye drop or through mass vaccination by water or spray. Viral vector recombinant vaccines in fowlpox and herpesvirus of turkeys have been designed to express ILTV immunogenic proteins and are administered to individual birds by in ovo, SC, or wing-web vaccination.

1.24. Malignant Catarrhal Fever (MCF)

Synonyms

Bovine malignant catarrh, Malignant head catarrh, Catarrhal fever, Epitheliosis.

Malignant catarrhal fever (MCF) is an infectious systemic disease that presents as a variable complex of lesions affecting mainly ruminants and rarely swine. It is principally a disease of domestic cattle, water buffalo, Bali cattle (banteng), American bison, and deer. In addition to these farmed animals, MCF has been described in a variety of captive ruminants in mixed zoologic collections. In some species, such as bison and some deer, MCF is acute and highly lethal, capable of affecting large numbers of animals. With occasional exceptions, the disease in cattle normally is seen sporadically and affects single animals. MCF is typically fatal; however, there are outbreaks in which several animals are affected, with evidence of recovery and mild or inapparent infections in some cases. It also occasionally presents as chronic alopecia and weight loss. Its distribution is essentially worldwide, mirroring that of the principal carriers, domestic sheep and wildebeest. MCF has long been a major problem in farmed deer operations and in recent years has emerged as a severe threat to the commercial bison industry.

Malignant catarrhal fever (MCF) is almost invariably fatal disease of cattle characterized by catarrhal inflammation of the nasal and oral mucosa, keratoconjunctivitis, encephalitis, rapid dehydration and generalized enlargement of lymphnodes. The disease is usually sporadic in nature. The disease is world-wide distribution and prevalent in both temperate and tropical zones. This disease is caused by ovine herpes virus -1 and alcelaphine herpes virus- 2 which are belonging to the family Herpesviridae. The disease is primarily a disease of cattle and buffalo. Inapparent infection has been noted in sheep and goat. Now the disease is increasingly encountered in deer. This disease is transmitted through wildbeast. The wildbeast develop viraemia which may persist up to 3 months and during that time they remain highly infective for cattle of all ages. Cattle acquire the infection through sub clinically affected sheep. The sheep are the indicator host and wild rabbits are the reservoir host for MCF.

Clinical Signs

Incubation period of the disease ranges from 2-8 weeks. As a whole the following four clinical findings have been outlined but it is not a rigid one and all the manifestations may follow in a case.

Sl.No.	*Form of the Disease*	*General Clinical Signs*
1	Peracute form	High rise of temperature, dyspnoea and iarrhea but with out any head and eye lesions
2	Head and eye form	Clinical course of around 9 days characterized by nervous syndrome like paralysis and convulsion prior to death
3	Intestinal form	
4	Inapparent (mild) form	

The disease as a whole is characterized by dullness, depression, anorexia and high rise of temperature ranging from 105-108°F. This is followed by ocular and nasal discharge. Discharges are initially mucoid in nature which soon become mucoprulent, stingy and contain blood flecks. There is acceleration of pulse and respiratory rate. Signs of dysponea may be evident. There is oedema of the eyelids leading to panopthalmitis. Changes in the epithelium of mouth cavity comprising of congestive changes, precisely on the gum, beneath the tongue, hard palate and oral papillae. Erosive and ultimate necrotic changes may follow in the oral mucosa giving rise to offensive odour from the mouth. Ocular lesions– photophobia and meiosis, corneal opacity, blindness. Cutaneous lesions (congestion, petechiation, bluish discolouration and thickening) localized or generalized. Prominent on the muzzle, skin of the hoof, scrotum, base of the horn and teat.

Diagnosis

Diagnosis of MCF is based on clinical signs, gross and histologic lesions, and laboratory confirmation. Primary differential diagnoses include bovine viral diarrhea/mucosal disease, rinderpest, infectious bovine rhinotracheitis, and East Coast fever (theileriosis). When CNS involvement is prominent, MCF can resemble rabies and the tickborne encephalitides. A history of contact with a carrier species (sheep, goats, or wildebeest) can be helpful, although recrudescent cases can be seen without such a history. Reliable and specific laboratory assays for antibody and for viral DNA are available. The test of choice for clinical diagnosis is PCR to detect viral DNA. Preferred tissues for testing are anticoagulated blood, kidney, intestinal wall, lymph node, and brain. Serology is used to survey healthy animals and is indicative only of infection—latent infection among susceptible animals may render serology alone inconclusive evidence of current disease. Several seroassays are available, including viral neutralization, immunoperoxidase, immunofluorescence, and ELISA. The polyclonal assays are hampered by cross-reactivity. The monoclonal-based competitive ELISA is currently the most specific and detects antibody against all of the known MCF group viruses. Only PCR can discriminate between the different viruses.

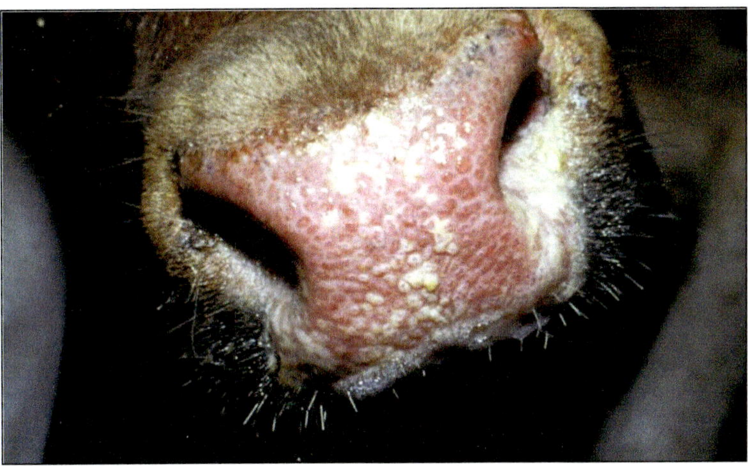

Figure 1.24. Malignant catarrhal fever.

Differential Diagnosis

Rinderpest, mucosal disease, infectious bovine rhinotracheitis.

Prevention and Control

Inactivated or live vaccines with suitable adjuvants induce antibodies against MCFV. In the absence of a vaccine, the only effective strategy is to limit contact between MCF susceptible species and the natural hosts of the virus. Sheep has been considered as a spreader of field outbreaks. Therefore, rigid separation of cattle from sheep is suggested. The feed used by ewes and lambs should not be provided to cattle. Avoid contact between reservoir host (wildebeest and wild rabbits) and cattle.

1.25. Mareks Disease (MD)

Synonyms

Range paralysis, skin leucosis, Neural leucosis, Neural lymphomatosis, pearl eye.

Chickens are the most important natural host for Marek's disease virus, a highly cell-associated but readily transmitted alphaherpesvirus with lymphotropic properties of gammaherpesviruses. Quail can be naturally infected, and turkeys can be infected experimentally. However, severe clinical outbreaks of Marek's disease in commercial turkey flocks, with mortality from tumors reaching 40 per cent –80 per cent between 8 and 17 wks of age, were reported in France, Israel, and Germany. In some of these cases, the affected turkey flocks were raised in proximity to broilers. Turkeys are also commonly infected with turkey herpesvirus (HVT), an avirulent strain related to Marek's disease virus that is commonly used as a Marek's disease vaccine in chickens. Other birds and mammals appear to be refractory to the disease or infection. Marek's disease is one of the most ubiquitous avian infections; it is identified in chicken flocks worldwide. Every flock, except for those maintained under strict pathogen-free conditions, is presumed to be infected. Although clinical disease is not always apparent in infected flocks, a subclinical decrease in growth rate and egg production may be economically important.

Marek's disease (MD) is a lymphoproliferative, highly contagious disease of poultry and caused by a highly cell associated gallid herpes virus, a DNA virus belonging to Herpes viridae family. There are three serotypes of the virus recognized. Serotypes 1 and 2 are designated as virulent and avirulent chicken isolates respectively. Serotype 3 designates the avirulent turkey herpes virus. Serotypes 2 and 3 and attenuated serotype-I virus are used for vaccine production. The virus remains stable for about 24 hours at 30°C. The Marek's disease virus (MDV) has been propagated and assayed in newly hatched chicks, tissue cultures (co-cultivation of lymphocytes with chicken kidney cells or duck embryo fibroblasts) and embryonated eggs. This disease is exists in poultry-producing countries throughout the world. The infection is transmitted through inhalation of infected material from the environment. Virus particle can persist for a considerable period of time in the dandruff of feather follicles, which are released in environment. The infective materials are oral, nasal and tracheal secretions and litter materials. The darkling beetle (*Alphitrbius diaperinus*) is acting as mechanical transmitter of the disease. The chickens are the most important natural host and MD is very rare and probably of no real importance in other species with the possible exception of quail. Chickens of 12-24 weeks of age are mostly susceptible to Marek's disease and generally it does not occur in chickens below 6 weeks of age and older birds above 24 weeks of age.

Clinical Manifestations

Incubation period-ranges from 3 weeks to 9 weeks. The disease appears in several forms.

(a) **Classical form or neural form:** Birds of 16-20 weeks age usually suffer. Signs are mostly concerned with the affection of nerves. Paralysis of legs, drooping wings. Nerves like sciatic nerve, brachial nerve, celiac and vagus nerve running through neck, thoracic and abdominal viscera are affected. Birds unable to stand remain in recumbent position, legs and wings may stretch in either direction. The "split leg" stance is the usual feature. Vents remain soiled with green iarrhea. Mortality rate is comparatively low and mostly noted at the onset of maturity.

(b) **Acute or visceral form:** Generally birds at the age of 3-4 weeks are affected. Depression, droopiness, unthirfitness, dehydration, emaciation and anaemia. Internal organs of the birds affected. Mortality rate may go as high as 60 per cent. Chicks may die suddenly without showing any clinical manifestation. Ovaries of the affected layers and pullets – looks like a cauliflower and mulberry respectively.

(c) **Transitional paralytic form:** Occurs in chickens at the age of 5-18 weeks of age. Sudden development of paresis or paralysis of the legs, wings and neck. Signs usually disappear within 24-48 hours.

(d) **Ocular form:** Blindness in birds due to mononuclear cell infiltration in the iris causing "grey eye" or "pearl eye".

(e) **Skin or cutaneous form:** Distinct white nodules on the skin and in extreme cases look like brownish nodules.

(f) **Muscular form:** Superficial and deep muscles like pectoral muscles affected. Muscles look lusterless, whitish grey and there are tiny white streaks to nodular tumours in the muscles.

Lesions

Affected nerves thickened to more than 2-3 times than normal. Striation and glistening appearance of nerve is lost and looks oedematous. Celiac, cranial, mesenteric, brachial and sciatic plexes and greater splanchnic nerves are mostly affected. Tiny whitish streaks to nodular tumours in muscles, Atrophy of bursa, Ovary- cauliflower like appearance. Pale, single or multiple nodular tumours in myocardium, Skin- whitish nodule, scab with brownish colour.

Diagnosis

Specimens to be collected, Skin, dander, feather tips of infected chickens, blood, Based on the clinical signs and postmortem lesions, Identification of the agent, Under field conditions, most chickens become infected with MDV during the first few weeks of life and then carry the infection throughout their lives, often without developing overt disease. The infection is usually detected by inoculating live buffy coat cells on to monolayer cultures of chicken kidney cells or duck embryo fibroblasts, in which characteristic viral plaques develop within a few days. Two serotypes of MDV are recognized – 1 and 2 – and a third serotype is represented by the related herpes virus of turkeys (HVT). Serotype 1 includes the virulent strains and serotype 2 the naturally avirulent strains. MD viral antigen can be detected in the feather tips of infected birds using a radial precipitin test.

Serological Tests

Antibodies to MDV develop within 1–2 weeks of infection and are commonly recognized by the agar gel immunodiffusion (AGID) test, the indirect fluorescent antibody test, and by other serological tests such as enzyme-linked immunosorbent assay, virus neutralization tests.

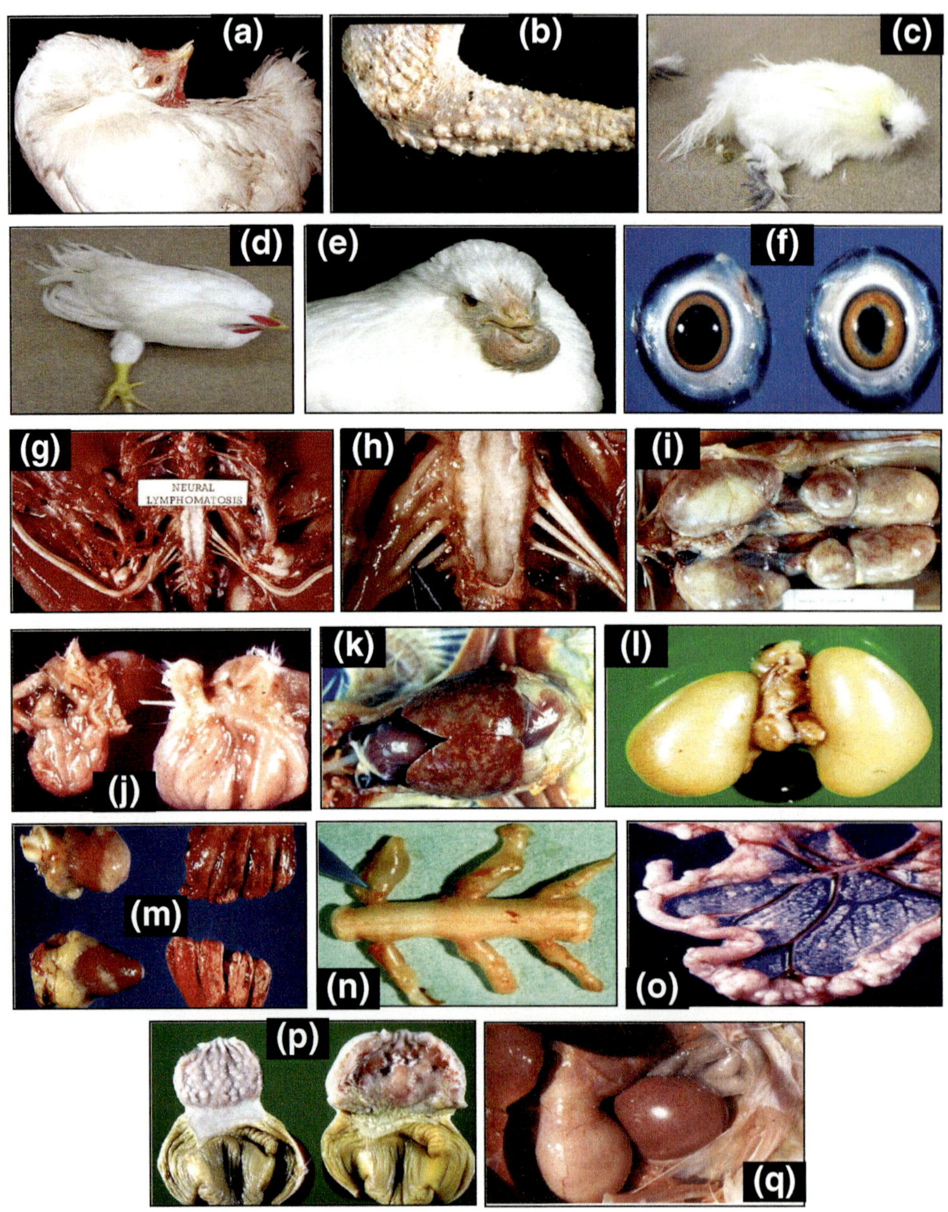

Figure 1.25

(a) Torticolis in MD, (b) Lymphoid infiltration in feather follicles- MD, (c) Leg paralysis – MD, (d) MD-Spastic paralysis, (e) MD-Swelling of wattle and lymphomatosis, (f) Lymphoid infiltration of iris-MD, (g) Schiatic plexus enlargement – Neural lymphomatois-MD, (h) Odema, loss of straitation of nerves-MD, (i) MD-Diffuse enlargement of kidneys, (j) MD-Bursa compared with normal (left), (k) MD-liver, (l) MD-Testes tumor, (m) Visceral lymphomatosis, (n) MD-Dorsal root ganglia enlargement, (o) MD-lymphoid tumours-intestine, (p) MD-Proventriculus compared with normal (left), (q) MD-Splenomegaly.

Prevention and Control

Vaccination is the central strategy for the prevention and control of Marek's disease. The efficacy of vaccines can be improved, however, by strict sanitation to reduce or delay exposure and by breeding for genetic resistance. Probably the most widely used vaccine consists of turkey herpesvirus (HVT), which has seen rapidly increased use as a backbone in recombinant vaccines featuring the insertion of genes from other poultry viruses, such as Newcastle disease virus, infectious bursal disease virus, or infectious laryngotracheitis virus. These recombinant vaccines offer protection against both Marek's disease virus and the inserted virus. Bivalent vaccines consisting of HVT and either the SB-1 or 301B/1 strains of Gallid herpesvirus 3 have been used to provide additional protection against challenge with virulent Marek's disease virus isolates. The most protective commercial vaccine currently available appears to be CVI988/Rispens, an attenuated Marek's disease virus strain that is also commonly mixed with HVT at vaccination. Because vaccines are administered at hatching and require 1–2 wk to produce an effective immunity, exposure of chickens to virus should be minimized during the first few days after hatching. Vaccines are also effective when administered to embryos at the 18th day of incubation. *In ovo* vaccination is now performed by automated technology and is widely used for vaccination of commercial broiler chickens, mainly because of reduced labor costs and greater precision of vaccine administration. Proper handling of vaccine during thawing and reconstitution is crucial to ensure that adequate doses are administered. Cell-associated vaccines are generally more effective than cell-free vaccines, because they are neutralized less by maternal antibodies. Under typical conditions, vaccine efficacy is usually >90 per cent. Since the advent of vaccination, losses from Marek's disease have been reduced dramatically in broiler and layer flocks. However, disease may become a serious problem in individual flocks or in selected geographic areas (*e.g.*, the Delmarva broiler industry). Of the many causes proposed for these excessive losses, early exposure to very virulent virus strains appears to be among the most important.

1.26. New Castle Disease

Synonyms

Ranikhet disease, Avian Pneumoencephalitis, Pseudo fowl pest, avian pest, Avian distemper, Vellaikalichal (Vernacular), Doyle's disease.

Newcastle disease is an infection of domestic poultry and other bird species with virulent Newcastle disease virus (NDV). It is a worldwide problem that presents primarily as an acute respiratory disease, but depression, nervous manifestations, or diarrhea may be the predominant clinical form. Severity depends on the virulence of the infecting virus and host susceptibility. Occurrence of the disease is reportable and may result in trade restrictions.

Newcastle disease is a highly contagious acute viral disease of birds characterized by respiratory signs (distress, coughing, sneezing), nervous signs leading to wing paralysis, inco-ordination, torticolis, swelling of head and chalky white iarrhea. It was first observed in 1926, in Java, Indonesia and in Newcastle-upon-Tyne,

England. The name Newcastle disease was coined by Doyle. In India in July 1927, the virus was recognized in Ranikhet by Edwards. Hence it named as Newcastle disease or Ranikhet disease. Nine serotypes of avian paramyxoviruses recognized but only avian paramyxovirus 1 is associated with clearly defined disease. This disease is caused by single stranded RNA virus namely Avian paramyxovirus type -1, Genus: Avula virus subfamily: Paramyxo virinae, family: Paramyxo viridae order: Mononegavirales. The genome of NDV codes for six proteins. They are NP – Nucleocapsid protein, P – Phosphorylated – Nucleocapsid associated, M – Matrix protein, F – fusion protein, forms the smaller of the surface projections, HN – haemagglutinin and neuraminidase – larger of the surface projections and L – RNA directed RNA polymerase associated with the nucleocapsid. The "HN" protein is responsible for attachment and release of virus from the host cell in addition to its serological identification. The "F" plays a major role in fusion of the virus and cell membrane and it has a critical role in pathogenesis. The Newcastle disease virus (NDV) causes agglutination of chicken and human 'O' erythrocytes. The agglutination reaction is not permanent and after 30 minutes as a result of loss of receptor the agglutination is lost due to the action of neuraminidase and this phenomenon is referred as elution. Only one serotype of NDV recognized, but many strains are there. All strains are immunologically identical. Some of the important virus strains are as follows.

Pathotype Strains

Velogenic Hertz 33, Texas GB, Mesogenic K, R 2 B, Lentogenic F, LaSota, Ulster 2C, Avirulent V4. The virus is comparatively stable virus and survives for long periods at ambient temperature, especially in faeces and can persist in houses (in faeces, dust, *etc.*) for up to 12 months. However it is sensitive to disinfectants, fumigants and sunlight. The virus is inactivated by temperatures of 56°C for 3 hours or 60° C for 30 min, acid pH, formalin and phenol, and is ether sensitive. This virus can be readily cultivated in embryonated eggs. The preferred route is allantoic cavity in 9-11 days old embryos. Virulent strains cause death of embryos in 24 hours with hemorrhages through out the body particularly in occipital region. Lentogenic strains do not cause death. Presence of virus is usually confirmed by HA and HI test using specific serum. The virus also grows readily in primary cell cultures like chicken embryo fibroblast and pig kidney cells and in BHK 21 cell line. Domestic chicken is the principal host. In addition to chickens, turkeys, pheasants, guinea fowl, ducks, geese, and pigeons, a wide range of captive and free ranging semi domestic and free-living birds, including migratory waterfowl, is susceptible. NDV has been reported at least 241 species of birds. In birds that survive, virus is shed in all secretions and excretions for at least 4 weeks. Transmission occurs by direct contact between birds by the airborne route via aerosols and dust particles by inhalation, ingestion of faeces or contaminated material, by inanimate objects, by movement of people, contaminated feed and water, by non-avian species like flying insects, fly (*Musca domestica*), ectoparasites (*Argus persicus*), endoparasites (*Ascardia galli, Eimeria tenella, etc.*) and by vaccine also (incomplete inactivation and exaltation). With lentogenic strains, tvertical transmission is important, and virus –infected chicks may hatch from virus-containing eggs. Some psittacine species may become persistently infected with velogenic virus and excrete it intermittently for more than 1 year without showing clinical signs. Virus may also be disseminated by frozen chickens, uncooked kitchen waste, foodstuffs, bedding, manure and transport containers.

Clinical Features

There are five forms of disease recognized.

(a) **Viscerotropic velogenic (Doyle's form or Asiatic form):** Very acute form with hemorrhagic lesions of the digestive tract. The infection caused by this also called as Asiatic or exotic ND.

(b) **Neurotropic velogenic (Beach's form):** Viruses causing disease characterized by high mortality, which follows neurological and respiratory disease.

(c) **Mesogenic (Beaudette's form):** Acute respiratory and some times lethal nervous infections of young chicks.

(d) **Lentogenic (Hitchner's form):** Mild or inapparent respiratory infections of chicks.

(e) **Asymptomatic enteric:** Inapparent intestinal infection, Incubation period is varies from 2 to 15 days (VVND – 2 to 6 days). Morbidity is usually high and up to 100 per cent. In chickens respiratory, circulatory, gastro-intestinal and nervous signs are seen. A combination of dyspnea, cyanosis of comb and wattles, and clonic muscular spasm is indicative. There is a loss of appetite, listlessness, abnormal thirst, huddling, weakness, and somnolence. Intestinal symptoms may include crop dilatation, presence of foamy mucus and fibrinous eexudates in the pharynx, a similar discharge from the beak, and yellow-green iarrhea. Nervous system involvement is indicated by paralysis of wings and/or legs, torticolis, ataxia or circular movements, bobbing-and-weaving movements of the head, and clonic spasms. In layers, there is a sudden decrease in egg production together with depigmentation and/or loss of shell and reduction in the albumen quality of eggs. In VVND, edema of the head, especially around the eyes may become apparent after birds have been sick for 2 or 3 days. This odema usually does not involve comb and wattle as in a case of HPAI. A dark ring sometimes forms around the eye, probably due to cyanosis and poor blood circulation in the odematous tissue. This 'black eye' appearance is especially visible in white chickens. Bile stained, greenish-dark iarrhea may be noted 2 to 3 days after onset of illness.

Lesions

Ecchymotic hemorrhages in the larynx, trachea, esophagus and throughout the intestine. The most prominent histological lesions are necrotic foci in the intestinal mucosa and lymphatic tissue and hyperemic changes in most organs, including the brain. Non-purulent encephalomyelitis in CNS is also seen. Virulent velogenic strains cause predominantly hemorrhagic lesions, in particular at the oesophagus/ proventriculus and proventriculus/gizzard junctions and in the posterior half of the duodenum, the jejunum, and ileum. These lesions are virtually pathognomic for velogenic strains. Hemorrhages with necrosis in the intestinal wall. In addition to this egg peritonitis, edematous, hemorrhagic or degenerated ovary is also seen.

Diagnosis

Samples to be collected from live birds of cloacal swabs, droppings, oro-nasal swabs. From dead birds of brain, bile, caecal tonsils, liver, spleen, lung, kidney and heart tissue or pooled organ samples, based on history and clinical signs. Samples taken from birds are inoculated into the allantoic cavity of 9–11-day-old embryonated fowl eggs. The eggs are incubated at 37°C for 4–7 days. The allantoic fluid of any egg containing dead or dying embryos, as they arise, and all eggs at the end of the incubation period are tested for haemagglutinating activity. Any haemagglutinating agents should be tested for specific inhibition with a monospecific antiserum to NDV. The NDV may show some antigenic cross-relationship with some of the other avian paramyxovirus serotypes, particularly APMV-3 and APMV-7. The pathogenicity of any newly isolated virus can be assessed by determining the intracerebral pathogenicity index (ICPI), Mean death time (MDT) and Intravenous pathogenicity index (IVPI). The most virulent viruses give ICPI values approaching the maximum score of 2.0, while lentogenic viruses give values of, or close to 0.0.

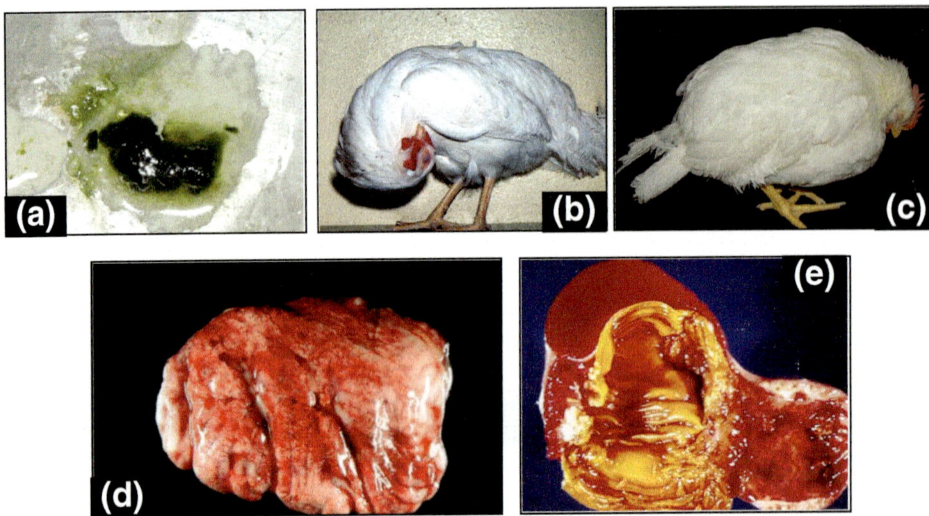

Figure 1.26

(a) ND-Greenish white diarrhea, (b) ND-Torricolis, (c) ND-Sign of severe depression, (d) ND-Extensive Haemorrhages in the lung, (e) ND-Haemorrhagic lesions in proventriculus and gizzard.

Serological Tests

The haemagglutination inhibition test is used most widely in NDV serology, its usefulness in diagnosis depends on the vaccinal immune status of the birds to be tested and on prevailing disease conditions. Demonstration of viral antigen on impression smears by IFT and other serological tests *viz.*, HI, ELISA and molecular techniques like RT-PCR are highly valuable.

Prevention and Control

Control is mainly by vaccination. There are three types of vaccines used for ND. Live Lentogenic-F, LaSota, Live mesogenic – Komarov, Roakin, Mukhteswar, R_2B, and inactivated vaccines. Live lentogenic vaccines are usually derived from field viruses that have been show to have low pathogenicity for poultry but produce an adequate immune response. Typical vaccine strains are HB1, LaSota, F, V4 or Ulster 2C viruses. These vaccines are given to young chicks through eyes or nostrils. They are very safe and only LaSota will produce mild post vaccinal reaction in certain flocks. This type immunization is also called as priming. Mesogenic strains are used only in areas where ND is epidemic and in village chickens. These vaccines are suitable only for secondary vaccination because of their high virulence. Normally mesogenic chickens, such as Komarov, Roakin, Mukhteswar and R2B are used as secondary vaccines after a primary vaccination with a lentogenic vaccine. Inactivated vaccines are produced by growing a ND virus in eggs, and then treating the infective allantoic fluid with an inactivating agent and adjuvant, such as formalin or betapropinolactone-and mineral oil as adjuvant. Inactivated vaccines are usually applied after an initial priming vaccination with a live vaccine. Vaccination is usually applied through water, aerosol spray, eye or nasal drops, or by injection. Broilers are vaccinated with Ranikhet disease F strain at 7, and 21 days. Layers are also vaccinated at 10 and 22 weeks (point of lay). In addition to vaccination usual biosecurity measures should be followed.

Ranikhet F strain	4-10 days	Intra ocular or intra nasal
Ranikhet disease F strain (Booster)	5-6 weeks	Intra ocular or drinking water
Ranikhet (R2B) strain	8-9 weeks	Subcutaneous
Ranikhet disease (Killed)	18-19 weeks	Intramuscular or subcutaneous

Control

National Level-Quarantine, slaughter and vaccination (Ring vaccination). Farm level- Strict hygienic practices and medical measures, by vaccination, Import restrictions on chickens and eggs. Quarantine of psittacine birds in the same air space as non-immune chickens.

Zoonotic Risk

All NDV strains can produce a transitory conjunctivitis in people, but the condition has been limited primarily to laboratory workers and vaccination teams exposed to large quantities of virus. Before poultry vaccination was widely practiced, conjunctivitis from NDV infection occurred in crews eviscerating poultry in processing plants. The disease has not been reported in people who rear poultry or consume poultry products.

1.27. Peste des Petits Ruminants (PPR)

Synonyms

Goat plague, Kata.

Peste des petits ruminants (PPR) is an acute or subacute viral disease of goats and sheep characterized by fever, necrotic stomatitis, gastroenteritis, pneumonia, and sometimes death. It was first reported in Cote d'Ivoire (the Ivory Coast) in 1942 and subsequently in other parts of West Africa. Goats and sheep appear to be equally susceptible to the virus, but goats exhibit more severe clinical disease. The virus also affects several wild small ruminant species. Cattle, buffalo, and pigs are only subclinically infected. People are not at risk.

Peste des petits ruminants (PPR) is a highly contagious, acute or sub acute viral disease of goats and sheep characterized by fever, erosive stomatitis, conjunctivitis, gastro enteritis and pneumonia. This disease was first described in 1942 in West Africa and it is closely related to rinderpest virus, canine distemper virus and human measles virus. Peste des petits ruminants virus (PPRV) is a single stranded, non-segmented RNA virus belonging to the genus Morbili virus, subfamily Paramyxovirinae, family Paramyxoviridae. It is primarily a disease of goats and sheep. Goats, particularly young ones, (4 months to 1 year of age) are usually more severely affected than sheep. The infection also occurs in wild ungulates. Cattle, buffaloes, camels and pigs are rarely susceptible. They do not exhibit clinical signs and are unable to transmit the disease to other animals. Cell culture systems are ideal for virus cultivation. The PPRV grows well in vero and lamb kidney cells. The CPE develops within 5 days and consists of cell rounding, aggregation and syncytia formation in lamb kidney cells. In Vero cells syncytia are rare and if present are very small. Intracytoplasmic inclusions and vacuolation of cells are also seen. Affected animal excrete the virus in all secretions and excretions. Transmission requires close contact between animals. Infection occurs mainly through inhalation of aerosols and by ingestion. There is no known carrier state. The spread is not dependant on vectors.

Clinical Manifestations

Incubation period is 6 days.

(a) **Acute form**: Fever and serous rhinorrhoea – Erosions in the mucous membranes lining the upper alimentary, upper respiratory and urogenital tracts for first 1-2 days followed by fever. Salivation profuse, tongue is continuously protruded and retracted. Rhinorrhea becomes mucopurulent often blocks the nostrils, iarrhea and pneumonia. Mucosal erosions coalesce, formation of ulcers.

(b) **Per acute form:** Follow incubation period that are often as short as 2 days. Profuse nasal catarrh precedes a sudden high fever with signs of depression, dyspnoea, anorexia and constipation, iarrhea, leucopaenia.

(c) **Predisposing Factors**: Predisposing factors for PPR infections are, history of recent movement or gathering together of sheep and/or goats of different ages, introduction of recently purchased animals, change in weather such as the onset of the rainy season or dry, cold periods, contact with trade or nomadic animals.

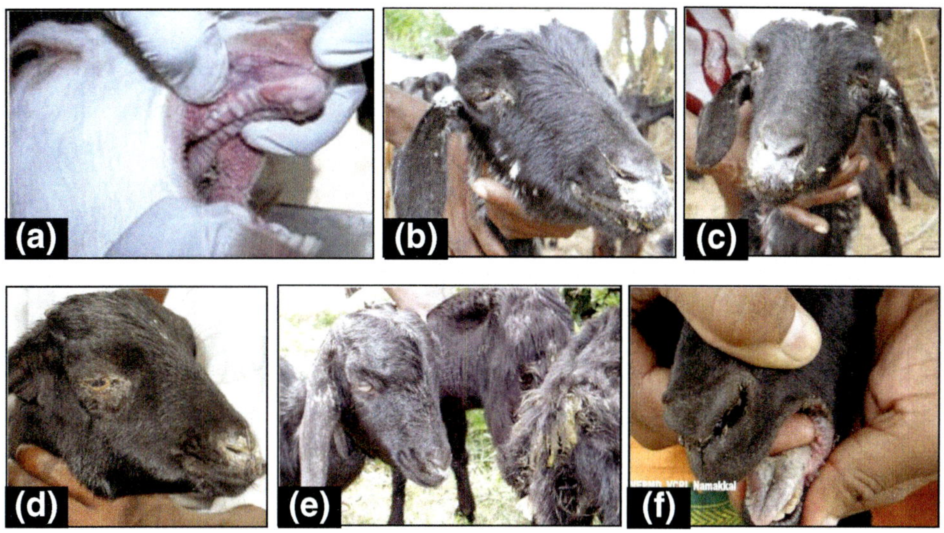

Figure 1.27

(a) Goat affected with PPR (b) PPR-Mucoprulent ocular and nasal discharge, (c) PPR-Muccoprulent nasal discharge, (d) PPR-Dried muccoprulent ocular and nasal discharge, (e,f) Goats affected with PPR.

Diagnosis

A presumptive diagnosis is based on clinical, pathologic, and epidemiologic findings and may be confirmed by viral isolation and identification. Historically, simple techniques such as agar-gel immunodiffusion have been used in developing countries for confirmation and reporting purposes. However, PPR virus cross-reacts with rinderpest virus in these tests. Virus isolation is a definitive test but is labor intensive, cumbersome, and takes a long time to complete. Currently, antigen capture ELISA and reverse transcription-PCR are the preferred laboratory tests for confirmation of the virus. For antibody detection (such as might be needed for epidemiologic surveillance, confirmation of vaccine efficacy, or confirmation of absence of the disease in a population), competitive ELISA and virus neutralization are the OIE-recommended tests. The specimens required are lymph nodes, tonsils, spleen, and whole lung for antigen or nucleic acid detection, and serum (from unclotted blood) for antibody detection, The virus neutralization test may also be used to confirm an infection if paired serum samples from a surviving animal yield rising titers of dikhuaaa 4-fold. PPR must be differentiated from other GI infections (*e.g.*, GI parasites), respiratory infections (*e.g.*, contagious caprine pleuropneumonia), and such other diseases as contagious ecthyma, heartwater, coccidiosis, and mineral poisoning.

Diagnosis

It is based on Classical clinical signs, Virus isolation and identification in cell cultures. Demonstration of viral antigen in buffy coat, body secretions, feces, lymphnode and tonsils by immunohistochemical methods, dot-ELISA, AGID and CIEP.

Note: Unlike rinderpest, PPR viral antigen is still high in tissues of animals dying from the disease.

Serology

Virus neutralization tests (VNT) and competitive Elisa's recommended serological tests by OIE. Complement Fixation Test and AGID are most commonly used. More recently cELISAs have been developed based on monoclonal antibodies specific for the N or H proteins of PPR and rinderpest viruses, and which enable differential diagnosis of the two viruses.

Differential Diagnosis

- **Rinderpest**: In Rinderpest both cattle and small ruminants are involved. The symptoms are very severe in cattle than small ruminants.
- **Pasteurellosis**: The disease is characterized by obvious respiratory signs, infrequent iarrhea, and a mortality rate rarely exceeding 10 per cent. The bipolar organisms can be readily demonstrated in smears.
- **CCPP**: There is no digestive system involvement, and the clinical signs and lesions are confined to the respiratory system and pericardium.
- **Bluetongue**: Sheep are mostly affected. Swelling of the lips, muzzle, oral mucosa and coronitis are more common.
- **Contagious ecthyma/ORF**: Proliferative necrotic lesions are seen in the lips rather than the whole oral cavity. The absence of nasal discharges and diarrhea also distinguish orf from PPR.

Prevention and Control

There is no treatment for PPR. Oxytetracycline and chlortetracycline are recommended to prevent secondary bacterial infections. Hyper immune serum which may be obtained from cattle hyper immunized against rinderpest can be used as therapy. Quarantine of the newly purchased animals, isolation of the affected animals, and following strict hygienic measures will helps to control the disease. Vaccines, Sheep or goats vaccinated with PPR vaccine at the age of 6 months and booster dose should be given once in a year. The tissue culture rinderpest vaccine at a dose of $10^{2.5}$ TCID50 protects goats for atleast 12 months against PPR. The vaccine is currently used in many African countries for vaccination against PPR. This vaccine is safe in pregnant goats. A homologus PPR tissue culture vaccine produced by attenuation in vero cells is commercially available. In southern India, a homologus PPR vaccine using AR-87 strain is used to control PPR in sheep and goats. This vaccine was developed at the Department of Veterinary Microbiology, Madras Veterinary College. Newly developed recombinant vaccinia or capripox viruses expressing the fusion (F) and Haemagglutinin (H) protein genes of the rinderpest virus are also effective against PPR.

1.28. Rabies

Synonyms

Hydrophobia, Lyssa, Mad dog disease.

Rabies is an acute, progressive viral encephalomyelitis that principally affects carnivores and bats, although any mammal can be affected. The disease is fatal once clinical signs appear. Rabies is found throughout the world, but a few countries claim to be free of the disease because of either successful elimination programs or their island status and enforcement of rigorous quarantine regulations. Globally, the dog is the most important reservoir, particularly in developing countries. Integrated veterinary management of local animal populations, by mass vaccination of dogs and community promotion of responsible pet ownership, is the most cost-effective, humane, long-term solution toward eliminating regional canine rabies in a One Health context.

Rabies is acute viral encephalitis of all warm-blooded animals characterized by altered behaviour, aggressiveness, progressive paralysis and in most species by death. It is an important disease of man and animals, which is usually transmitted through the bite of rabies animals to other animals or human result in rapid fatal encephalomyelitis after a somewhat lengthy incubation period. The disease in man is called hydrophobia because the patient exhibits fear of water, being incapable of drinking though subject to intolerable thirst. Rabies in animals is not called hydrophobia because they do not have this peculiar feature. Fox, wolf, coyotes and jackal are extremely susceptible. Guinea pig, Hamster, Bat, Mongoose, mice, rabbit, skunk and cattle are highly susceptible. Dog, sheep, goat, horse and human are moderately susceptible. Poultry and opossum are resistant. At the present time rabies occurs in most parts of the world except in Japan, UK, New Zealand, Antarctica, Australia, Hawaii islands and Switzerland. In India the incidence is very high. Rabies virus belongs to the Rhabdo virus group, one of the RNA helical enveloped virus group. It appears as filamentous, bell shaped or bullet shaped and approximately 60-175 nm in size. The virion is rounded at one end and flat or truncated at the other. It is surrounded by a fringe of short pointed projections. Rabies virus can agglutinate RBCs of day old chicks and goose at 0-4°C and pH 6.2.The virus is deficient in neuraminidase activity. The nucleic acid consists of single stranded RNA. It is found in nerve tissue, saliva, salivary glands, pancreas, less often in urine and lymph and rarely in blood, milk and other body fluids of infected animals. It is readily inactivated by sunlight, drying in air, 40-70 per cent alcohol, quaternary ammonium compounds, tincture-iodine, carbolic acid and any lipid solvents. The virus is very resistant to autolysis and putrefaction. The virus will persist for months in infected nervous tissue in 50 per cent glycerol. The virus survives at 4°C for weeks. It can be preserved at –70°C or by lyophilization. Rabies virus grows very well in human diploid cell line WI-38 and MRC-5, BHK21, Vero and Chicken embryo fibroblast. Cytopathic effects are not apparent. In continuous lines of human diploid cells and BHK21 infected with rabies, almost 100 per cent of the cells are infected and there is a marked CPE. Five or six day's old embryonated hen's eggs are preferred for growth of virus by yolk sac route. The virus also grows in CAM route and produce miliary pock lesions. The strains that have been adapted in egg are Flurry strain, Keller strain. Low egg passage (LEP) strains can be obtained by 40 to 50 passages. High egg passage (HEP) strains can be obtained by 180 passages. Duck eggs are commonly used for preparation of vaccine. Rabies can be cultivated in a wide range of laboratory animals such as hamsters, mice, guinea pig and rabbits in the order of decreasing susceptibility by intracerebral or intramuscular routes. In usual circumstances the only risk of rabies virus transmission is by the bite or scratch of a rabid animal, although in bat caves, where the amount of virus may be very high and the extremely high humidity may stabilize the virus transmitted by aerosol infection. In rare circumstances the virus can pass through the intact mucous membrane. The amount of virus required and to initiate infection varies considerably and depends upon the susceptibility of the patients. Susceptible wild living animals particularly foxes, wolf, jackals constitute the most important residual focus of rabies infection the most prevalent and most difficult to control. Because they carry 10^6 infectious units of virus/ml of saliva. Domestic dog is still the most important source of infection. Although virus titers in the saliva of confirmed case of rabies in dog varies widely. The saliva is believed to be infective in only 50-60 per cent of the rabid dogs at the time of bite and the presence of virus is greatly evident in a few days before death. The factors, which influence the course of infection, include the virulence, invasiveness and concentration of inoculated virus, the amount of nervous tissue near the site of wound, the degree of trauma and the type of animal inflicting the bite. Blood licking bats in chiroptera family constitute an important reservoir in central and South Africa and they frequently infect cattle, man by biting at nights. In a report from Ethiopia in 1964, the isolation of true rabies virus was obtained from the saliva of dog, which remains clinically healthy 4 years after the sample had been taken.

Clinical Manifestations

The incubation period in natural outbreak of dog rabies averages from 3-8 weeks. But it may be as short as 10 days to as long as one year. The clinical features divided into three phases.

(a) **Prodromal form**: During the prodromal period, which lasts 1-3 days, animals show only vague CNS signs, which intensify rapidly. Dog has a change in the temperament aimless snapping and barking at imaginary objects.

(b) **Furious form**: By about 3rd day after the onset of illness the dog enters the furious stage which lasts for 3-7 days. During this stage dog becomes irritable, restless, nervous, deprived appetite, aggressive, and often dangerous as it loses all fear of humans and bites at anything that gains its attention. There is usually exaggerated response to light and sound. Dog exhibit characteristic change in its barking and may howl in an unusual tone due to the paralysis of laryngeal muscle. Salivation and frothing at the mouth becomes progressively more profound. Terminally, there are often convulsive seizures, coma and respiratory arrest, with death occurring

2 to 14 days after the onset of clinical signs. If it does not die it passes into paralytic stage.

(c) **Dumb or paralytic form**: In cases when the furious phase is extremely short or absent the animal rapidly enters the paralytic or dumb stage; where the dog is rarely irritable and seldom bites. Paralysis of the throat and masseter muscles, dropping of the lower jaw or lower jaw paralysis is the clinical signs common in dogs. In dumb form animals are not vicious and rarely attempt to bite. The paralysis progresses rapidly to all parts of the body, and coma and death follow in a few hours.

Note: Veterinarians/Owners frequently examine the mouth of dogs and livestock searching for foreign body or administer medication with their bare hands, thereby exposing themselves to rabies. In cats the clinical signs are similar to those of dogs but lost for 2-4 days before death occurs.

Cattle

Among farm animals, cattle are most commonly affected. In the paralytic form, knuckling of the hind fetlocks, sagging and swaying of the hindquarters while walking, often deviation or flaccidity of the tail to one side, are common signs. Decreased sensation over the hindquarters is one of the best criterions for the detection of rabies. There is drooling of saliva, tenesmus, pumping of anus and followed by recumbency seen in later stages. In furious rabies, the animal alert, hypersensitive, violently attack, loud and coarse bellowing, sexual excitement and collapses suddenly. Cattle are very restless, excited and aggressive with salivation, abdominal pain, diarrhoea and rectal straining. Paralysis of hind quarters occurs followed by death in 3-6 days after the first signs of illness. In sheep and goat the symptoms are similar to cattle.

Sheep

Clinically the picture is similar to cattle. Sexual excitement, violent attack, vigorous wool pulling, sudden falling and salivation are characteristic. Goats are commonly aggressive, and continuous bleating is common.

Horse

Muzzle tremors and pharyngeal paresis are common. In addition to these abnormal postures, frequent whinnying, kicking, biting, colic, sudden onset of lameness in one limb followed by recumbency, high stepping gait, blindness, recumbency, paddling, convulsions and terminally paralysis.

Pigs

Tendency to attack, twitching of the nose, rapid chewing movements, excessive salivation, walk backward and terminally paralysis.

Isolation and Identification of Virus

Confirmatory diagnosis must be obtained by animal inoculation or other means. Animal inoculation: For isolation of virus, the brain or other tissue specimens are prepared as 10 per cent suspension. Suckling mice or hamsters of 3-6 weeks age are generally used for isolation and identification. Route of inoculation is intracerebral. Infected mice almost always develop clinical symptoms with in 17 days of inoculation. The clinical signs to look far in mice are ruffled fur, arching of back, flaccid paralysis of legs. To establish a positive diagnosis the mouse brain are removed and examined microscopically for negribodies. The confirmatory diagnosis can be obtained by serum neutralization test in mice or by Immunofluorescence. Rabies virus can be cultured in human diploid cells, neuroblastoma and BHK21. A 5 or 6 day old embryonated hen's eggs are preferred for growth of virus by yolk sac route.

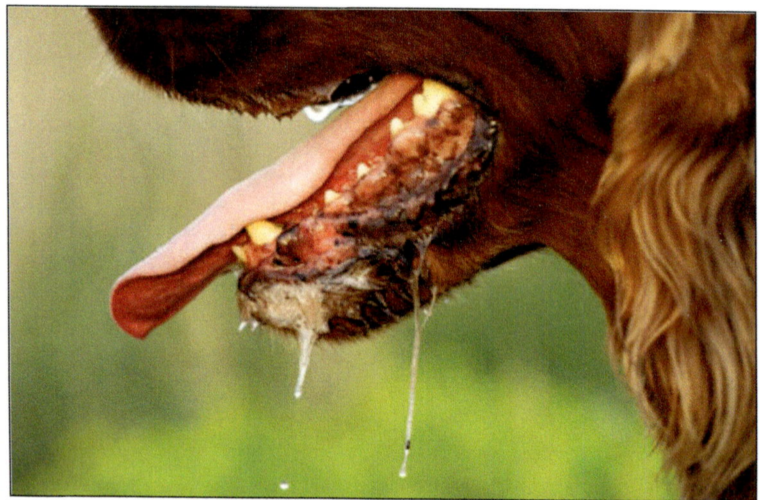

Figure 1.28. Rabies foaming at mouth.

Diagnosis

Sample to be collected from live animals of saliva, corneal/Conjunctival smear or dead animals, the whole carcass or the severed head of the animal suspected to have died of rabies. Alternatively, the brain may be removed carefully and two portions, one in 50 per cent glycerol saline and the other in Zenker's fixative, sent for biological test and microscopy, respectively. The brain tissue selected should include portions of hippocampus, cerebellum, cerebral cortex, and placed in 50 per cent glycerol saline to preserve the virus. No refrigeration is required. Glycerinated tissues are generally unsuitable for immunofluorescence staining for which smears fixed in acetone free methyl alcohol and dried at room temperature without blotting should be sent.

Demonstration of Negribodies

Negribodies are abundantly present in pyramidal cells of ammon's horn and purkinje cells of cerebellum. They can be demonstrated in impression smears either by Seller's method (for unfixed sections) or Mann's method (fixed sections). Seller's method has the advantage that fixation and staining is done simultaneously. Negribodies are intracytoplasmic, magenta red or cherry red spherical or oval bodies with characteristic basophilic inner granules. They are varying in size from 3-27μ. They are inclusions of aggregates of nucleocapsids and they are specific to rabies infection.

Note: Animal should not be killed for the demonstration of negri bodies. They can be demonstrated in only 80-85 per cent cases. It should be differentiated from intranuclear inclusions produced by Infectious Canine Hepatitis and Canine Distemper.

Demonstration of Virus Antigen

Demonstration of viral antigen in ammon's horn, cerebellum, corneal/ conjunctival impression smear, skin biopsy (from facial area) and in submaxillary salivary glands by fluorescent antibody technique (FAT) is the most widely used, confirmatory test for the diagnosis of rabies since it provides rapid reliable and highly specific means of detecting the viral antigen. This test is recommended by both WHO and OIE. By serology, Immunoperoxidase test, ELISA, Rapid fluorescence focus inhibition test (RFFIT), Virus neutralization test, Rapid rabies enzyme immuno diagnosis test (RREID) based on the use of antinucleocapsid lgG are highly useful, RT-PCR amplification technique is 1000 times more sensitive than other tests.

Treatment

There is no specific treatment for rabies. Dogs usually die after showing clinical signs. The site of bite should be washed with water or soap. Alkali prevents multiplication of virus. Sodium bicarbonate or caustic soda may be used. Then the wound is treated with 2 per cent quaternary ammonium compound or tincture iodine or 40-70 per cent alcohol. Wound may also be cauterized with carbolic acid or nitric acid. Antirabies serum may be applied topically or infiltrated around the wound. Treatment with antirabies serum is also effective. Antirabies serum is prepared by hyperimmunisation of horses. It should be given as early as possible after exposure and in any case within five days, after which it may not be beneficial. The dose recommended is 40 I.U. per kg body weight.

Prophylaxis

- **Nervous tissue vaccine:** This is a flurry type vaccine. These are prepared from brain tissues of sheep inactivated through 1 per cent phenol. These are made as 5 per cent and 20 per cent suspension.
- **Pasteur's cord vaccine:** This vaccine is prepared by drying over caustic potash for varying period's pieces of infected rabbit spinal cord.
- **Semple vaccine:** This vaccine was developed by Semple (1911) at the Central Research Institute, Kasauli. It is a 5 per cent or 20 per cent suspension of sheep brain infected with fixed virus and inactivated with phenol at 37°C.
- **Beta Propinolactone vaccine:** This is a modification of Semple vaccine in which BPL is used as the inactivating agent instead of phenol.
- **UV treated vaccines (Webster):** Inactivated vaccines prepared from brain of infected animals, which were exposed to UV rays.

- ✰ **Non - nervous tissue vaccine**
- ✰ **Duck egg vaccine:** This is fixed virus adapted for growth in duck eggs and inactivated with BPL. This has been discontinued because of its poor immunogenicity. *Live attenuated chick embryo vaccine: Two* types of vaccines are available. *Avianized or chick embryo vaccine.* This is made through passaging the virus in chicken embryo. Low egg passage (LEP) (40 to 50 passages) is completely safe for dogs. Avianized live virus vaccine is a single dose vaccine. Age of first vaccination is 3 months, dose 3 ml i/m. Immunity 3 years. Repeat after 3 years. High Egg Passage (HEP) vaccine at 180 passage level used for cattle and cats. *Tissue culture vaccine,* The first cell culture vaccine was the human diploid cell strain (HDCS) vaccine developed by Koprowsky, Wiktor and Plotkin. It is a purified and concentrated preparation of fixed rabies virus (Pitman – Moore Strain) grown on human diploid cells (WI 38 or MRC 5) and inactivated with betapropinolactone. It is highly antigenic and free from side effects. Its only disadvantage is high cost. Nowadays more economical, primary chicken embryo and vero cell culture adapted, vaccines are available. The avianized live virus vaccine is a single dose vaccine. Age of first vaccination is 3 months, dose 3 ml i/m. Immunity 3 years. Repeat after 3 years. In tissue culture vaccine, age of first vaccination is 3 months. Revaccination should be done after 6 months and then at yearly intervals. Dose 5 ml s/c in the neck or flank region.
- ✰ **Subunit vaccine:** The glycoprotein subunit on the virus surface, which is the protective antigen has been cloned and recombinant vaccines produced. They are still in the experimental stage.
- ✰ **Pre exposure vaccination-** Pre exposure vaccination schedule for dogs starts at 12th week age – first dose, 28 days later – second dose, one year later- third dose, three years later- fourth dose.
- ✰ **Post exposure immunization:** 0, 3, 7, 28, 60, 90 days after exposure.

Control (as per the WHO recommendations)

Notification of suspected cases, and destruction of dogs with clinical signs and dogs bitten by a suspected rabid animal. Compulsory immunization of dogs, sterilization and vaccination of stray dogs by using baits, epidemiological surveillance, education of public, development of cost effective vaccine.

Comprehensive guidelines for control in dogs have been prepared internationally by the World Health Organization and in the USA by the National Association of State Public Health Veterinarians (NASPHV). They include the following: 1) notification of suspected cases, and euthanasia of dogs with clinical signs and dogs bitten by a suspected rabid animal; 2) reduction of contact rates between susceptible dogs by leash laws, dog movement control, and quarantine; 3) mass immunization of dogs by campaigns and by continuing vaccination of young dogs; 4) stray dog control and euthanasia of unvaccinated dogs with low levels of dependency on, or restriction by, people; and 5) dog registration.

The Compendium of Animal Rabies Control, compiled and updated regularly by the NASPHV, summarizes the most current recommendations for the USA and lists all USDA-licensed animal rabies vaccines marketed in the USA. Many effective vaccines, such as modified-live virus, recombinant, and inactivated types, are available for use throughout the world; in the USA, no modified-live rabies virus vaccines are currently marketed (for any species). Recommended vaccination frequency is every 3 yr, after an initial series of two vaccines 1 yr apart. Several vaccines are also available for use in cats, and a few for use in ferrets, horses, cattle, and sheep. Because of the increasing importance of rabies in cats, vaccination of cats is critical. No parenteral vaccine is approved for use in wildlife. Protective immunity from the commercially available vaccines for domestic species has not been definitively demonstrated in wildlife species.

Until recently, the control of rabies in wildlife populations relied on population reduction of wildlife in an attempt to reduce the contact rate between susceptible animals; however, this proved difficult and often not publicly acceptable, ecologically sound, economically warranted, or programmatically effective. In Europe and Canada, use of oral vaccines distributed in baits to control fox rabies has been widespread and effective. The disease in foxes has been eliminated from most of Western Europe and curtailed significantly in Ontario. Use of a vaccinia-rabies glycoprotein recombinant virus vaccine in the USA has successfully eliminated coyote rabies in southern Texas and has limited the western expansion of raccoon rabies from the eastern USA. The license limits use of the vaccine to state or federal rabies programs; it is not available to private veterinarians or for individual animal use. Together with other vaccines, it is also being used to assist in the control of dog rabies in developing countries.

Zoonotic Risk

Rabies has the highest case fatality of any infectious disease. When a person is exposed to an animal suspected of having rabies, the risk of rabies virus transmission should be evaluated carefully. Risk assessment should include consideration of the species of animal involved, the prevalence of rabies in the area, whether exposure sufficient to transmit rabies virus occurred, and the current status of the animal and its availability for diagnostic testing. Wild carnivores and bats present a considerable risk where the disease is found, regardless of whether abnormal behavior has been observed. Insectivorous bats, though small, can inflict wounds with their teeth and should never be caught or handled with bare hands. Bat bites may be ignored or go unnoticed, so direct contact with bats could be considered a risk of virus exposure. Any wild carnivore or bat suspected of exposing a person to rabies should be considered rabid unless proved otherwise by laboratory diagnosis; ideally, this includes bats in direct contact with people, such as those found in rooms with sleeping or otherwise unaware persons. Wildlife, including wolf hybrids, should never be kept as pets; if one of those animals exposes a person or domestic animal, the wild animal should be managed like free-ranging wildlife.

Any healthy domestic dog, cat, or ferret, whether vaccinated against rabies or not, that exposes (bites or deposits saliva in a fresh wound or on a mucous membrane) a person should be confined for 10 days; if the animal develops any signs of rabies during that period, it should be euthanized and its brain promptly submitted for rabies diagnosis. If the dog, cat, or ferret responsible for the exposure is stray or unwanted, it may be euthanized as soon as possible and submitted for rabies diagnosis. Since the advent of testing by immunofluorescence microscopy, there is no value in holding such animals to "let the disease progress" as an aid to diagnosis.

Internationally, the World Health Organization recommends several types of cell-culture vaccines for human groups at risk. In the USA, guidelines for human rabies prevention follow recommendations prepared by the Advisory Council on Immunization Practices. Preexposure immunization is strongly recommended for people in high-risk groups, such as veterinary staff, animal control officers, rabies and diagnostic laboratory workers, and, under certain circumstances, some travelers working in countries in which canine rabies is enzootic. Pre-exposure vaccine is administered on days 0, 7, and 21 or 28. However, pre-exposure prophylaxis alone cannot be relied on in the event of subsequent rabies virus exposure and must be supplemented by a limited postexposure regimen (two doses of vaccine, IM, on days 0 and 3). For healthy, unvaccinated patients bitten by a rabid animal, postexposure prophylaxis consists of wound care, local infiltration of rabies immune globulin, and vaccine administration on days 0, 3, 7, and 14. When provided in a timely and appropriate manner, modern postexposure prophylaxis virtually assures human survival.

1.29. Rift Valley Fever

Synonyms

Enzootic hepatitis.

Rift Valley fever (RVF) is a peracute or acute, mosquito-borne, zoonotic disease of domestic and wild ruminants in Africa, Madagascar, and the Arabian Peninsula. Large outbreaks of clinical disease are usually associated with heavy rainfall and localized flooding. During epidemics, the occurrence of abortions in livestock and deaths among young animals, particularly lambs, together with an influenza-like disease in people, is characteristic. However, infections are frequently subclinical or mild. Rift valley fever is an acute arthropod-borne disease of sheep, cattle and goats, causing high mortality among young lambs, calves and kids and abortion in pregnant females. Many species can be infected by Rift Valley fever virus (RVFV), including humans. Horses and pigs are resistant to this disease. This disease found through out Africa. Recent outbreaks have occurred in Saudi Arabia and Yemen considerable humans have succumbed. This disease is caused by single stranded RNA virus belonging to the genus Phlebovirus, family Bunyaviridae. Rift Valley fever occurs in Africa and the Middle East in sheep, goats, cattle, camels, antelopes and humans. This disease is transmitted by mosquitoes (*Aedes* spp.), by contact and also by aerosol.

Etiology and Epidemiology

RVF virus belongs to the genus *Phlebovirus* and is a typical Bunyavirus. An enveloped spherical particle of 80–100 nm in diameter, it has a three-segmented, single-stranded, negative-sense RNA genome with a total length of ~11.9 kb. Each of the segments, L (large: 6.4 kb), M (medium: 3.9 kb), and S (small: 1.7 kb), is contained in a separate nucleocapsid within the virion. Remarkably little genetic diversity has been found between RVF virus isolates from many countries, and no significant antigenic differences have been demonstrated, but differences in pathogenicity are seen. The disease is endemic in many tropical and subtropical regions of Africa, Madagascar, and the Arabian Peninsula. Thought to have been originally confined to the Rift Valley region of eastern and southern Africa, the virus has recently expanded its range, with major outbreaks having occurred in Egypt since 1977, West Africa since 1987, Madagascar since 1990, and the Arabian Peninsula in 2000. Particularly large epidemics with large numbers of human cases occurred in Egypt in 1977–1978 and in Kenya in 2006–2007. It is considered a threat to regions further afield, where competent mosquito vectors are present. Sporadic, large epidemics have occurred at 5–10 yr intervals in drier areas of eastern Africa, and less frequently in southern Africa. Outbreaks are usually associated with periods of abnormally heavy rainfall or, in some cases, with localized flooding due to dam building or flood irrigation. During interepidemic periods, the virus may remain dormant in eggs , floodwater, breeding aedine mosquitoes in the dry soil of small, ephemeral wetlands (dambos or pans). In some areas, this transovarial transmission is believed to be the most important interepidemic survival strategy of the virus; however, inapparent cycling of the virus between vectors and wild or domestic mammalian hosts has been shown to occur in many areas. RVF virus may also spread by movement of viremic animals and possibly by wind-borne mosquitoes. When emergence of infected mosquitoes, or introduction of virus to an area, coincides with abnormally wet conditions and the presence of a highly susceptible host population, a large epidemic may ensue when the virus is amplified in ruminants and spread locally by many species of mosquitoes or mechanically by other insects. The incidence of RVF peaks during the late rainy season. In areas with cold winters, both the disease and vectors may disappear after the first frost. In warmer climates where insect vectors are present continuously, seasonality is not seen.

People are readily infected through blood aerosols from infected animals during slaughter, or by exposure to infected animal tissues, aborted epticae, mosquito bites, and laboratory procedures. Therefore, veterinarians, farm epticaem, and abattoir workers are particularly at risk. People can also act as amplifying hosts and introduce the disease (via mosquitoes) to animals in uninfected areas.

Clinical Manifestations

The incubation period is up to 3 days in sheep and goats and in newborn animals, it can be as short as 12 hours. Infection is most severe in young animals, and is characterized by a high fever, anorexia, weakness, and rapid death. Some affected animals may have nasal discharge and hemorrhagic diarrhea. Hepatic necrosis is the primary lesion, and is especially extensive in younger animals and fetuses. Adult animals are less severely affected. Abortion is the most prominent sign in pregnant animals (up to 100 per cent). In adult animals, hepatic necrosis can be more focal and may only be visible microscopically. Mortality rate may exceed 70 per cent in young animals but is considerably less in adults. Humans may become infected by mosquitoes and through contact with diseased tissues. Infections are "flu-like", and can infrequently be severe and fatal. Cattle are less severely affected than sheep.

Diagnosis

RVF should be suspected when abnormally heavy rains and flooding are followed by widespread occurrence of abortions and mortality among newborn animals characterized by necrotic hepatitis, concurrent with influenza-like disease in people handling animals or their products. The necropsy of infected animals poses considerable risk to the operator and should be performed only by trained personnel, using appropriate personal protective equipment. The virus can readily be isolated from tissues of aborted epticae and the blood of infected animals. The viral titer in these tissues is often high enough to use organ suspensions as antigen for a rapid diagnosis in neutralization, complement fixation, ELISA, agar gel diffusion tests, or staining of organ impression smears; however, these tests should be supplemented by isolation in suckling mice or hamsters injected intracerebrally or in cell cultures such as baby hamster kidney (BHK21), monkey kidney (Vero), chicken embryo–related (CER) and mosquito cells, or primary kidney and testis cell cultures of lambs. Detection of viral nucleic acid by PCR is possible, and reverse transcriptase-PCR tests have been described. Virus can be demonstrated in organ sections using immunohistochemical stains. All conventional serologic tests can be used to detect antibody against RVF virus and are helpful in epidemiologic studies. In some areas, however, serologic surveys may be complicated by cross-reactivity between RVF virus and other phleboviruses; virus neutralization tests are the most specific in this situation. An IgM ELISA can demonstrate recent infection using a single serum sample.

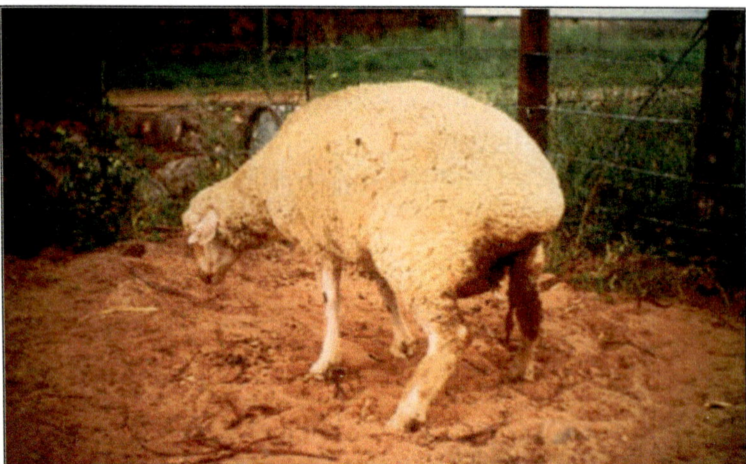

Figure 1.29. Rift valley fever.

Wesselsbron disease and other insect-borne viral diseases tend to occur under the same climactic conditions. RVF mortality associated with hepatic lesions should be distinguished from hepatotoxic plant and algal intoxications; bacterial epticaemias such as pasteurellosis, salmonellosis, and anthrax; and other viral infections such as Nairobi sheep disease and peste des petits ruminants. When abortion is the only finding, other important diseases such as brucellosis, leptospirosis, chlamydiosis, campylobacteriosis, *Coxiella burnetii* infection, and salmonellosis should be eliminated

Differential Diagnosis

Agents or poisoning caused by poisonous plants such as *Seneciao* sp, *Crotalaria* sp, *Lasiospermum*, pasteurellosis, salmonellosis, anthrax, RP, and PPR.

Prevention

Modified live virus and killed virus vaccines are used in countries where the disease is endemic. The modified live vaccine should not be used in pregnant animals. Mosquito control reduces the chances of infection. In countries where the disease does not occur, outbreaks are dealt with by strict quarantine and slaughter.

Zoonotic Risk

Because RVF virus can cause a severe and potentially fatal disease in people, those involved in the livestock industry should be made aware of the potential dangers of exposure to RVF-infected animals and tissues. Appropriate protective measures should be taken when investigating cases of abortion, handling potentially infected animals, and collecting diagnostic samples.

1.30. Rinderpest

Synonym

Cattle plague.

Historically, rinderpest virus was a scourge that wrought economic havoc throughout Africa, Asia, and Europe. The need to combat rinderpest provided the impetus for the establishment of the first modern veterinary school in Lyon (France) in 1762. After several decades of success in eradicating rinderpest from Europe, the disease recurred unexpectedly in Belgium in 1920, and renewed efforts to eradicate it resulted in the creation of the World Organization for Animal Health (OIE) in 1924. Shortly after the creation of the Food and Agriculture Organization (FAO) of the United Nations in 1946, the OIE and FAO signed a cooperation agreement in 1952. Since then, the two organizations (FAO and OIE) have been major participants in several global campaigns to combat rinderpest, which culminated in global eradication of the disease in 2011. In fact, the last reported rinderpest outbreak occurred in Kenya in 2001, but a 10-yr active surveillance period was necessary before global eradication could be declared. Rinderpest is only the second viral disease, after smallpox, to have been successfully eradicated worldwide. The successful eradication of rinderpest shows that smallpox eradication in 1980 was not an unrepeatable feat and should provide a certain degree of confidence to the international community that concerted, science-based efforts can result in future successes. Rinderpest virus is biologically similar to the virus of peste des petits ruminants, which has been targeted by the OIE and FAO as the next animal disease for global eradication. Rinderpest was a disease of cloven-hoofed animals characterized by fever, necrotic stomatitis, gastroenteritis, lymphoid necrosis, and high mortality. In epidemic form, it was the most lethal plague known in cattle. All wild and domesticated species of the order Artiodactyla were variably susceptible to rinderpest, although dissemination of the virus largely depended on continual transmission among domesticated cattle, domesticated buffalo, and yaks. The virus also infected goats and sheep, leading to under-diagnosis of the clinically similar peste des petits ruminants in regions where the two diseases coexisted.

Rinderpest or cattle plague is an acute, highly contagious virus disease, primarily of cattle and to a lesser degree of sheep, goats and wild ruminants. In India "Hill Zebu cattle" are more susceptible than "Plain zebu cattle". This disease is characterized by necrosis, and erosions of the mucosa in the respiratory and digestive tracts. Early constipation, usually preceded by dehydration and prostration, is followed by avoured. Rinderpest is caused by a negative-strand RNA virus of the Morbili virus genus within the family Paramyxoviridae. Rinderpest is enzootic in northern equatorial Africa, the Middle East countries. Rinderpest eradicated in India. The virus strains are of a single serotype, but represent various pathotypes, *i.e.*, they vary in virulence, pathogenicity. The virus is immunologically related to measles, and canine distemper viruses. The virus is usually transmitted from sick to susceptible animals in aerosols and normally the contact has to be close because the infectious droplets are large and short-lived. Transmission through ingestion of virus contaminated food or water is rare. The virus grows in sheep, goats, rabbits, hamster and white mice. It can be grown in chick embryos by intravenous or CAM route. Cytopathogenic effect (CPE) is produced by the virus in susceptible cells from cattle, sheep, goats, chick embryos, pigs, hamsters and man. Cytopathogenic effect consists of large, well defined multinucleated giant cells known as "syncytia". Infected cell cultures have stellate or spindle shaped cells with large fine anastamosing intracellular processes. The virus multiplies in the cytoplasm of the host cells like verocells (African green monkey kidney cells). Both intra cytoplasmic and intranuclear inclusion bodies are present.

Clinical Manifestations

In enzootic areas, where most animals could have been exposed to the virus and develop a certain degree of immunity, it may be longer. It is an acute febrile disease with morbidity in susceptible populations reaching 100 per cent and mortality 90-100 per cent. The normal route of infection is through nasopharyngeal mucosa. The course of the disease comprises of 4 stages.

- **I stage: Incubation period:** 2-9 days. It depends according to the strain and dose of the virus. The virus multiplies rapidly in the lymphoid tissue, lungs, bone marrow and intestines. Active proliferation of the virus in the tissue results in fever.
- **II stage: Prodromal phase:** There is first rise in temperature – 105-107°C (41-42°C) and lasts for about 3-5 days until the appearance of lesions in the mouth. Animal shows depression, restlessness and anorexia. Muzzle is dry, starry coat and initial constipation noticed, Leucopenia with onset of fever and persists till death.

- ☆ **III stage: Mucosal phase:** Mouth lesions on the inner lips and adjacent gums. Visible mucous membranes are congested. The mouth lesions are avoure foci with necrotic centers and shallow erosions with bleeding. Ulcers with bran like deposits noticed. Smacking as in FMD is not common. Animal is restless and shows excess thirst. Temperature is high and recedes after that avoured begins. Rapid dehydration, marked weakness and severe progressive emaciation leads to death.
- ☆ **IV stage: Diarrhoeic phase:** About three days after the appearance of the mucosal ulcers fever regresses and profuse avoured develops. The dark fluid faeces often contain mucus, necrotic debris and blood. Dehydration and wasting soon become evident. Severely affected animals may collapse and die within 12 days of the onset of clinical signs. In surviving animals convalescence lasts several weeks.
- ☆ **V stage: Convalescent phase:** Mouth lesions start healing. Rapid regeneration of the affected epithelium noticed. Slow recuperation of general health. Mortality in cattle, sheep and goats and pigs is 90 per cent.

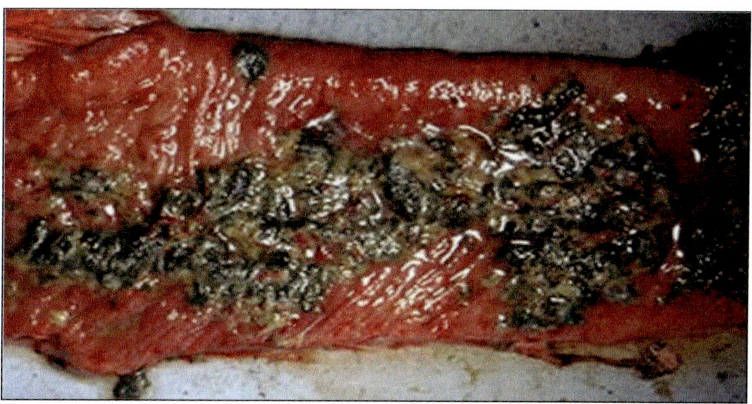

Figure 1.30. Rinderpest.

Diagnosis

Clinical and pathologic findings were sufficient for diagnosis in endemic areas and after initial laboratory confirmation of an outbreak. In areas where rinderpest was uncommon or absent, laboratory tests had to be used to differentiate it from bovine viral diarrhea in particular, as well as East Coast fever, foot-and-mouth disease, infectious bovine rhinotracheitis, and malignant catarrhal fever. Viral isolation and detection of specific viral antigens in affected tissues using an immunodiffusion test was the standard, but simpler, more rapid and more discriminating tests, such as immune capture ELISA and reverse transcription-PCR (RT-PCR), were avoured toward the end of the eradication campaign. The RT-PCR technique allowed phylogenetic characterization of the virus and helped trace the origin of strains in new outbreaks. A simple lateral flow penside test for field use also proved useful in the final stages of the eradication campaign. In the

10-yr period between occurrence of the last outbreak and the official declaration of eradication, active rinderpest surveillance in recent endemic areas included the testing of all susceptible cloven-hoofed animals presenting with erosive stomatitis.

Differential Diagnosis

Haemorrhagic septicemia, FMD, Mucosal disease, Bovine Viral Diarrhoea.

Prevention and Control

Laprinised vaccine: Immunity last for 1-7 years.

Goat tissue vaccine: Immunity last for 13 years or life long.

In countries where Rinderpest is exotic, confirmed outbreaks are controlled by the slaughter and disposal of all affected and in contact animals, as well as by appropriate quarantine and animal movement controls. All outbreaks of rinderpest in virgin areas have been due to the importation of live infected animals. Prevention in such areas is therefore largely dependent upon vigilant control of the introduction of live animals from potentially infected areas. Contaminated areas should be physically cleaned of all animal waste and soiled bedding and treated with disinfection solutions of high (>10) or low (<3) pH containing solvents to destroy the virus envelope. Solutions of caustic soda and Lysol have the highest virucidal activity against virus contaminated with organic matter. Attenuated tissue culture (bovine kidney cells, vero cells) Kabete "O" strain of RPV produced a totally safe and effective attenuated virus which has been the principal vaccine used to combat rinderpest through out the world during the past 40 years. It induces a life-long immunity, inexpensive and simple to produce and stable in freeze dried form. The only drawback of the vaccine is that after reconstitution in normal saline it has a working life of only a few hours in the hot climates. Recombinant vaccines in which genes expressing RPV immunizing antigen are incorporated into more thermostable pox viruses have been developed and used for differentiating vaccinated animals with the infected animals and thus helps in eradication of disease. In endemic areas calves at the age of 6-12 months vaccinated for RP. Annual vaccination of all cattle will produces highest levels of herd immunity.

1.31. Sheep Pox

Synonyms

Ovine pox, Variola ovina.

Sheeppox (or sheep pox, known as *variola ovina* in Latin, *clavelée* in French, *Pockenseuche* in German) is a highly contagious disease of sheep caused by a poxvirus different from the benign orf (or contagious ecthyma). Sheep pox is the most severe of all the pox diseases of animals. Sheep pox is a contagious pox disease of sheep caused by sheep pox virus and characterized by febrile condition and generalized development of pock lesions in the areas denied of wool. It is considered as one of the most dangerous pox virus infections among animals. This disease also affects the mucous membranes of the respiratory and gastrointestinal tracts. Sheep pox virus is a DNA virus belonging to the family Poxviridae, subfamily chorodopox virinae, genus Capripox. The disease is prevalent in many areas of Middle East countries, Africa, Asia and Mediterranean countries. The disease is widely prevalent in different parts of India. The sheep are the naturally susceptible host to this virus. Young sheep are more susceptible than older ones. In the young lambs the disease may flare up in an epidemic proportion. Transmission takes place due to direct contact of the infected animals with the healthy one. Droplet infection through nasal inhalation is an important way of disease transmission. Wounds and abrasion of the skin augment spread from one animal to other. Dog, cat, bird and animal handlers may mechanically transport the infective materials from one place to other. The scabs contain the virus and the virus may remain active on the wool or infected pens for as long as 6 months. On inhalation the virus enters the lungs. Transplacental transmission from ewe to the foetus results in the birth of lambs with pox eruptions.

Clinical Manifestations

Incubation period is 4-8 days after natural infection. The disease may appear in three clinical forms; Malignant form; Mild (benign) form; Abortive form.

(a) **Malignant form**: Most common, Lacrymation, salivation, serous nasal discharge, swelling of the eye lids, congestion of mucous membranes. High fever with pock lesions on the eye lids, lips, nostrils, ears, cheeks, inner side of the thigh, scrotum and prepuce, vulva, under the tail, chest region and buccal mucosa. Lesions first appear as macules, then turn into papules, which transform into large vesicles followed by necrotic changes in the vesicles results in scab formation. If lambs are affected mortality is 50 per cent. Death occurs due to respiratory embarrassment.

(b) **Mild (benign) form**: Common in adult sheep, Common form of the disease in indigenous breeds of sheep

(c) **Abortive form**: Pregnant ewes abort, foetus show pock lesions, in lactating ewes- mastitis due to lesions in the udder.

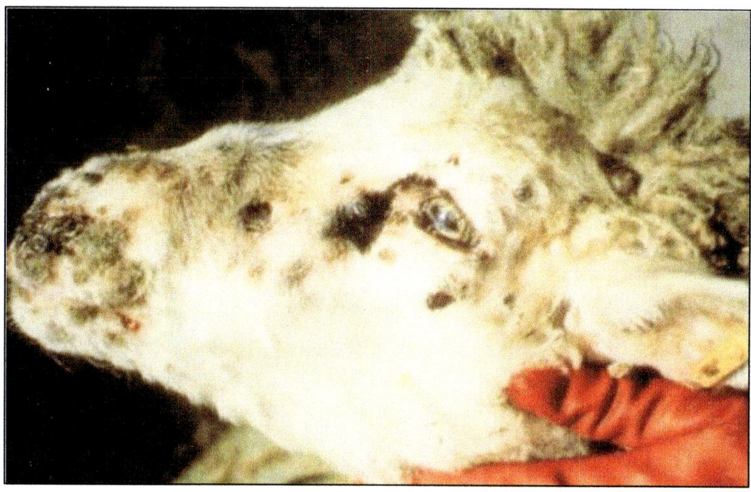

Figure 1.31. Pox lesions around nostrils and eye.

Lesions

Characteristic papules, vesicles, pustules and scabs on cutaneous surface. Lesions in the mucosa of respiratory and alimentary tract especially in the trachea.

Diagnosis

Samples- vesicles and vesicular fluid, scabs, based on characteristic lesions on the skin and infected cells show intracytoplasmic acidophilic inclusion bodies.

Animal Inoculation Test

The lymph or skin materials of the affected sheep inoculated on the scarified skin surface of the healthy sheep. Development of the disease in the inoculated sheep – positive reaction. Other tests are CFT, AGID, counter mmune electrophoresis.

Differential Diagnosis

FMD, ORF or contagious ecthyma.

Prevention and Control

Ovination

The lymph of the vesicle applied in scarified areas or the lymph is inoculated by intradermal injection on the ventral surface of the tail – oldest method of immunization.

Vaccination

Inactivated vaccines are commonly used for vaccination. First vaccination is given to the sheep at the age of 3 months. There after annual boosters are recommended. The vaccine is administered intradermally. At the site of inoculation a local reaction should develop. All vaccinated animals should be checked after a week for positive reaction. If the reaction is not developed the animal should be revaccinated.

1.32. Swine Vesicular Disease

Swine vesicular disease (SVD) is typically a transient disease of pigs in which vesicular lesions appear on the feet and snout and in the mouth. SVD is usually mild in nature and may infect pigs subclinically. However, the disease is of major economic importance, because it must be differentiated from foot-and-mouth disease, eradication is costly, and embargoes on export of pigs and pork products are often imposed on nations not free of SVD. Pigs are considered the only natural host of the virus, although it can infect sheep in close contact with infected pigs and infection of one laboratory worker was reported. SVD has been reported only in Europe and Asia, having been first identified in Italy in 1966 and subsequently in Hong Kong, Japan, Taiwan, and 16 other countries in Europe. Although SVD virus was eradicated from Japan in the mid-1970s and most European countries by the mid-1980s, it has remained endemic in Italy and caused sporadic outbreaks of disease in other European countries during the 1990s and in Portugal in 2003, 2004, and 2007. This disease is caused by Swine vesicular disease virus (SVDV) of

Entero virus genus, Family Picornaviridae. The SVD virus is closely related to the human enterovirus, Coxsackie B-5 virus. This disease was first reported in feeder pigs in Italy in 1966. It has since been reported in Great Britain (declared free in 1980), several European countries, and Asia. There have been reports of aseptic meningitis in humans caused by SVDV. Spread is by direct contact and fomites. Several outbreaks have been traced to uncooked or insufficiently cooked pork in garbage.

Clinical Manifestations

Clinically indistinguishable from foot-and-mouth disease (FMD), vesicular stomatitis (VS), and vesicular exanthema (VE). Epithelial tissue is initially involved, followed by viraemia with generalized infection of lymphoid tissues. The first signs – reduced feed intake, lameness and tenderness of the feet, fever up to 106°F, and the formation of vesicles on the feet, snout, tongue, mouth, nostrils, and teats. The prognosis is favorable, but in most countries infected animals are slaughtered.

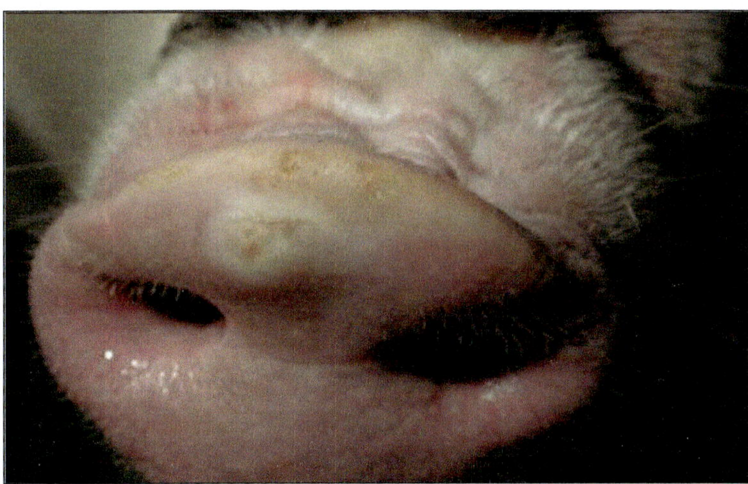

Figure 1.32. Subacute lesion on the snout of a gestating sow.

Diagnosis

Diagnosis is confirmed by laboratory tests on epithelial samples, feces, or serum. Virus detection is by antigen-detection ELISA, virus isolation, or reverse-transcriptase PCR. Serology is by antibody-detection ELISA or virus neutralization test, but low specificity may be a concern, particularly in older animals. In clinical cases, the preferred specimens are lesion material collected in phosphate-buffered saline. Subclinical infection may be detected by testing of pen-floor feces using reverse-transcriptase PCR or virus isolation.

Prevention

Vaccines are not available to prevent SVD. SVD is a reportable disease and, if it is suspected strict measures of control including quarantine and slaughter are implemented.

Control

Countries free of the disease can remain so by controlling the import of pigs and pork products or by ensuring that pork products are treated (heat or otherwise) to kill the virus. Feeding of garbage to pigs may be banned or regulated to ensure thorough cooking. Any suspected outbreak should be reported to the appropriate authorities. If SVD does occur, control is by zoosanitary measures, including restrictions on pig movement. There are no commercially available vaccines. Extensive serosurveillance is necessary to detect subclinically infected herds, and seroreactor herds must be followed up by clinical inspection and fecal virus testing. The virus is extremely resistant in the environment and is stable over a wide pH range (2.5–12); thus, disinfection of premises, trucks, and equipment must be thorough. The most effective disinfectants are strong alkalis, although hypochlorites or acid-containing iodophors can be used when organic material is not present.

1.33. Vesicular Stomatitis

Synonyms

Sore mouth, Pseudo foot and mouth disease, Mouth thrush, sore nose.

Vesicular stomatitis is a viral disease caused by two distinct serotypes of vesicular stomatitis virus—New Jersey and Indiana. Vesiculation, ulceration, and erosion of the oral and nasal mucosa and epithelial surface of the tongue, coronary bands, and teats are typically seen in clinical cases, along with crusting lesions of the muzzle, ventral abdomen, and sheath. Clinical disease has been seen in cattle, horses, and pigs and very rarely in sheep, goats, and llamas. Serologic evidence of exposure has been found in many species, including cervids, nonhuman primates, rodents, birds, dogs, antelope, and bats.

It is an infectious viral disease of cattle, horse, pig characterized by vesicular lesion containing serous fluids in the mouth, foot, interdigital space, udder and teats. Vesicular stomatitis virus belongs to number of closely related, antigenically distinct members of the genus *Vesiculovirus,* RNA virus belonging to Rhabdo viridae family. There are three serotypes of the virus named as Indiana strain, NewJersey strain and Trinidad strain or Eocal strain. The strains can be separated from each other by serum neutralization and complement fixation test. The Indian serotype is comprised of four sub types. New Jesrsey strain is more virulent over other strains. This febrile disease affects mainly horses, donkeys and cattle and pigs. Other susceptible species include camels, several wildlife species and humans. Vesicular stomatitis is clinically similar to foot and mouth disease. The disease is limited to the western hemisphere and the infection is endemic in Central America and in regions of South America. Outbreaks of the disease occur every two to three years in tropical and subtropical regions, with clinical cases most common at the end of the rainy season and early in the dry season. The virus can be biologically transmitted by black flies and mechanically by Culicoides, houseflies. The saliva and vesicular fluid from clinically affected animals are highly infective but infectivity diminishes rapidly and may be lost within 1 week after the vesicle rupture.From this source, virus may be transmitted by fomites, such as contaminated feed, milking machine and restraint devices. Recovered cattle act as convalescent carrier for 38 days to 5 months.

Clinical Features

The incubation period is up to five days. Subclinical infection is common. Affected animals, which are usually more than one year old, become febrile. Vesicles develop on the tongue and on oral mucous membranes, often accompanied by profuse salivation. Secondary lesions may occur on the coronary band and teats. Lameness is often a prominent feature of the disease in pigs. Mastitis may develop in cows with severe teat lesions. In the absence of secondary infection, lesions generally heal within two weeks. Following infection, animals develop high levels of neutralizing antibodies but the duration of protection is variable.

Cattle

The incubation period is 3-15 days. There is a sudden appearance of mild fever and the development of vesicles on the dorsum of the tongue, dental pad, lips and the buccal mucosa. Development of vesicles is usually accompanied by ropy salivation. Vesicles ruptured followed by erosive necrotic lesion. Subclinical infection is common. Affected animals, which are usually more than one year old, become febrile. Secondary lesions may occur on the coronary band and teats. Mastitis may develop in cows with severe teat lesions. In the absence of secondary infection, recovery is rapid, affected animals are clinically normal in 3-10 days. Cross-protection between vesicular stomatitis Indiana virus and vesicular stomatitis New Jersey virus is limited.

Horses

There is fever, depression and drooling of saliva. Affected horse may rupture their lips on troughs. Vesicles coalesce, rupture and formation of shallow ulcers. Lesions are also seen in coronary band and teats.

Pigs

Lameness is more common.

Diagnosis

Specimens for isolation of virus–epithelium from lesions and vesicular fluid. Prompt laboratory confirmation is required because of similarities between vesicular stomatitis, foot-and-mouth disease and swine vesicular disease. If horses present with vesicular lesions, infection with vesicular stomatitis virus should be considered. Antigen detection- CFT or ELISA. Virus isolation in suitable cell lines, in embryonated eggs or in suckling mice by intracerebral inoculation. FAT, EllSA, CFT or the virus neutralization tests are suitable for identification of the isolates. Electron microscopy can be used to identify virus in specimens or tissue culture. Serological tests- CFT, the virus neutralization test, competitive ELISA or lgM-specific capture ELISA. Because levels of complement fixing and IgM79 antibodies persist for only short periods, assays based on procedures involving these antibodies can be used to confirm recent infections in endemic areas.

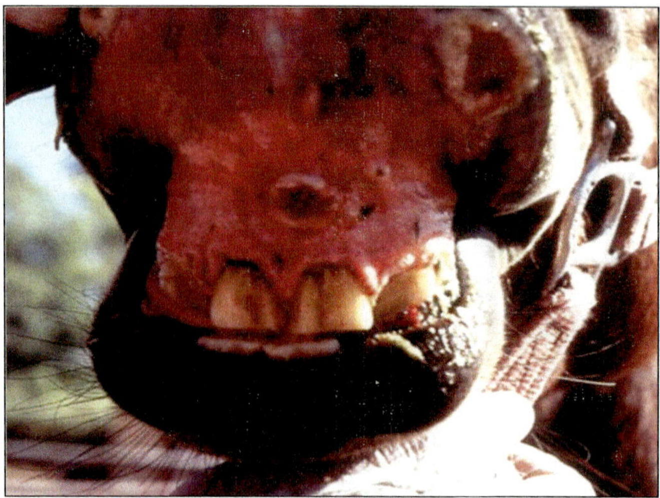

Figure 1.33. Vesicular stomatitis.

Treatment, Control, and Prevention

No specific treatment is available or warranted. Cachexia can be avoided by providing softened feeds. Cleansing lesions with mild antiseptics may help avoid secondary bacterial infections. Management factors suggested to reduce risk of exposure to the virus include limiting time on pasture during insect season, providing shelters or barns during insect feeding times, and implementing other procedures that reduce animal contact with insects, such as application of insecticides. This should include application to the inner surface of the pinna, where black flies feed. If livestock need to be kept on pasture during outbreaks of vesicular stomatitis, then keeping them pastured away from moving surface water (such as streams, irrigation canals, or rivers) may reduce the risk of exposure to *Vesiculovirus*. Affected animals should be isolated, and movement of other animals from the affected premises restricted. Vesicular stomatitis is a reportable disease in most areas, including the USA, so state and federal animal health officials must be notified when it is suspected. Commercially produced vaccines are not available in the USA, but vaccines for livestock are available in some Latin American countries.

Veterinarians act as a part of the surveillance network as they examine animals involved in shows, exhibitions, races, and interstate or international movement in order to write a health certificate (*i.e.*, certificate of veterinary inspection). When practitioners observe suspect cases of vesicular stomatitis, they should report to both their state and federal animal health officials. Reporting will prompt a regulatory investigation. Mucosal swab and serum samples from suspected animals are submitted for testing to veterinary diagnostic laboratories.

Zoonotic Risk

The vesicular stomatitis viruses are zoonotic and may cause self-limiting influenza-like disease (headache, fever, myalgia, and weakness) lasting 3–5 days in people working in close contact with the virus (*e.g.*, laboratory exposure, direct contact with lesions in infected animals). Rarely, people can develop vesicles on the buccal and pharyngeal mucosa, lips, and nose. More severe signs, including encephalitis, are rare.

Chapter 2

Bacterial Diseases

Bacterial diseases include any type of illness caused by bacteria. Bacteria are a type of microorganism, which are tiny forms of life that can only be seen with a microscope. Other types of microorganisms include viruses, some fungi, and some parasites. Millions of bacteria normally live on the skin, in the intestines, and on the genitalia. The vast majority of bacteria do not cause disease, and many bacteria are actually helpful and even necessary for good health. These bacteria are sometimes referred to as "good bacteria" or "healthy bacteria."

Harmful bacteria that cause bacterial infections and disease are called pathogenic bacteria. Bacterial diseases occur when pathogenic bacteria get into the body and begin to reproduce and crowd out healthy bacteria, or to grow in tissues that are normally sterile. Harmful bacteria may also emit toxins that damage the body.

2.1. Fowl Cholera

Synonym

Avian Pasteurellosis.

Fowl cholera is a contagious bacterial disease that affects domestic and wild birds worldwide. It usually occurs as a septicemia of sudden onset with high morbidity and mortality, but chronic and asymptomatic infections also occur.

Etiology and Transmission

Pasteurella multocida, the causal agent, is a small, gram-negative, nonmotile rod with a capsule that may exhibit pleomorphism after repeated subculture. *P. multocida* is considered a single species although it includes three subspecies: *multocida, xudat,* and *gallicida*. Subspecies *multocida* is the most common cause of disease, but *xudat* and *gallicida* may also cause cholera-like disease. In freshly isolated cultures or in tissues, the bacteria have a bipolar appearance when stained with Wright's stain. Although *P. multocida* may infect a wide variety of animals, strains isolated from nonavian hosts generally do not produce fowl cholera. Strains that cause fowl cholera represent a number of immunotypes (or serotypes), which complicates efforts at widespread prevention using bacterins. The organism is susceptible to ordinary disinfectants, sunlight, drying, and heat. Turkeys and waterfowl are more susceptible than chickens, older chickens are more susceptible than young ones, and some breeds of chickens are more susceptible than others.

Chronically infected birds and asymptomatic carriers are considered to be major sources of infection. Wild birds may introduce the organism into a poultry flock, but mammals (including rodents, pigs, dogs, and cats) may also carry the infection. However, the role of these as a reservoir has not been thoroughly investigated. Dissemination of *P. multocida* within a flock and between houses is primarily by excretions from the mouth, nose, and conjunctiva of diseased birds that contaminate their environment. In addition, *P. multocida* survives long enough to be spread by contaminated crates, feed bags, shoes, and other equipment. The infection does not seem to be egg-transmitted.

Prevalence of Infection

It is seen worldwide and was one of the first infectious diseases to be exudates by Louis Pasteur in 1880.

Predisposing Factors

Predisposing factors include high density and concurrent infections such as respiratory viruses.

Source of Infection

Carrier birds, excretions, carcasses of the infected birds, feeds, water are acting as important source of infection. Rats, cats and possibly pigs act as reservoirs. Infection usually spread through conjunctival, oral, nasal eexudates, faeces, contaminated soil, equipment and people.

Host Affected

All avian species are susceptible. Ducks, geese, water fowl and turkeys are more susceptible than chicken. Mostly growers and adult birds are being affected than young ones. Caged chickens are less affected by *Pasteurella multocida.*

Pathogenesis

The disease can range from acute septicaemia to chronic and exudates infections and the morbidity and mortality may be up to 100 per cent. Many of the lesions are related to vascular disturbances. Hyperemia is especially evident in the vessels of the abdominal viscera. Petechial and ecchymotic hemorrhages are common, particularly in subepicardial and subserosal locations. Increased amounts of peritoneal and pericardial fluids are frequently seen. The liver may be swollen and often develops multiple, small, necrotic foci.

Clinical Signs

It has been divided into peracute, acute, chronic and localized infection.

(a) **Peracute:** No clinical signs noticed and dead birds are found dead with good with bodily condition.

(b) **Acute**: The incubation period is usually 5-8 days; affected birds are dull, depressed, and anorectic. Mucus discharge from orifices; cyanosis of mucous membrane; foetid diarrhea.

(c) **Chronic:** Birds survived from acute form of disease are due to low virulent infection manifests depression, conjunctivitis, dyspnoea, lameness, toriticolis (twisting of the neck) and swollen wattles.

Necropsy Findings

(a) **Per acute and acute form**: These forms show marked congestion of carcass, multiple petechiation in all visceral organs, multiple pin-point necrotic foci in the liver. Free yolk found in the body cavity in layer birds.

(b) **Sub acute**: Edema of lungs in turkeys, pneumonia and focal perihepatitis and yolk peritonitis. Purulent pneumonia (especially in turkeys). Cellulitis of face and wattles. Purulent arthritis. Lungs with a consolidated pink 'cooked' appearance in turkeys.

(c) **Chronic**: Caseous arthritis of hock and foot joints. Swelling and induration of both wattles. Caseous exudates in the middle ears.

Diagnosis

Although the history, signs, and lesions may aid diagnosis, *P. multocida* should be isolated, characterized, and identified for confirmation. Primary isolation can be accomplished using media such as blood agar, dextrose starch agar, or trypticase soy agar. Isolation may be improved by the addition of 5 per cent heat-inactivated serum. *P. multocida* can be readily isolated from viscera of birds dying from peracute/acute fowl cholera, whereas isolation from suppurative lesions of chronic cholera may be more difficult. At necropsy, bipolar microorganisms may be demonstrated by the use of Wright's or Giemsa stain of impression smears obtained from the liver in the case of acute cholera. In addition, immunofluorescent microscopy and *in situ* hybridization have been used to identify *P. multocida* in infected tissues and eexudates.

PCR has been used for the detection of *P. multocida* in pure and mixed cultures and clinical samples. This method may help identify carrier animals within flocks. However, the specificity and sensitivity of the PCR must be improved. *P. multocida* can be subgrouped by capsule serogroup antigens into five capsular types (A, B, D, E, and F) and into 16 somatic serotypes. Somatic serotyping is important to choose the right bacterins for prevention. However, conventional serotyping suffers from problems with reproducibility and reliability, and the methods are quite laborious. Recently, a multiplex PCR has been developed that can differentiate between different somatic serotypes. This will be of great value as a diagnostic tool and enable more efficient vaccine development in the future. Serologic testing can be done by rapid whole blood agglutination, serum plate agglutination, agar diffusion tests, and ELISA. Serology may be used to evaluate vaccine responses but has very limited value for diagnostic purposes. Several bacterial infections may be confused with fowl cholera based solely on the gross lesions. *Escherichia coli*, *Salmonella xudate*, *Ornithobacterium rhinotracheale*, gram-positive cocci, and *Erysipelothrix rhusiopathiae* (erysipelas) may all produce lesions indistinguishable from those caused by *P. multocida*.

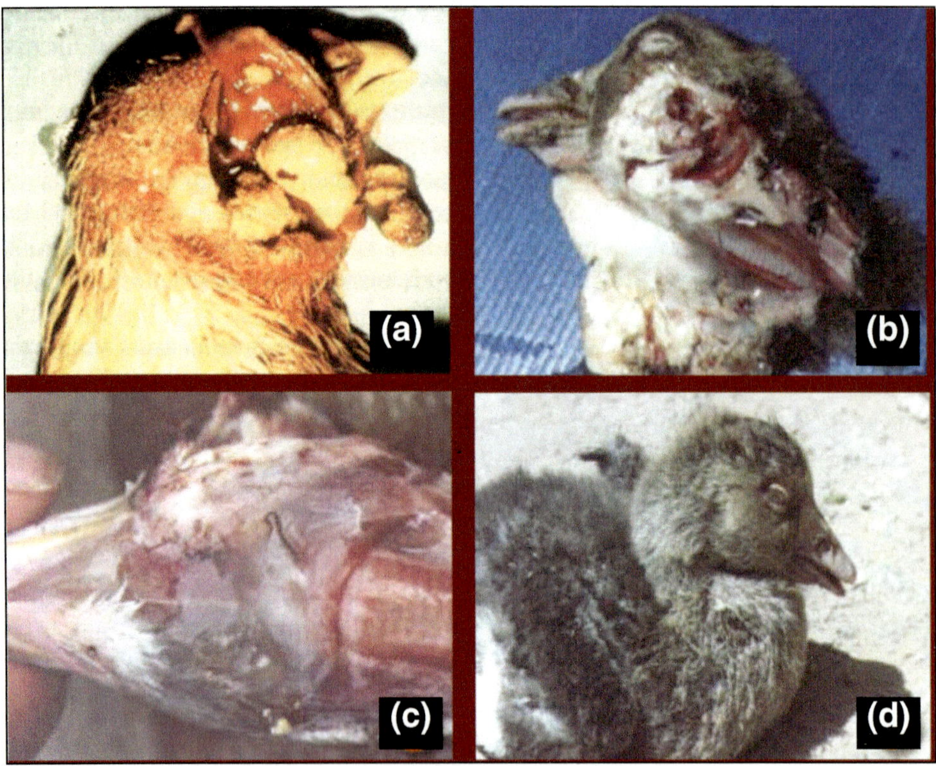

Figure 2.1

(a) Cheesy eexudates in infraorbital sinus, (b) Caseous eexudates located in the head region (subcutis), (c) Geese, submandibular edema, (d) Geese, swollen head.

Sample Collection

Impression smears from liver, heart and lung. *P. mutocida* inoculated lab animal will die in 24-48 hrs.

Differential Diagnosis

Salmonellosis; Pullorum disease; Fowl typhoid.

Treatment

A number of drugs will lower mortality from fowl cholera; however, deaths may resume when treatment is discontinued, showing that treatment does not eliminate *P. multocida* from a flock. Eradication of infection requires depopulation and cleaning and disinfection of buildings and equipment. The premise should then be kept free of poultry for a few weeks.

Sulfonamides and antibiotics are commonly used; early treatment and adequate dosages are important. Sensitivity testing often aids in drug selection and is important because of the emergence of multiresistant strains. Sulfaquinoxaline sodium in feed or water usually controls mortality, as do sulfamethazine and sulfadimethoxine. Sulfas should be used with caution in breeders because of potential toxicity. High levels of tetracycline antibiotics in the feed (0.04 per cent), drinking water, or administered parenterally may be useful. Norfloxacin administered via drinking water is also effective against fowl cholera. However, many countries do not allow the use of quinolones in food-producing animals, including poultry, because of the risk of development of drug resistance. Penicillin is often effective for sulfa-resistant infections. In ducks, a combined injection of streptomycin and dihydrostreptomycin can be effective.

2.2. Actinobacillosis

Synonyms

Wooden tongue, Timber tongue and Big head disease.

Actinobacillosis refers to a group of diseases caused by gram-negative coccobacilli in the genus *Actinobacillus*. Although there are >22 different bacterial species in this genus, only four (*A. pleuropneumoniae, A. suis, A. equuli* and *A. lignieresii*) are frequently associated with disease in animals. It is a chronic and infectious disease of cattle and sheep featured by inflammation of soft tissues of the head, neck, oro-pharyngeal lymphnodes, oesophageal groove and nasal cavity.

Etiology

Actinobacillosis is caused by *Actinobacillus lignieresi.* It is a small, rod shaped, motile, gram negative, aerobic organism and appears as single or in short chain. The organism is susceptible to ordinary environment and disinfectants. The organism may live for year in lyophilized culture. Blood and serum is required for growth of the organism.

Epidemiology

Prevalence of Infection

The disease is worldwide in distribution. Its occurrence is sporadic and prevalent in India.

Predisposing Factors

Eruption of permanent teeth in young animals favors the organism to penetrate sub-epithelial tissues. Other diseases causing vesicular and erosive stomatitis predispose animals for Actinobacillosis.

Source of Infection

Infection is spread through discharges from infected animals. Grazing on infected pastures.

Transmission

Feeding of animals with contaminated feeds. Through injury and abrasion made by sharp objects permit the entry of organisms through oral mucosa. External parasites help the development of cutaneous actinobacillosis.

Host Affected

Cattle, buffalo and sheep are found susceptible. Horses, pigs and human beings are also affected by the natural infection. Intra-peritoneal injection of guinea pigs with suspected materials demonstrates "Strauss reaction" and death. Young animals of 2-5 years of age are found more affected.

Pathogenesis

The organism is a normal inhabitant of digestive and respiratory tract; nevertheless, they gain into nasal and buccal mucosa and into dependent lymphnodes following trauma or injury of them. Unlike *Actinomyces* spp., this organism has affinity to soft tissues of head and neck and occasionally invades into bony tissues. In localized infection, inflammatory and granulomatous tissue changes occur followed by necrosis and suppuration with discharge of pus to the exterior and spread into adjacent lymphnodes. Infection of tongue interferes in prehension and mastication. Theoretically, inflammatory changes occur at an earlier stages and deformity of the tongue occur at a later stages.

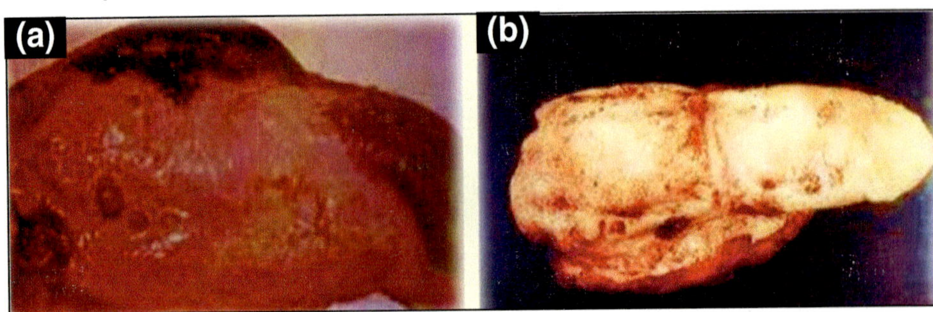

Figure 2.2

(a) Actinobacillosis- Yellow lump granules burst out of wooden tongue, (b) Actinobacillosis – Swollen tongue

Clinical Findings

Cattle

Affected tongue appears like wood and hence the disease has got the name wooden or timber tongue. Inflammation of tongue followed by ulceration. Ulceration of tongue leads to drooling of saliva, difficulty in mastication. Animals unable to eat in spite of a good appetite and loose body weight. Enlarged abscess in inter and sub-mandibular lymphnodes open and discharge pus. Affection of retropharyngeal region interferes with breathing and causes loud snoring. Abscess in posterior margin of soft palate produces dyspnoea. Discharge of nodules from subcutaneous tissues and mediastinal lymphnodes. Swelling in mediastinal lymphndoes imparts a pressure on esophageal groove and produce tympany. Affected lymphnodes are normally evinces pain. The organism also produces infection in liver, rumen, reticulum, peritoneum and lungs. In testis produces granulomatous lesion.

Sheep

Tongue is usually not affected in this species. Lesion seen in cutaneous portion of lower jaw, face and extending into sternum. Affected lymphnodes have yellowish greenish pus discharging from the openings. Bilateral nasal discharges noticed. Affected sheep die due to starvation.

Chronic Form

Accumulation of fibrous tissue affects prehension and mastication. Death in sheep due to in-anition may occur.

Necropsy Findings

The tongue becomes hard by proliferation of fibrous tissues. Lesions of soft tissue appeared as thick walled abscesses filled with thick tenacious pus. Firm, pale nodules containing in the center with minute yellow "sulfur granules".

Diagnosis

Based on clinical signs and lesions. Identification of gram negative coccobacilli in stained pus. Examination of rosettes formation in granules (less than one mm in diameter). Press cheesy mass on a glass drop slide with 10 per cent KOH solution and observe rosette mass under microscope with out staining.

Differential Diagnosis

Actinomycosis, Tuberculosis, Bovine leukosis, Granuloma or abscess due to pseudomonas, Ataphlococcus infection.

Treatment

X-Ray radiation for 10 consecutive weeks along with antibiotics and Sodium Iodide is beneficial. Lugols Iodine injected into the lesion may be useful. Oral feeding of cattle with Iodine 10 gm/1000 lb bw daily for 2-4 weeks until iodism signs appears (anorexia, salivation and depression). Administration of Sodium Iodide @70 mg/kg bw (10-20 per cent) solution in slow i/v and repeated after 7-10 days. Administration of streptomycin sulphate @5 g/day i/m for 3-5 days.

2.3. Actinomycosis

Synonyms

Lumpy Jaw.

Members of the genus *Actinomyces* are gram positive, anaerobic, non-acid-fast rods, many of which are filamentous or branching. Branches are <1 μm in diameter, as opposed to fungal filaments, which are >1 μm in diameter. Although they are normal flora of the oral and nasopharyngeal membranes, several species are associated with diseases in animals. Actinomycosis is a chronic, sporadic disease, affecting cattle followed by pigs and horses. Rarefying osteomyelitis of the bone in skull, enlargement of mammary gland, inflammation of bursa of the ligamentum nuchae is the prominent problem develops in cattle, pigs and horses. In association with *Brucella abortus* it causes "Fistulous withers" and "Poll evil" in horses.

Etiology

The disease is caused by *Actinomyces bovis.* As cultured organism has both bacterial and fungus features it is ascribed as fungal like bacteria. The organism is associated with *Coryenebacterium pyogenes* and *Staphylococcus. A. xudate* causes actinomycosis in human, but *A. bovis* and *A. xudate* are considered as different organism. There is no evidence for *A. bovis* causing infection in human.

Epidemiology

Prevalence of Infection

The disease is world wide in distribution. It is recorded from various regions in India. Incidence is higher in straw and silage fed cattle, because, these coarse materials injure the buccal mucosa and spread the infection further in to the other parts of the body. Its occurrence is sporadic and prevalent in India.

Predisposing Factors

Eruption of permanent teeth in young animals favors the organism to penetrate sub-epithelial tissues.

Source of Infection

Other diseases causing vesicular and erosive stomatitis predispose animals for Actinobacillosis. Infection is spread through discharges from infected animals. Grazing on infected pastures.

Transmission

Organism also exists as normal inhabitant in the oral cavity. Infection occurs through abraded injury or wounds induced by coarse feed stuff. Infection spread through dental alveoli at the of time of eruption of teeth. Alimentary tract harbor *A. bovis* from where it invades subcutaneous tissues through injury made by sharp object. Animal to animal transmission occurs but animal to human transmission is rare.

Host Affected

Infection is sporadic and more common in cattle of 2-5 years old. The disease rarely affects pigs, horses and goats. Chronic actinomycosis prevails in horses and dogs.

Pathogenesis

Pathogenesis developed purely by physical activity. The organisms does not produce toxin. *A. bovis* produces lesions in cervico-facial region, mandible and subcutaneous tissues of the lower jaw in cattle. Infection of rumen leads to ruminitis and indigestion which results in partial starvation. Serologically and clinically active cases of pulmonary actinomycosis have been recorded in cattle. Primarily the jawbone and then alimentary mucosa is affected. But rarely, the organism enters the haematogeous route. Rarefication and osteomyelitis of jaw bone interfere with mastication and prehension.

Clinical Signs

Cattle

The disease is sporadic and occasionally endemic in this species. Initially hard, painless, distinct swelling at the level of central molar teeth of the mandible or maxilla causes problem in mastication, and digestion. Partial block in trachea causes dyspnoea, followed by development of painful granulomatouss swelling, which breaks through skin and discharge through one or more openings. Invasion and damage to bony tissues causes proliferative osteitis. Oral cavity exhibits loose teeth or missing teeth as a result halitosis, hyper salivation and dysphagia is noticed. Occasionally eexudates with passage of undigested food materials is seen. Distended stomach, allotriophagia is observed. It has more prolonged course than Actinobacillosis and leading to suppurative granulomatous mass on superficial layer of jaw and ensues the formation of sinus tract. Discharges from abscess are sticky, mucoid, purulent and honey like eexudates containing minute hard, yellowish white sulphur granules. Infection spread to adjacent bones and lymphatic channels in case of prolonged infection. Localization of infection in testis of bull, brain and lungs occurs. Old lesions heal, however, fresh lesion develops.

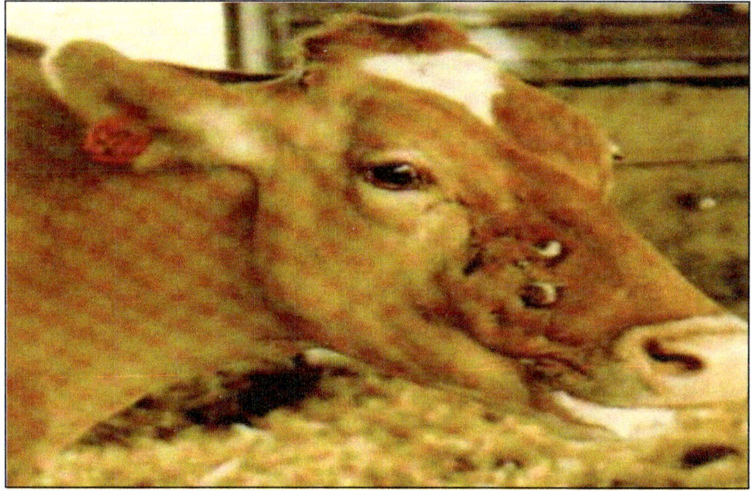

Figure 2.3. Actinomycosis (Lumpy Jaw), granulomatous masses have broken through the skin in the upper jaw.

Horses

Bursa between the nuchal ligament and primary thoracic spine and bursa between the nuchal ligament and atlas axis are affected. *A. bovis* and *Br. abortus* jointly develops suppuration and granulation leads to poll evil and Fistulous withers.

Pigs

Rarely suffer from extensive granulomatous lesions of the skin over the udder and become emaciated. Wasting due to visceral actinomycosis rarely occurs.

Dogs

Chronic pyogranulomatous lesion appears on the skin of sub-mandibular, abdomen and thoracic region.

Necropsy Findings

Rarefication of bones is widespread infection. Softening and liquefaction of pus gradually spread to cortex and rarefies it and which in turn forms a sub-perioisteal bone. Oesophagus and anterior wall of the reticulum containing pockets of pus and spread to causes chronic local peritonitis. Lumpy jaw is an important manifestation of a suppurative osteomyelitis of the mandible. Affected bone is filled with distinct granulation tissues and nodules. Miliary nodules present in udder and lungs. In sows infected udder is indurated and fibrosed with suppuration. Mild abomasitis and enteritis occurs.

Diagnosis

Based on clinical signs and necropsy findings. Isolation and identification of organism. Stained pus containing sulphur granules of *A. bovis.* Tissue section show cellular change. The granules of *A. bovis* exhibit the grit, non-acid fast branched filaments while stained by brown modification of Gram's stain. In a glass slide, a small drop of pus and water is mixed and examined under low power microscope. It reveals irregular club shaped filamentous gram positive bacteria.

Sample Collection

Pus from unopened lesion must be aspirated by a syringe and examined the visible granules by naked eye

Differential Diagnosis

Foreign body problem, chronic peritonitis, cutaneous or mammary disease, borreliosis are main sympotoms.

Treatment

Early lesion can be reduced using iodine and sulphur therapy. Streptomycin is used successfully. Surgical correction of abscess can be done. Administer Sodium Iodide 5-8gm in 250-500 ml distilled water I/V. Isoniazide 20 ml/kg body weight for 10 days @ 10-20 mg/kg body weight daily orally for 30 days. Response in advanced case is poor. Combination of Streptomycin with iodide and surgical drainage may provide good response. Cryotherapy with liquid nitrogen is found to be effective for treating abscess and rarefication.

2.4. Anthrax

Synonyms

Spleenic fever, Milzbrand, Charbon, Wool sorters disease and malignant carbuncle.

Anthrax is a zoonotic disease caused by the sporeforming bacterium *Bacillus anthracis*. Anthrax is most common in wild and domestic herbivores (*e.g.*, cattle, sheep, goats, camels, antelopes) but can also be seen in people exposed to tissue from infected animals, to contaminated animal products, or directly to *B. anthracis* spores under certain conditions. Depending on the route of infection, host factors, and potentially strain-specific factors, anthrax can have several different clinical presentations. In herbivores, anthrax commonly presents as an acute septicemia with a high fatality rate, often accompanied by hemorrhagic lymphadenitis. In dogs, people, horses, and pigs, it is usually less acute although still potentially fatal. *B. anthracis* spores can remain viable in soil for many years. During this time, they are a potential source of infection for grazing livestock but generally do not represent a direct risk of infection for people. Grazing animals may become infected when they ingest sufficient quantities of these spores from the soil. In addition to direct transmission, biting flies may mechanically transmit *B. anthracis* spores from one animal to another. The latter follows when there have been rains encouraging a high fly hatch and reporting has been delayed on the index ranch, such that there are 4–6 moribund or dead cattle for the flies to feed on. Feed contaminated with bone or other meal from infected animals can serve as a source of infection for livestock, as can hay muddy with contaminated soil. Raw or poorly cooked contaminated meat is a source of infection for zoo carnivores and omnivores; anthrax resulting from contaminated meat consumption has been reported in pigs, dogs, cats, mink, wild carnivores and people.

It is a peracute, acute and septicaemic disease of cattle and sheep leading to sudden death. The extensive enlargement of the spleen given this disease the name spleenic fever. It is a zoonotic disease spread from infected animals to human during processing of wool and hides.

Etiology

Bacillus anthracis is a pathogenic strain causing anthrax in both human and animals. It is a non-motile, capsulated, aerobic, spore forming, gram positive, organism. Appears as straight, very large rod shaped, arranged in a small short chain. The organism has two virulent factors such as, a capsule containing poly D-glutamic acid, which resists the phagocytosis induced by the host immune cells and is coded by the virulent plasmid pxo2, and the triple toxins such as edema factor-1, lethal factor-11 and the protective antigen factor- 111 and these are coded by the plasmid pXo1. The organism produces spores when exposed to external environment and can live for a prolonged period outside the host in the environment.

Epidemiology

Prevalence of Infection

The disease is reported to be recognized from sub Saharan Africa and has worldwide distribution. The prevalence of the disease depends upon the nature of soil and climatic condition, because, the climatic parameter helps to forecast the "anthrax year". If the infection is restricted to a particular area is called as "anthrax belts" or enzootic region. During heavy and prolonged rainfall, following a draught, or dry summer, in warm weather and in the temperature at which (>60°F/15°C) formation of spores, vegetative proliferation with the production of disease or the outbreak occurs. In African countries, every summer with a heavy rain fall is followed by a devastating occurrence of anthrax. In India it is enzootic.

Economic Impact

Mortality, reduced milk yield and the expenses incurred for vaccination leads to severe economic loss.

Predisposing Factors

pH of the infected soil, infected wool, materials, hides and other materials. In wet soil and in stagnant water spores are concentrated and suspended. Alkaline soil (pH 9.0) under warm climate preserve the organism to develop anthrax but acid soil destroys the organism. Blood transfusion may also spread the disease. Contaminated bone meal, pasture contaminated with tannery effluents, fodders grown on infected soil, turning up of soil, blood and other discharges from infected animals are the major source of infection. Calciumrich alluvial soil, organic and poorly drained soils have the risk of causing endemic infection.

Source of Infection

Contaminated soil, environment, infected excretions and secretions from animals.

Transmission

Ingestion, inhalation and contamination of wound by spores are prime mode of spread. Injury to oral mucosa permits the invasion of the organism. Inhalation plays less important role in animals contrast to more spread in human being and is responsible for causing wool sorters disease. Mechanical transmission through Tabanid fly bite occurs.

Host Affected

Cattle and sheep are highly susceptible as compared to goat and horses. Human is less susceptible than cattle. Pigs, dogs and cats are relatively resistant. But once affected the case fatality rate is high in farm animals and pigs. Hippopotamus, Cape buffalo and elephants die in large numbers due to anthrax. Persons working in wool and hide industries are mostly affected. Predators act as carrier for this infection.

Pathogenesis

Discharges and materials containing anthrax bacilli when exposed to air, spores are produced. The spores are very resistant in the external environment but the un-germinated spores are considered not harmful it become vegetative form inside the host. The organism is resistant to phagocytosis due to the presence of poly D glutamic acid containing capsule, and triple toxin factors such as edema factor-I, lethal factor-II and protective antigen-III. Primarily, spores proliferate in the regional draining lymphnodes, subsequently, travels via lymphatic vessels and reach the blood stream and cause septicemia followed by massive invasion into all body tissues. The lethal toxin of *B. anthracis* causes edema, tissue damage, and death as a result of shock, acute renal failure and terminal anoxia. The blockage of capillaries initiating death is commonly known as "Log Jam" theory. As per the evidence atleast $3x10^6$ bacteria/ml blood is necessary for causing death. In pigs, exudatest of the organism occurs in the lymphnode of the throat following invasion through upper part of the digestive tract eventually lead to a fatal septicaemia. Shock acute renal failure and terminal anoxia leads to death.

Clinical Signs

Cattle and Sheep

(a) **Peracute form**: Sudden death without any premonitory signs. Upon close observation following signs will be seen. Fevers, muscle tremor, dyspnoea, congestion of mucous membrane are noticed. Animal collapses and die due to terminal convulsions. After death, oozing of blood from nostrils, mouth, anus and vulva is noticed.

(b) **Acute form**: Incubation period of the disease is 1-2 weeks. The course of this form is about 48 hours. Fever (42°C), severe depression, listlessness, congestion and heamorrhage of deep mucous membrane, increased heart rate and rapid respiration observed. Affected cattle with mouth breathing due to oxygen hunger. Abortion, decrease in milk yield, blood stained or deep yellow color milk, eexudates, local edema of the tongue, throat, sternum, perineum and flank occur.

Pigs

Acutely and sub-acutely infected animals show high temperature, appears dull, anorectic with distinct inflammatory edema in throat and face. Painless swelling causes obstruction which leads to swallowing and respiration difficulty. Blood stained froth present at the mouth. Petechial eexudates of skin, dysentery without any edema of throat occurs.

Pulmonary Form

In baby pigs, it develops lobar pneumonia and exudative pleuirisy through inhalation of dust which leads to death in a day or two. Occassionally, affected individuals may be alive for several days after infection.

Horse

Always horses are affected with acute infection by ingestion and leads to septicaemia, enteritis and colic. Painful, edematous and subcutaneous swellings appear in throat over the lower neck, floor of the thorax, abdomen, prepuce and mammary gland. There is a high fever, severe depression, dyspnoea due to swelling of the throat or colic due to intestinal irritation. The course of the disease is about 48-96 hours.

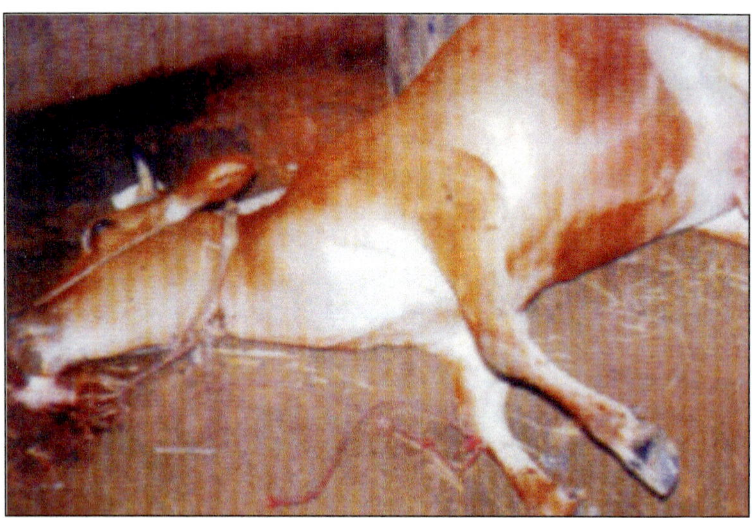

Figure 2.4. Anthrax- Oozing blood – nasal orifices.

Zoonosis

It is a fatal disease of human beings. *B. anthracis* is an agent of bio-terrorism and listed as category A disease by OIE. Occupational hazard by inhalation of spores occurs mostly while sorting out wool and processing of hides.

Necropsy Findings

Absence of rigor mortis with gaseous decomposition, quick assumption of the characteristic saw horse posture. Un-clotted tarry colored blood oozes out through natural orifices. There is a soft and enlarged spleen with a black berry jam consistency and is important feature of anthrax. The carcass eexudates of anthrax should not be opened before confirmation made by peripheral blood smear examination. In horses and pigs enlargement of local lymphnodes, lesions in the soft tissues of the neck and pharynx are important and it is called as pharyngeal form of anthrax.

Diagnosis

Based on clinical signs and necropsy findings. Isolation and identification of organism. Haematological and blood chemistry examinations should not be conducted because of the risk for human exposure. The square ended blue bacilli (chain) with metachromatic pink capsule detected by microscopic examination after staining with ripened polychrome methylene blue stain is called as 'McFadyean's reaction'. In early stages bacilli may not be present in blood, so, culture can be done or the materials like infected fluid can be injected into guinea pigs would give proper diagnostic result. Fluorescent antibody technique using monoclonal antibody can be done to detect the disease. In decomposed carcass vegetative bacilli may not be present; in such a condition diagnosis is difficult so that the protective antigen is detected by xudat-chromatography test. It has a high specificity but does not give positive results in recently vaccinated cattle. Isolation of bacilli from infected soil is difficult but real time quantitative PCR and Nested PCR have been found highly sensitive. In human cutaneous anthrax is diagnosed by Immunohistochemical detection of the bacilli in the skin biopsies. Gelatin stab culture: The growth resembles an 'inverted fir tree appearance' with slow liquefaction commencing from the top. Nutrient agar media: The 5 per cent blood agar show 'medusa head colonies'.

Ascolis Test

To demonstrate the antigen in severely decayed carcass and the skin in which tube containing positive serum is overlayed with suspected sample develops a white precipitation ring at the junction of the two liquids.

B. anthracis
Gram stain.
Cells : Squared end
Endospores: Ellipsoidal shape, Central in sporangium.
Spores are highly refractile to light and resistant to staining.
B. anthracis
Incubation at 5 per cent CO_2 tension increases the production of poly-D-glutamyl acid production by capsule thereby mucoid colonies.
B. anthracis
McFadyean's reaction: Cells in short chains with plenty of disintegrated capsular material. White blood cells stained blue.
B. anthracis: Medusa Head Colonies.
Anthrax Spore Vaccine
It is a nonpathogenic, noncapsulated variant vaccine strain Sterne 34F2 of *B. anthracis* spore vaccine in saponin, in India.

Sample Collection

Unopened carcass, blood, edema fluid in sealed leak proof containers and direct smears from tip of the ears. In live animals, organism may be detected in a stained peripheral blood smear, edema fluid, lymphnode needle puncture smear, amputated tail or ears and jugular vein aspiration, *etc.* If anthrax is suspected then shipping of diagnostic samples via air or courier is not permitted.

Differential Diagnosis

Lightening strike, peracute blackleg, malignant edema, bacillary hemoglobinuria, hypomagnesemia.

Treatment, Control and Prevention

Anthrax is controlled through vaccination programs, rapid detection and reporting, quarantine, treatment of asymptomatic animals (postexposure prophylaxis), and burning or burial of suspect and confirmed cases. In livestock, anthrax can be controlled largely by annual vaccination of all grazing animals in the endemic area and by implementation of control measures during epizootics. The nonencapsulated Sterne-strain vaccine is used almost universally for livestock immunization. Vaccination should be done at least 2–4 wk before the season when outbreaks may be expected. Because this is a live vaccine, antibiotics should not be administered within 1 wk of vaccination. Before vaccination of dairy cattle during an outbreak, all of the procedures required by local laws should be reviewed and followed. Human anthrax vaccines currently licensed and used in the USA and Europe are based on filtrates of artificially cultivated *B. anthracis*.

Early treatment and vigorous implementation of a preventive program are essential to reduce losses among livestock. Livestock at risk should be immediately treated with a long-acting antibiotic to stop all potential incubating infections. This is followed by vaccination ~7–10 days after antibiotic treatment. Any animals becoming sick after initial treatment and/or vaccination should be retreated immediately and revaccinated a month later. Simultaneous use of antibiotics and vaccine is inappropriate, because available commercial vaccines for animals in the USA are live vaccines. Animals should be moved to another pasture away from where the bodies had lain and any possible soil contamination. Suspected contaminated feed should be immediately removed. Domestic livestock respond well to penicillin if treated in the early stages of the disease. Oxytetracycline given daily in divided doses also is effective. Other antibacterials, including amoxicillin, chloramphenicol, ciprofloxacin, doxycycline, erythromycin, gentamicin, streptomycin, and exudatestd also can be used, but their effectiveness in comparison with penicillin and the tetracyclines has not been evaluated under field conditions.

In addition to therapy and immunization, specific control procedures are necessary to contain the disease and prevent its spread. These include the following: **1)** notification of the appropriate regulatory officials; **2)** rigid enforcement of quarantine (after vaccination, 2 wk before movement off the farm, 6 wk if going to slaughter); **3)** prompt disposal of dead animals, manure, bedding, or other contaminated material by cremation (preferable) or deep burial; **4)** isolation of sick animals and removal of well animals from the contaminated areas; **5)** cleaning and disinfection of stables, pens, milking barns, and equipment used on livestock; **6)** use of insect repellents; **7)** control of scavengers that feed on animals dead from the disease; and **8)** observation of general sanitary procedures by people who handle diseased animals, both for their own safety and to prevent spread of disease. Contaminated soils are very difficult to completely decontaminate, but formaldehyde will be successful if the level is not excessive. The process generally requires removal of soil.

Human infection is controlled through reducing infection in livestock, veterinary supervision of animal production and slaughter to reduce human contact with potentially infected livestock or animal products, and in some settings either pre- or postexposure prophylaxis. In countries where anthrax is common and vaccination coverage in livestock is low, people should avoid contact with livestock and animal products that were not inspected before and after slaughter. In general, consumption of meat from animals that have exhibited sudden death, meat obtained via emergency slaughter, and meat of uncertain origin should be avoided. Routine vaccination against anthrax is indicated for individuals engaged in work involving large quantities or concentrations of *B. anthracis* cultures or activities with a high potential for aerosol production. Laboratory workers using standard Biosafety Level 2 practices in the routine processing of clinical samples are not at increased risk of exposure to *B. anthracis* spores. The risk for workers who come into contact with imported animal hides, furs, bone meal, wool, animal hair, or bristles has been reduced by improvements in industry standards and import restrictions. Routine preexposure vaccination is recommended for people in this group only when these standards and restrictions are insufficient to prevent exposure to anthrax spores. Routine vaccination of veterinarians in the USA is not recommended because of the low incidence of animal cases. However, vaccination may be indicated for veterinarians and other high-risk individuals handling potentially infected animals in areas where there is a high incidence of anthrax cases.

The CDC has recommended that those at risk of repeated exposure to *B. anthracis* spores in response to a bioterrorism attack should be vaccinated. Those groups include some emergency first responders, federal responders, and laboratory workers. Vaccination in anticipation of a terrorist attack is not recommended for other populations.

For people, postexposure prophylaxis against *B. anthracis* is recommended after an aerosol exposure to *B. anthracis* spores. Prophylaxis may consist of antibiotic therapy alone or the combination of antibiotic therapy and vaccination; if vaccine is available (most human vaccines are not live). Although there is no approved regimen, the CDC has suggested that antibiotics may be discontinued after three doses of vaccine have been administered according to the standard schedule (0, 2, and 4 wk). Because of availability and ease of dosing, doxycycline or ciprofloxacin may be chosen initially for antibiotic chemoprophylaxis until the susceptibility of the infecting organism is determined. Penicillin and doxycycline are approved by the FDA for treatment of anthrax in people and have traditionally been considered the drugs of choice. Both ciprofloxacin and ofloxacin have demonstrated *in vitro* activity against *B. anthracis*. Although naturally occurring *B. anthracis* resistance to penicillin is infrequent, it is reported; resistance to other antibiotics has been noted. Antibiotics are effective against the germinated form of *B. anthracis* but are not effective against the spore form of the organism. Spores may survive in the mediastinal lymph nodes in the lungs for months without germination in nonhuman primates.

There are currently no approved vaccination regimens for postexposure prophylaxis after *B. anthracis* exposures. Although postexposure chemoprophylaxis using antibiotics alone has been effective in animal models, the definitive length of treatment remains unclear. Antibiotic chemoprophylaxis may be switched to penicillin VK or amoxicillin in children or pregnant women once antibiotic susceptibilities are known and the organism is found to be susceptible to penicillin.

The safety and efficacy of anthrax vaccine in children or pregnant women has not been studied; therefore, a recommendation for use of vaccine in these groups cannot be made. Although the shortened vaccine regimen has been effective when used in a postexposure regimen that includes antibiotics, the duration of protection from vaccination is not known. The existing evidence suggests that vaccine protection is adequate for 12 months. If subsequent exposures occur, additional vaccinations may be required.

There are no definitive recommendations for postexposure prophylaxis after cutaneous or GI exposures of people to *B. anthracis*. Based on the slow progression of disease, low fatality rate, and ease of antibiotic treatment of cutaneous anthrax, and the general low risk of cutaneous disease after natural exposure, postexposure prophylaxis is not recommended after direct cutaneous exposure to contaminated animals or animal products. However, immediate washing of the exposed areas is advised. Those exposed should be advised of the signs of cutaneous anthrax (*i.e.,* an inflamed but painless area with or without circumferential small vesicles, enlargement of the regional lymph nodes) and should seek medical assistance if illness develops. Because of the high fatality rate and rapid progression of GI anthrax, serious consideration should be given to initiating postexposure antibiotic prophylaxis for those who consume contaminated undercooked or raw meat. There is no current indication for vaccination after either cutaneous exposure or ingestion.

2.5. Botulism

Synonyms

Equine grass tetany, Equine dysantonomia, Limber neck and Shaker foal syndrome.

Botulism is a rapidly fatal motor paralysis caused by ingestion of the toxin produced by *Clostridium botulinum* types A-G. The spore-forming anaerobic organism proliferates in decomposing animal tissue and sometimes in plant material. *Clostridium botulinum* produces potent neurotoxins during their vegetative transformation. The vegetative cells multiply rapidly and elaborate a stable and highly lethal toxins types such as B, C and D which when ingested or absorbed by tissues develops botulism. Preformed toxin is the main source for intoxication. Botulism causes toxaemia and flaccid paralysis in human, animals and birds.

Etiology: Botulism is in most cases intoxication, not an infection, and results from ingestion of toxin in food. There are seven types of *C. botulinum*, differentiated on the antigenic specificity of the toxins: A, B, C_1, D, E, F, and G. Types A, B, and E are most important in people; C_1 in most animal species, notably wild ducks, pheasants, chickens, mink, cattle, and horses; and D in cattle. In horses, the most common type in North America and Europe is type B (>85 per cent of USA cases), and in the western USA type A has been reported in only two outbreaks, both in people, known to have been caused by type F. Type G, isolated from soil in Argentina, is not known to have been involved in any outbreak of botulism. The usual source of the toxin is decaying carcasses or vegetable materials such as decaying grass, hay, grain, or spoiled silage. Toxins of all types have the same pharmacologic action. Like tetanus toxin, botulinum toxin is a zinc-binding metalloprotease that cleaves specific proteins in synaptic vesicles. Motor neuron surface receptors vary for the different botulinum toxins, explaining some of the species differences in susceptibility to the different toxins.

The exact incidence of botulism in animals is not known, but it is relatively low in cattle and horses, probably more frequent in chickens, and high in wild waterfowl. Probably 10,000–50,000 birds are lost in most years, with losses reaching 1 million or more during the great outbreaks in the western USA. Most affected birds are ducks, although loons, mergansers, geese, and gulls also are susceptible. Dogs, cats, and pigs are comparatively resistant to all types of botulinum toxin when challenged orally; however, there are recent individual case reports mentioning botulism in dogs.

Most botulism in cattle occurs in South Africa and South America, where a combination of extensive agriculture, phosphorus deficiency in soil, and *C botulinum* type D in animals creates conditions ideal for the disease. The phosphorus-deficient cattle chew any bones with accompanying bits of flesh they find on the range; if these came from an animal carrying type D strains of *C. botulinum*, intoxication is likely to result. Any animal eating such material also ingests spores, which germinate in the intestine and, after death of the host, invade the musculature, which in turn becomes toxic for other cattle. Type C strains also cause botulism in cattle in a similar fashion. This type of botulism in cattle is rare in the USA, although a few cases have been reported from Texas under the name of loin disease, and a few cases have occurred in Montana. Hay or silage contaminated with toxin-containing carcasses of birds or mammals and poultry litter fed to cattle have also been sources of type C or type D toxin for cattle ("forage botulism"). Big bale silage and haylage seem to be a particular risk and result in botulism problems if fermentation fails to produce a low and stable pH (<4.5). Botulism in sheep has been encountered in Australia, associated not with phosphorus deficiency as in cattle, but with protein and carbohydrate deficiency, which results in sheep eating carcasses of rabbits and other small animals found on the range. Botulism in horses often results from forage contaminated with type C or D toxin. In six out of eight outbreaks of equine botulism associated with type A, the source of infection was confirmed to be hay or silage.

Toxicoinfectious botulism is the name given the disease in which *C. botulinum* grows in tissues of a living animal and produces toxins there. The toxins are liberated from the lesions and cause typical botulism. This has been suggested as a means of producing the shaker foal syndrome. Gastric ulcers, foci of necrosis in the liver, abscesses in the navel and lungs, wounds of the skin and muscle, and necrotic lesions of the GI tract are predisposing sites for development of toxicoinfectious botulism. This disease of foals and adult horses appears to resemble "wound botulism" in people. Type B toxin is often implicated in botulism in horses and foals in the eastern USA. Toxicoinfection is also suggested as a cause of equine grass sickness.

Botulism in mink usually is caused by type C strains that have produced toxin in chopped raw meat or fish. Type A and E strains are occasionally involved. Botulism has not been reported in cats but occurs sporadically in dogs. Type C toxin is usually responsible, but there have been reports in which type D was incriminated.

Epidemiology

Prevalence of Infection

Spores survive in the environment for long period. The disease is distributed worldwide, including India.

Predisposing Factors

Heat and moisture favors the germination of spores.

Source of Infection

The proliferation of organism occurs in decaying vegetable or animal matters. The toxin is stable particularly in bones. In sheep, due to dietary deficiency of protein or net energy. Phosphorus deficient cattle or sheep chew and ingest dead carcass, bones, debris and get highest possible infection. Meat and milk containing toxin causes public health hazard.

Transmission

The spread of infection by ingestion of contaminated material or birds or blow flies are possible. Spread of infection through injury.

Host Affected

Cattle and sheep are susceptible for type C and D while horses are susceptible for type B toxin. Pigs, dogs and cats found to be resistant. Human is also susceptible for bolutinum toxins.

Pathogenesis

Botulism toxins are neurotoxins absorbed by the intestinal tract or the wound and traverse through the blood stream to peripheral cholinergic nerve terminals and neuromuscular junction, post ganglionic parasympathetic nerve endings and peripheral ganglia. The toxin has heavy chain bind to the receptors and translocated into the cells and the light chain of the toxin blocks the release of acetylcholine at the neuromuscular junction/motor nerve endings. Toxins produce functional flaccid paralysis. Animal dies due to respiratory paralysis.

Types of Botulism

Carrion associated botulism: Multiplication of the organism in the feed produce toxin and is mostly consumed by phosphorous deficient and protein deprived animals. Wound botulism: The organisms produce toxins directly in the wounds. Toxico-infectious botulism: The organism grows and produce toxin in alimentary tract. Forage botulism: Most cases of botulism are associated with the ingestion of preformed toxin in forages.

Clinical Signs

Cattle and Horses

Incubation period is 3-17 days. After exposure to toxic material even within a day the exudates signs may appear. It may be depends on the amount of toxin released and ingested. The toxico-infectious botulism can also be a cause for "equine grass tetany" (equine dysantonomia).

(a) **Peracute**: No rise of temperature or clinical signs seen. Animals die immediately.

(b) **Acute**: One of the most important signs is the development of progressive symmetric, muscular paralysis of the limb muscles and the muscles of jaw, tongue, throat and muscle weakness. Paralysis starts in the mid quarters and proceeds to the forequarters, followed by head and neck. Muscle weakness, an obvious muscle tremor and fasciculation may be enough to cause limb tremor. Colic in horse is an important sign. Partial or complete paralysis of muscles of locomotion.

(c) **Sub acute**: Restlessness, respiratory distress, discinlination to rise, pronounced roaring sound and persists up to 3 months in some animals. In-coordination, stumbling, knuckling, ataxia, inability to rise or to lift the head, mydriasis and ptosis occur early. Difficulty to take hay for 3 weeks. Mydriasis is prominent in type-C botulism in horses. Sternal recumbancy, turning of head on the ground or into the flank. Reduced tongue tone, paralysis, tongue hangs out from mouth, difficulty in chewing, or swallow and drooling of saliva is prominent. Depression of rumen motility and constipation present. Paralysis of chest muscles results in terminal abdominal type respiration. Animals are alert and consciousness until at the end or death.

Foals

Toxico-infectious botulism in foals by type-B toxin. In young foals of up to 8 months highest prevalence occurs. The multiplication of organism in the intestine and production of toxins causes the disease called "shaker foal syndrome". Type–B toxin has been isolated from feces of naturally infected animals. Muscle tremor is a prominent early signs. If the foal walks, show stiff gait, stilted gait, dragging of toes and drooling of saliva from mouth. Attempts to eat hay but regurgitate it through nostrils. Constipation occurs consistently. Rapid progression to severe muscular weakness, prostration, loss of condition and unable to rise. Prostrate foals are bright and alert have normal sense, pain perception, dilation of pupils with a sluggish exudates light reflex and in later period, complete cessation of peristaltic movement. Temperature varies from slightly elevated to depress. Death occurs in 72 hours after the onset of signs due to respiratory failure.

Sheep

Affected sheep do not show typical flaccid paralysis. Stiffness while walking, in-coordination and excitability in the early stages noticed. Head held on one side or bobbed up and down while walking (Limber neck). Lateral switching of tail, salivation and serous, nasal discharge are common. Terminal abdominal respiration, limb paralysis followed by rapid death.

Pigs

Affected pigs show staggering, recumbancy, vomiting, eexudates dilatation, flaccid paralysis of the muscle, anorexia and adypsia.

Dogs

In dogs, symptoms develop more quickly, within 12-36 hours after exposure to the toxin. There is generalized weakness, paralysis which spread from the hind limbs to the forelimbs. In addition increased respiratory effort, facial nerve paralysis, and difficulty in swallowing. The disease progresses to fatal respiratory failure.

Zoonosis

Botulism toxin is an agent of bio-terrorism. Meat and milk containing toxins should not be used for human consumption. Human get infections by eating improperly cooked meat, its products and milk.

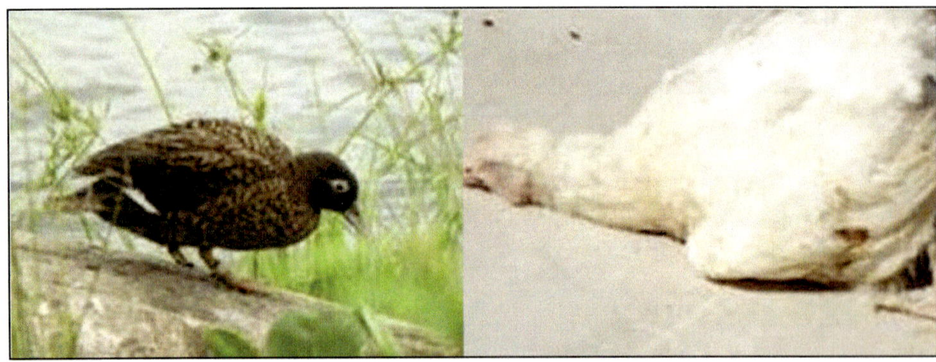

Figure 2.5. *Clostridium botulinium*- Sick Birds.

Necropsy Findings

Non-specific sub-endocardial, sub-epicardial haemorrhages and congestion of intestines found. Non specific perivascular haemorrhages in the corpus stratum, cerebellum and cerebrum present.

Diagnosis

Based on clinical signs and necropsy findings. Demonstration of toxin in serum, feed, intestinal contents and from wounds. In foals arterial blood analysis shows exudates, hypercapnia, hypoxemia and desaturation of Haemoglobin. Repeated arterial blood gas analysis should be conducted during first 48 hours of treatment. Demonstration of spores of *Cl. botulinum* in feed. Mice: Injected with toxin and neutralized with polyvalent antitoxin. But the sensitivity is low in mice as compared to ruminants and horses to botulism toxin. In chronic/sub-acute condition, ELISA is used for the detection of type C and D in cattle.

Samples Collection

It is taken from suspected contaminated feed material, liver, rumen contents serum, *etc.* and Formalin fixed brain.

Differential Diagnosis

Ruminants

Parturient paresis in cattle. Hypocalcaemia in sheep. Tick paralysis. Rabies. Organophosphate or carbomate poisoning. Louping ill.

Horses

Equine protozoan myelitis. Equine encephalomyelitis. Hepatic encephalopathy. Rabies.

Treatment

Early administration of antitoxin before complete recumbancy. Supportive therapy includes fluid therapy, parenteral feeding, nasal in-sufflation with oxygen and mechanical ventilation. Although it is expensive, a single dose of specific or polyvalent antiserum administrated early in course with 30,000IU for a foal and 70,000IU for adult horses may increase the survival rate. Antimicrobials for treating secondary complications such as aspiration pneumonia. Avoid the use of drugs that may deplete the neuromuscular junction of acetylcholine such as neostigmine and that procaine penicillin, tetracyclines, aminoglycocides potentiate neuromuscular weakness. Muzzling is essential to prevent aspiration pneumonia. Frequent turning to prevent the development of muscle necrosis and decubital ulcers.

2.6. Brucellosis

Synonyms

Bang's disease, Mediterranean fever, Undulant Fever and Malta fever.

Brucellosis is caused by bacteria of the genus *Brucella* and is characterized by abortion, retained placenta, and to a lesser extent, orchitis and infection of the accessory sex glands in males. The disease is prevalent in most countries of the world. It primarily affects cattle, buffalo, bison, pigs, sheep, goats, dogs, elk, and occasionally horses. The disease in people, sometimes referred to as undulant fever, is a serious public health problem, especially when caused by *B. melitensis*. It is an important Zoonotic disease, causes a significant reproductive losses through abortions, placentitis, epididymitis and orchitis in infected animals. Brucellosis is caused more often by *B. abortus*, less frequently by *B. melitensis* and occasionally by *B. suis*.

Etiology

Brucella is a Gram negative, non-motile, facultative intracellular, coccobacillary/ short, rod shaped organism. They are strict aerobes and grow very slowly (fastidious) on blood agar. *Chlamidophila* and *Coxiella exudates* are indistinguishable from Brucella. Some species of this genus and their host specificity has been listed below:

Brucella abortus - Cattle, bison and buffalo, human. *Brucella melitensis, B. ovis* – Sheep and goats. *B. suis* –Pigs. *B. canis* –Dogs. *B. maris* – Marine mammals. *B. neotomae* –Rodents (found in this species but not causing the clinical disease). *B. pinnipdedialis* –Pinnipeds (seals, sea lions and walruses). *B. cetaceae* –Cetaceans (whales, porpoises and dolphin). There are five biovars in *B. suis* and three for *B. melitensis* and nine for *B. abortus* present. *B. suis* contains more diverse isolates and broader host range as compared to any other species of *Brucella*. *B. abotus*, *B. melitensis*, *B. suis* and *B. canis* causes brucellosis in human. In addition, some species of *Brucella* has been used in biological warfare.

Epidemiology

Prevalence of Infection

It is worldwide in distribution. Brucellosis is endemic in India.

Source of Infection

Brucella species have also been found in secretions and excretions which include urine, feces, hygroma fluids, saliva, nasal and ocular discharge. After the first full term abortion, cattle become an asymptomatic chronic carriers, and continue to shed the organism in milk and uterine discharges. Dogs may or may not show clinical signs but shed the specific organism in later stage of pregnancies. In ruminants, udder colonizes the organisms after parturition and the in the uterus during pregnancy.

Transmission

Brucllosis occurs by ingestion, inhalation while having direct contact with food and other materials contaminated with brucella in addition the organism spread to skin injury and conjunctival route. Mostly, *Brucella abortus*, *B. melitensis* are shed through bull semen for a long period but venereal spread is seems to be uncommon. The venereal route is the primary route of transmission for *B. ovis*, *B. suis* and *B. canis* and occurs frequently. General spread of infection occurs through ingestion, mucous membranes, broken skin. The infection spread also from milkers and farmers hands but long-term shedding not occurs normally in ruminant's milk.

Host Affected

Cattle, bison, buffaloes, sheep, goats, pigs, dogs, marine mammals, rodents, pinnipeds such as seals, sea lions and walruses, cetaceans such as whales, porpoises, European otter and dolphins are affected. Sheep and goats acts as reservoir for *B. melitensis* and deer as a maintenance host for *B. ovis*. Wildlife reservoirs which include feral pigs, bison, elk and European hares maintain the organisms complicate the eradication processes of *B. abortus* and *B. suis*. *B. abortus*, *B. melitensis* and *B. suis* affects horses, camels, moose, chamois, alpine ibex, raccoons, opossums, dogs, coyotes, foxes and wolves (accidental hosts). Dogs are the only species known to be naturally infected with *B. canis*, although antibodies to this organism have been found in other carnivores.

Pathogenesis

Following entry, the bacteria are swallowed by neutrophils, monocytes and macrophages. Within the phagocytic cells they proliferate intracellularly and remain in lymphnodes if not killed by the host immune cells and get eexudates in regional lymphnodes. Brucella primarily eexudates in the organs rich in sugar, erythritol *i.e.*;

breast, uterus, epididymis and testes, *etc.* Within the phago-lysosome B. abortus releases 5′ –guanosine and adenine which inhibits the de-granulation of peroxidase-containing granules and thus inhibit the myeloperoxidase-peroxide-halide system of bacterial killing. The intracellular persistence of the brucella leads to granuloma formation in organs and tissues are due to hypersensitivity reactions, mostly type-IV. The organism is distributed from lymphnodes to lympho-reticular organs such as spleen, bone marrow, liver and testes where they develops granulomas or microabscesses which resulted in abortion in the thierd term pregnancy.

Clinical Signs

Cattle

The disease in cattle, water buffalo, and bison is caused almost exclusively by *Brucella abortus*; however, *B. suis* occasionally is isolated from seropositive cows but does not appear to cause clinical signs and is not contagious from cow to cow. In some countries, the disease in cattle is caused by *B. melitensis*. The syndrome is similar to that caused by *B. abortus*. *B. melitensis* is not present in the USA. Infection spreads rapidly and causes many abortions in unvaccinated cattle. In a herd in which disease is endemic, an infected cow typically aborts only once after exposure; subsequent gestations and lactations appear normal. After exposure, cattle become bacteremic for a short period and develop agglutinins and other antibodies; some cattle resist infection, and a small percentage of infected cows spontaneously recover. A positive serum agglutination test usually precedes an abortion or a normal parturition but may be delayed in ~15 per cent of cows. The incubation period may be variable and is inversely related to stage of gestation at time of exposure. Organisms are shed in milk and uterine discharges, and the cow may become temporarily infertile. Bacteria may be found in the uterus during pregnancy, uterine involution, and infrequently, for a prolonged time in the nongravid uterus. Shedding from the vagina largely disappears with the cessation of fluids after parturition. Some infected cows that previously aborted shed brucellae from the uterus at subsequent normal parturitions. Organisms are shed in milk for a variable length of time—in most cattle for life. *B. abortus* can frequently be isolated from secretions of nonlactating udders. Natural transmission occurs by ingestion of organisms, which are present in large numbers in aborted exudates, fetal membranes, and uterine discharges. Cattle may ingest contaminated feed and water or may lick contaminated genitals of other animals. Venereal transmission by infected bulls to susceptible cows appears to be rare. Transmission may occur by artificial insemination when *Brucella*-contaminated semen is deposited in the uterus but, reportedly, not when deposited in the midcervix. Brucellae may enter the body through mucous membranes, conjunctivae, wounds, or intact skin in both people and animals. Brucellae have been recovered from eexudates and from manure that has remained in a cool environment for >2 mo. Exposure to direct sunlight kills the organisms within a few hours.

Brucella abortus: Abortion in second half to full term pregnancy, still births, weak calves, retained fetal membrane, reduction in lactation noticed. Once aborted animals become symptomatically normal for the further pregnancy but actively shed the organism in uterine discharge and in milk in the subsequent parturition. In bulls, epididymitis, seminal vesiculitis, orchitis, testicular abscess, infertility, in both sexes, unilateral or bilateral hygroma and arthritis following longterm infection. Rarely causing death of fetus.

Sheep and Goats

Brucella melitensis infection in certain breeds of sheep causes clinical disease similar to that in goats. However, *B. ovis* produces a disease unique to sheep, in which epididymitis and orchitis impair fertility—the principal economic effect. Occasionally, placentitis and abortion are seen, and there may be perinatal mortality. The disease was first described in New Zealand and Australia and has since been reported from many sheep-raising areas of the world. *B ovis* infection among sheep in the USA is rare. There is no evidence that the disease is present in any other animal species. Rare natural and experimental infections in farmed red deer stags have been reported in New Zealand.

Rams as young as 8 weaks have been infected experimentally by various nonvenereal routes. The disease can be transmitted among rams by direct contact. Active infection in ewes is unusual but has developed after mating with naturally infected rams. Contaminated pastures do not appear to be important in spread of the disease. Infection frequently persists in rams, and a high percentage shed *B. ovis* intermittently for several years.

Primary manifestations are lesions of the epididymis, tunica, and testis in rams; placentitis and abortion in ewes; and occasionally perinatal death in lambs. Lesions may develop rapidly. In rams, the first detectable abnormality may be a marked deterioration in semen quality associated with the presence of inflammatory cells and organisms. An acute systemic phase is rarely seen in naturally occurring infections. After regression of the acute phase—which may be so mild as to go unobserved—lesions may be palpated in the epididymis and scrotal tunics. Epididymal enlargement may be unilateral or bilateral. The tail of the epididymis is involved more frequently than the head or body, and the most prominent lesion is spermatoceles of variable size containing partially inspissated spermatic fluid. The tunics frequently become thickened and fibrous, and extensive adhesions develop between them. The testes may show fibrous atrophy; these lesions are usually permanent. In a few cases, palpable lesions are transient, while in others, organisms may be present in semen over long periods without clinically detectable lesions.

Because not all infected rams show palpable abnormalities of scrotal tissues (and not all cases of epididymitis are due to brucellosis), the remaining rams must be examined further. Rams shedding organisms, but having no lesions, must be identified by culture of semen. Repeated examinations may be necessary to identify intermittent shedders. Microscopic examination of stained semen smears may also be helpful; fluorescent antibody examination is a highly specific diagnostic aid. Serologic tests used for eradication of disease and certification of animals include indirect ELISA, complement fixation, hemagglutination inhibition, indirect agglutination, and gel diffusion.

Incidence and spread of the disease may be reduced by regular examination of rams before the breeding season and culling of those with obvious genital abnormalities. Because susceptibility in rams increases markedly with age, it is advantageous to keep a young ram flock and isolate noninfected rams from older, possibly infected rams.

Immunization of weaner rams with attenuated (Rev. 1) *B. melitensis* has been recommended in some countries. Because infection in ewes apparently originates almost exclusively from service by infected rams, lamb losses through infection of ewes may be controlled economically by restricting vaccination to rams. There is no recommended vaccination in the USA.

Chlortetracycline and streptomycin used concurrently have effected bacteriologic cures. However, treatment is not economic except in especially valuable rams, and even if infection is eliminated, fertility may remain impaired.

The signs of brucellosis in goats are similar to those in cattle. The disease is prevalent in most countries where goats are a significant part of the animal industry, and milk is a common source of human brucellosis in many countries. The causal agent is *Brucella melitensis*. Infection occurs primarily through ingestion of the organisms. The disease causes abortion at approximately the fourth month of pregnancy. Arthritis and orchitis may occur. Diagnosis is made by bacteriologic examination of milk or an aborted fetus or by serum agglutination tests. The disease can be eliminated by slaughter of the herd. In most countries where *B. melitensis* is endemic, vaccination with the Rev. 1 strain is common. Rev. 1 is an attenuated strain of *B. melitensis* and is administered by SC or intraconjunctival routes. *B. melitensis* is highly pathogenic for people.

Brucella melitensis: It causes abortions in second weeks to fifth weeks of pregnancy, still birth, weak offspring, retained fetal membrane, re-invasion during subsequent pregnancies, reduction in milk yield, absence of mastitis. In acute cases, orchitis, epididymitis in males which results in infertility. Arthritis develops in both males and females.

Brucella ovis: It affects only sheep not goats. Epididymitis (unilateral occasionally bilateral), orchitis, impaired infertility and in rams, poor quality semen, atrophied testes, *etc.* Ram shed *B.ovis* for long periods while it is asyptomatic. Abortion and placentitis but mortality in ewes is not common.

Pigs (Porcine and Rangiferine Brucellosis)

Clinical manifestations of brucellosis in pigs vary but are similar to those seen in cattle and goats. Although the disease is often self-limiting, it remains in some herds for years. Brucellosis caused by *Brucella suis* rarely occurs in domestic animals other than pigs. Epidemics of brucellosis in people have been reported among packing-house workers, and the usual source is infected pigs. The prevalence in the USA is sometimes high among feral pigs. The incidence of swine brucellosis among domesticated animals in the USA is very low. Currently there are no known infected domestic swine herds.

Brucella suis: It is causes abortion at any time in pigs, weak and still birth piglets, vaginal discharge, infertility, metritis is occasional. Temporary or permanent orchitis and sterility in boars common. Infected boars are persistent carriers. Biovar-2 in hares produces nodules in internal organs, reproductive organs, subcutaneous tissues, muscles, and that may be purulent in nature. Biovar-4 causes abortion, retained placenta, metritis, mastitis and in male orchitis, lameness, arthritis, bursitis, tenosynovitis, and/or hygromas and subcutaneous abscess in caribou and reindeer.

Dogs

Brucella canis: It produces abortion in 7-9 weeks of gestation followed by a mucoid, serosanguineous/gray green vaginal discharge that persists for up to 6 weeks. Early embryonic death, resorption in a few weeks after mating, and may be mistaken for a failure to conceive. Pups born alive, weak, later develop disease. Epididymitis, scrotal edema, orchitis, poor sperm quality, unilateral or bilateral testicular atrophy in chronic infection and lymphadenitis is common. Lethargy, decreased appetites, poor performance, loss of alertness, discospondylitis of the thoracic and lumbar vertebrae cause stiffness, lameness, back pain, uveitis, endophtholmitis, polygranulomatous dermatitis, endocarditis, and meningoencephalitis without fever noticed.

Horses

Horses can be infected with *Brucella abortus* or *B. suis*. Suppurative bursitis, most commonly recognized as fistulous withers or poll evil, is the most common condition associated with brucellosis in horses. Occasionally, abortion has been reported. It is unlikely that infected horses are a source of the disease for other horses, other animal species, or people. Brucellosis in horses is very rare in the USA because of elimination of the disease in cattle.

***Brucella abortus* and *B. suis*:** It causes inflammation of supra spinous or supra atlantal bursa and leads to "fistulous withers" or "poll evil". The bursal sacs become distended or thick wall, rupture leading to secondary inflammation. In chronic cases, nearby ligaments and dorsal vertebral spines may become necrotic. Rarely it cause abortion in horses.

Zoonosis

Brucellosis is an occupational hazard. Veterinarian, butchers, farmers and some animal handlers dealing with shandy and exhibition animals, exposed to infection while contact with infected animals. Ingestion of un-pasteurized milk and other dairy products, aerosol laden particles contact with laboratory cultures, tissue samples, accidental injection of live brucellosis vaccines spread the disease. It is a serious, debilitating and chronic disease develops a systemic infection in human. Although, human to human transmission is rare, the disease occurrence has been reported following blood transfusion, bone marrow transplantation or sexual contact. Transmission due to crossing of placental barrier and ingestion of breast milk leads to young ones. In clinical cases, acute febrile illness with non-specific flu like signs such as fever, head ache, malaise, back pain and muscular pain noticed.

Drenching sweats particularly at night, spleenomegaly, hepatomegaly, cough and pleuritic chest pain are sometimes seen.

Necropsy Findings

B. abortus, B. melitensis and B. suis develops autolysis of fetus, subcutaneous edema, blood stained fluid in body cavity in ruminants, enlargement of spleen, liver, lung, pneumonia and fibrinous pleuritis, placentitis. Cotyledeons becomes red, yellow, normal or necrotic. In cattle, small ruminant's inter-cotyledonary parts typically leathery, with focal thickening and exudates. In adult granulomatous to purulent lesion in mammary gland, superficial lymphnodes, lymphoid tissues, bones, joints and other tissues and organs lesions found. Mild to severe endometritis after an abortion, in male unilateral or bilateral epididymitis or orchitis. Hygroma of knee joint, fetlock, hock, stifles, haunch, nuchal ligaments and thoracic spines *etc.* are noted *B. suis:* Purulent nodules in hares present. *B. ovis:* Fibrous atrophy of the testes noticed *B. canis:* Atrophy of testes, subcutaneous edema, congestion, hemorrhage in abdominal region, duodenum, sero-sanguineous fluid, degenerative lesion in liver, spleen, kidneys, and in intestines. Enlargement of retropharyngeal and inguinal lymphnodes, scrotal edema, dermatitis, epididymitis, orchitis, prostatitis, testicular atrophy, fibrosis, metritis and vaginal discharge are seen in adult animals.

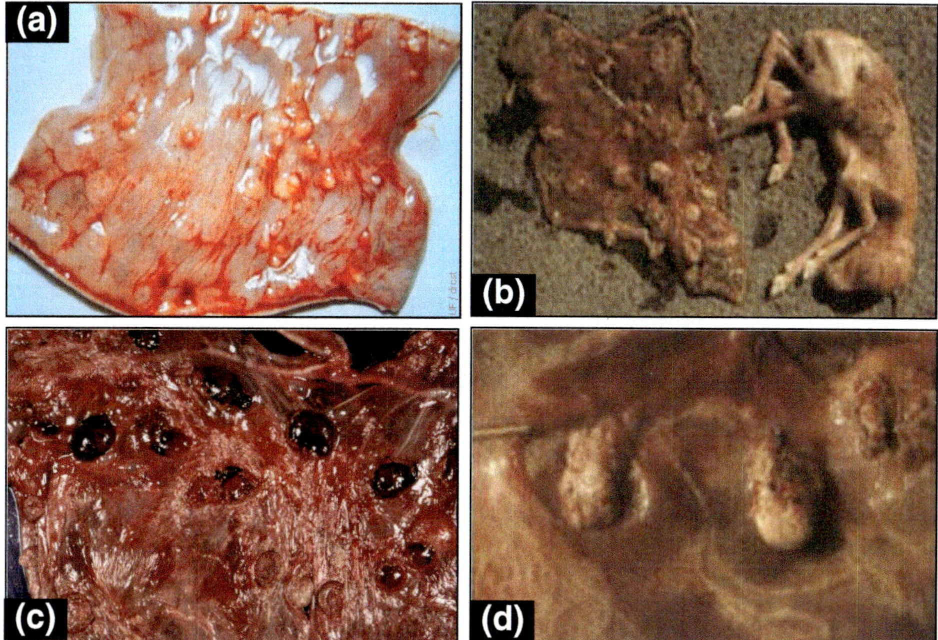

Figure 2.6

(a) *B. suis* – placenta, (b) *B. melitensis,* (c) *B. ovis,* (d) *B. melitensis* – necrotic cotyledons- aborted.

Diagnosis

Based on clinical signs and exudates findings. Identification of organism by Stamp's modification Ziehl Neelsen method. Stained smears reveals coccobacilli or short rods, arranged in a single chain, but sometimes in pairs or in small groups. Isolation of organism by culture. Immunostaining demonstrate the presence of *Brucella* spp. in a clinical specimen. PCR techniques can also be used for diagnosis.

Rose Bengal Plate Agglutination Test

It is a very sensitive, qualitative, antibody screening test for Brucellosis. But sometimes the test result may become positive in response to animal vaccinated with S19 vaccine, and false positive serological reactions. Hence, the test result should be confirmed with some other confirmatory test. False negative reactions occur due to prozoning. Antigen for this test is prepared from killed B.abortus S99 or S1119-3 cells.

Complement Fixation Test

It is an international trade test. It is a very specific and widely used confirmatory test for testing animals meant for export and import. It gives positive result in S19 vaccinated animals. Cows vaccinated with *B. abortus* S19 between 3 and 6 months are usually considered to be positive if the sera gives positive fixation at a titre of 30 or great ICFTU/ml when the animals are tested at an age of 18 months or older. *Indirect Enzyme Linked Immuno Sorbent Assay:* It is a test of international trade. *Fluorescent polarization assay:* It is a simple and international trade test. Its sensitivity and specificity (99 per cent) is similar to the C-ELISA.

Intradermal Brucellin Skin Test

It is a screening test of un-vaccinated herds in which purified standarfdized Brucellin INRA antigen is used. This inoculation may stimulate temporary anergy in the cellular immune response. An interval of 6 weeks is required to re-conduct this test in the same animal.

Serum Agglutination Test

It is an antibody detection test. Its specificity is improved with addition of EDTA to the antigen. The antibody titre of 1 : 40 is considered as positive in animals infected for the first time in uninfected area and 1 : 80 is considered positive for animals maintained in an endemic area. **Milk Ring test:** It is a simple, qualitative, antibody detection test in which 1 or 2 ml of milk from either bulk milk take for herd screening or individual animal diseas.

Gamma Interferon Test

It is a test of choice for detection of cell mediated immune response. Most human infections are diagnosed by serology. Tests used include serum agglutination, a modified Coombs' (antiglobulin) technique, ELISAs and Western blot. Blood, uterine discharge, foetal stomach content, hygroma fluid and milk.

Differential Diagnosis

Trichomoniasis, Leptospirosis, Campylobacteriosis, IBRT.

Treatment

No treatment is advised in animals. Long term antibiotics treatment is adviced in human with combination of antibiotics.

2.7. Campylobacteriosis

Synonyms

Traveler's exudates.

Campylobacter spp are spiral, microaerobic, gram-negative bacteria that cause gastroenteritis in people and animals. Several *Campylobacter* spp are zoonotic. Many domestic animals develop acute gastroenteritis after ingestion of *Campylobacter* spp, including dogs, cats, calves, sheep, pigs, ferrets, mink, monkeys, and several species of laboratory animals. Infection with *C. jejuni* is one of the most common causes of gastroenteritis in people worldwide and is the most extensively studied *Campylobacter* species. Campylobacteriosis is a venereal disease causing infertility, repeat breeding, abortion in early stages of exudates, and gastrointestinal problems in cattle, sheep, goats and humanbeings.

Etiology

Campylobacter and *Arcobacter* are now included in the family campylobacteriaceae. It has been identified that *C. jejuni* and *C. coli* is responsible for >95 per cent of campylobacter infections. However, *C.upsaliensis, C. lari, C. fetus subsp fetus, C. fetus subspecies venerealis, C. jejuni* has been isolated from human patients with exudates. Campylobacter is a small gram negative, microaerophilic, curved to spiral, rods shaped organism that possess a single polar flagellum. They have a characteristic corkscrew, rapid carting and or spinning kind of motility.

Epidemiology

Prevalence of Infection

Outbreaks occur following introduction of infected bulls or cows into the breeding farms and the presence of increased number of estrus cows in the herd. Prevalence has reported in human and poultry but the rate of prevalence varies between countries and regions. Prevalence mostly seen in dairy cattle.

Predisposing Factors

Contaminated soil and housing environmentm, introduction of nfected carriers, transport.

Source of Infection

Both young and older bulls have been identified as carriers for upto 18 weeks post infection, but older bulls are remaining as permanent carrier that has been attributed to the highest proliferation of *C. fetus* in the major site of epithelial crypts of the penis, in contrast, *C.fetus* concentration is very less in preputial fluid. Environment – soil, air, water (swimming water, recreational streams, disinfected effluent, puddles, pond water, surface waters), protozoans, wild birds and wildlife. Environmental contamination of pen, farm equipment. Infected eggs, hatchery waste and poutry house litters.

Transmission

Spread of infection occurs during coitus from infected cow to bull and vice versa. Bulls below five years of age rarely infected.

Host Affected

Cattle are highly susceptible for venereal campylobacteriosis as compared to sheep and goats. Sheep and goats affected by reproductive and gastrointestinal form of campylobacteriosis. Human are affected by gastrointestinal and nervous form of infection. Poultry species are affected mainly with gastrointestinal form of infection. Domestic and farm animals including pet dogs and cats, wild birds, farm animals (cattle, sheep, pigs, ducks, turkeys) insects (beetles, flies), rodents (mice, rats) are also affected.

Pathogenesis

Naturally infected bulls transmit *C. fetus subspecies venerealis* from one female to another, without any quality changes in semen and breeding ability. The organism establishes infection in the prepuce. In cows, in cervicovaginal area, during estrus, no uterine infection develop, due to presence of abundant neutrophils in the uterus at the time of estrus which prevent colonization of the organism within the uterus. But in the later stage of the estrus the organism invade and establish the infection in the uterus. Within 10 days following mating, the organism establishes infection in the mucous membrane of the vagina and cervix which leads to mild vaginitis, cervicitis and endometritis. Due to the presence of abundant neutrophils during the estrous period, spread of the infection is limited to endometrium until the progesterone phase. At this phase adhesion molecules keep the organism exudates in the intra-luminal location, so that in the absence of IgA/IgG2, no opsonization of the organism occurs. However, during di-oestrus period, neutrophils are fewer and so the organisms multiply in the reproductive tract and colonize the *C.fetus* subsp. *venerealis* in the endometrium. The pathogenic nature of the organism increased because of a protective surface antigen or anti-phagocytic macrocapsule comprising a paracrystalline array of (surface array protein) protein which exudates IgA, IgG, and IgM, following colonization of campylobacter. IgG is an important agglutinin/ opsonin secreted by the uterus of convalescent animals helps neutrophils and macrophages in the phagocytic process, while IgA found primarily in the cervico-vaginal mucus, immobilize *C. fetus* subsp. *venerealis* within this organ of convalescent animals which leads to carrier status. After conception if cows infected it may carry the organism. As there is insufficient stimulation of antigen the organism is restricted to the epithelial surface. Antigenic variation of the bacteria might be an additional factor enhancing the persistence of the carrier status in bulls as well as in cows.

Clinical Signs

Bovine Campylobacteriosis

It is mainly characterized by infertility, repeat breeding, early embryonic deaths, increased conception rate and abortion in the late pregnancy. Reddening of cervix and extension of mild mucopurulent exudates from uterus into cervix and vagina occurs. In contrast, infected heifers which have natural immunity quickly conceive, but remain as carrier for months.

Subacute or Chronic Form

Moderate problems may develop but resistant to infection due to an anamnestic immune response, where as the newly introduced. Susceptible females develop more acute form of disease. Highly susceptible animals show high prevalence and cause abortion.

In Poultry

C. jejuni in poultry is invasive in nature. Watery droppings, soiling of vent and feathers. In severe cases blood spots in droppings. Dehydration, depression, and death is noticed.

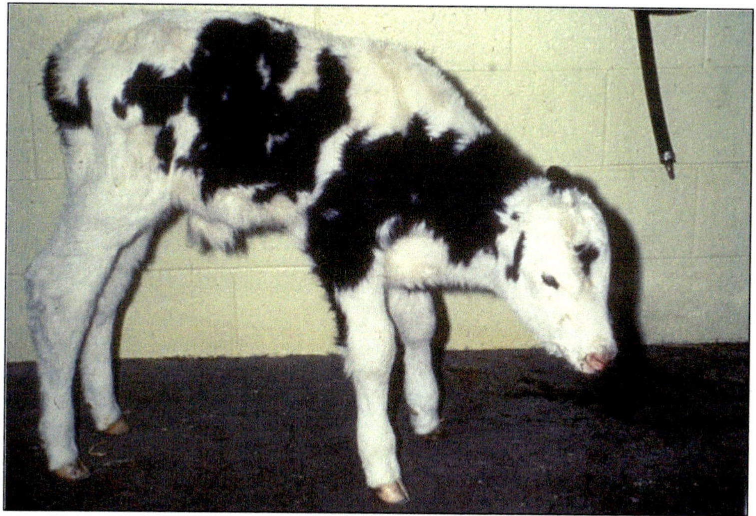

Figure 2.7. Campylobacteiosis – dehydrated calf.

Zoonosis

In India, *Campylobacter fetus* subspecies *jejuni* was isolated from 14.8 per cent of healthy population in rural South India. It produces exudates's exudates in human beings.

Necropsy Findings

Diffuse and mild infiltration with inflammatory cells, desquamation of the superficial epithelium observed. Periglandular fibrosis is restricted to cystic glands.

The endometritis has been identified by the presence of infiltrated plasma cells and foci of lymphocytes in the stroma. Not many abnormalities in the prepuce and penile mucosa of the bulls.

Diagnosis

Based on clinical signs and necropsy findings. Isolation and identification of organism. Serum agglutination, cervical mucus agglutination, fluorescent antibody and culture tests have been is used, however each test has certain limitations.

Serum Agglutination (SA) Test

It is not a reliable test and and antibodies are rarely found in the blood stream.

Cervical Mucus Agglutination Test (CMA)

It is a convenient and accurate method for herd level bovine campylobacteriosis, though this test is widely used there is a chances for false positive (Metestral bleeding or rough manipulation of the vagina during collection) and false negative (when cervical mucus dilutes the agglutinins) results. It takes 60 days following infection for the mucus to become positive on test. In individual animals the stage of estrus cycle and the time of exposure to the disease must be known to identify the infection. Around ten (selected) to twenty animals are enough to diagnose at farm level. Fluorescent antibody test used to detect antibody.

Sample Collection

Cervical mucus, reproductive discharges, aborted materials, blood and serum.

Differential Diagnosis

Infectious bovine rhinotracheitis, brucellosis, trichomoniasis, leptospirosis, listeriosis.

Treatment

Macrolide antibiotics (erythromycin, clarithromycin, or azithromycin) are the most effective drugs for *Campylobacter jejuni.* Fluoroquinolone antibiotics (ciprofloxacin, levofloxacin, gatifloxacin, or moxifloxacin) can also be used, but the organism is resistant to drugs.

2.8. Contagious Bovine Pleuropneumonia (CBP)

Contagious bovine plueuropneumonia is highly contagious and generally accompanied by pleurisy. It is present in Africa, with minor outbreaks occurring in the Middle East. The USA has been free of the disease since 1892, the UK since 1898, and Australia since 1973. The last outbreak of CBPP in Europe was seen in Portugal in 1999. Little is known about the disease in Asia, but China claims that its last outbreak was in 1995. Contagious bovine pleuropneumonia (CBPP) is primarily a disease of cattle caused species of *Mycoplasma*. It is characterized by fever, agalactia, anorexia, depression, coughing, thoracic pain, back arched back, dyspnoea, expiratory grunt, pleuritic friction rubs, dull areas of lung, edema of throat and dewlap.

Etiology

CBPP is caused by *Mycoplasma* mycoides susbspecies *mycoides* small colony (MmmSc). Six closely related members of this species affects cattle, sheep and goats but it is not spread to other species. The organism is pleomorphic. The organism can be grown in a special media and embryonated hens eggs.

Epidemiology

Prevalence of Infection

It is reported to be endemic in most parts of Africa.

Economic Impacts

It is the most economically important disease in cattle in Africa and has been imposed directly due to mortality, decreased milk yield, vaccination, disease surveillance and research program, and less due to quarantine, loss of trade, and fatal nature of the disease. Indirectly, the losses occurs via loss of weight, working ability, delayed marketing, decreased fertility, long quarantine period, loss of trade and fatal nature of the disease.

Predisposing Factors

The disease is mainly influenced by the environment including disinfectants, heat, and drying but the organism unable to survive in the environment without a host. Stress due to starvation, exhaustion, inter current disease can cause the sequestrum to break down and convert the animals into and active cases. The infected animals carry potential organism for at least 3 years period.

Sources of Infection

Large numbers of viable organism are passed through urine. The organism is isolated from semen, preputial washings, milk, urine frozen embryos of cows and bulls. Placenta and urine are infective for a long period. Chronic carriers are less infective than clinical cases. In Asia, CBPP has been reported in India, Bangaladesh, Myanmar. Sporadic outbreaks have been recognized in Middle East was attributed to importation of cattle from Africa.

Transmission

Direct and repeated contacts between sick and healthy animals. Inhalation of infective droplets from active or carrier animals is the principal route of infection. Though the distance one meter between animal is usually considered to be sufficient, but the disease is reported to spread over 45 m distance. Aerosol and indirect transmission occurs.

Host Susceptible

Cattle are the only species predominantly affected by the organism. However, natural infection also occurs in a wide variety of animals such as buffalo, yak, bison, reindeer, and antelopes. In sheep and goats infection causes local cellulitis without pulmonary movement. No difference in susceptibility of *Bos xudat* and *Bos indicus* cattle.

Pathogenesis

Cattle may need at least 8 months period (longer incubation period) before they infected and to show the signs and so require longer period of quarantine. The disease spread principally through inhalation of infected droplets. The organism possess carbohydrate cell capsule and produce hydrogen peroxide. It develops an acute lobar pneumonia, pleurisy and invades the lungs of cattle to cause mycoplasmemia resulting in localization in numerous other sites including kidneys, brain, leads to high morbidity and mortality. Thrombosis in pulmonary vessels prior to the development of pneumonic lesions and there is no general increase in blood coagulability and no generalized tendency to spontaneous thrombosis. Galactan is associated with pathogenicity of the organism but its mode of action is uncertain. Galacan can cause necrosis, and a connective tissue response in cattle similar to the sequestrum in chronically infected animals. Following infection the organism is isolated from bulls semen. Death results from anoxia and toxaemia.

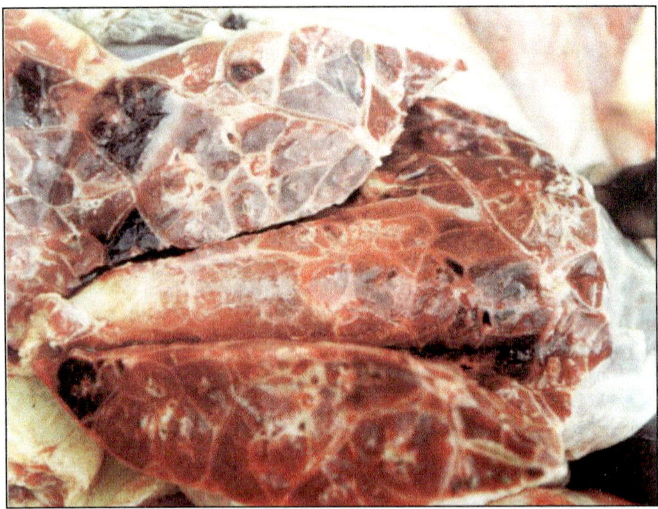

Figure 2.8. Contagious bovine plueuropneumonia, marbelled lung.

Clinical Signs

(a) **Per acute form**: Affected cattle may die in a week after the onset of respiratory distress.

(b) **Acute form:** The incubation period is 3-6 weeks and may exceed 6 months sometimes. It is characterized by sudden onset of high fever 40 degree celcius, a fall in milk yield, anorexia and cessation of rumination. Severe depression, animals stand apart or lag behind other group. Cough at the initial period during exercise, thoracic pain, disinclined to move, standing with the elbow out, arched back, extended head, shallow and rapid respiration with expiratory grunting. Pain evinced on percussion of chest. Auscultation reveals a pleuritic friction, sounds in early stages, dullness, fluid sounds, moist gurgling, noise in later stages of infection.

Edematous swelling of throat, and dewlap, swelling on large movable joints, in calves valvular endocariditis, myocarditis noticed. In fatal cases death occurs at a variable course from several days to 3 weeks.

(c) **Chronic and sub acute form:** Recovered animals may be clinically normal but in some animals inactive sequestrum forms in the lung with a necrotic centre of sufficient size to produce toxaemia causing unthriftiness. A chronic cough, mild respiratory distress. During exercise this sequestra commonly break down when the animal is exposed to environmental stress and cause an acute attack of disease.

Necropsy Findings

Lesions limited to thoracic cavity, lungs and the lesion is unilateral. The pleural cavity contains large quantity of clear, yellow brown fluid containing pieces of fibrin. This fluid is ideal for culture of the organism. Caseous fibrinous deposits are present on the parietal and visceral surfaces of the lungs. The interlobular septae are prominently distended with amber colored fluid surrounding distended lymphatics. This fluid distinctly outlines the lobules which vary in color with red, gray or yellow hepatisation. Consolidation of lungs with a typically marbled appearance is characteristic. In chronic or advance case a sequestrum of necrotic lung varying size from 1-10 cm in diameter. Which may be surrounded by a fibrinous capsule? The sequestrum rupture and are drained by a bronchus. This could be a source for aerosol infection to cattle; this may pave way for epidemics in closed herds. In calves exudative peritonitis, arthritis, bursitis and fibrinous anrthritis of carpal and tarsal joints present.

Diagnosis

Diagnosis is based on clinical signs and the characteristic gross pathologic lesions of the lungs. Complement fixation, latex agglutination, or competitive ELISA tests can be used to aid definitive diagnosis. Confirmation is often by isolation of the mycoplasma followed by growth inhibition or immunofluorescence test using hyperimmune rabbit sera against the mycoplasma, or increasingly by PCR. Confirmation of serologic reactions can be made by immunoblotting test. As soon as an outbreak is suspected, slaughter and necropsy of presumptively infected cattle is advisable.

Sample Collection

Blood, serum, nasal discharge, pleural fluid, pulmonary tissue.

Differential Diagnosis

Foot and Mouth Disease, Rinderpest, Haemorrhagic Septicemia, Theileriosis, Ephemeral fever, Pulmonary abscesses, Farcy, Actinobacillosis, Echinococcus (Hydatidosis).

Treatment

There is no specific treatment available. However, use of antibiotics has been found effective for controlling the secondary bacterial infection that may aggrevate the infection. Tilmicosin and danafloxacin are effective for both in terms of mycoplasmastatic and mycoplasmacidal activity. Florofenicol and tetracycline are for intermediate and spectinomycin is ineffective against some strains.

2.9. Contagious Caprine Pleuroneumonia (CCP)

Synonyms

Pleuropneumonia contagiosa and Abunini disease.

Contagious caprine pleuropneumonia is a highly fatal disease that occurs in goats in the Middle East, Africa, and Asia. It was seen for the first time on European soil in Thrace, Turkey, in 2002, but does not appear to have spread to neighboring countries, Greece and Bulgaria. Outbreaks have recently been reported in sheep and captive wildlife, including gazelles and small ruminants. It is a classical and contagious disease of goats resembles the contagious bovine pleuropneumonia. It develops pleuropneumonia in sheep and goats.

Etiology

It is caused by *M. capricolum* subsp. *capripneumoniae*. The causative agent is previously known as *Mycoplasma* strain F38. It is difficult to differente from *M. mycoides* subsp *xuda*. Mycoplasma mycoides subspecies Caprae, *M. mycoides* subspecies *mycoides*, *M. galactiae*, *M. arginini* and *M. capricola* have been considered as the principal cause of pleuropneumonia in kids upto 6 months.

Epidemiology

Prevalence of Infection

It is widespread in tropical countries. Reported from Chennai, Assam, Mumbai, Haryana, Uttarpradesh, Bihar, West Bengal in India. It is a fatal disease of goats distributed in about 38 countries in Asia and Africa. Infectivity is high with a morbidity rate 100 per cent. Mortality rate is 60-100 per cent.

Economic Impact

The direct losses of the disease result from its high mortality, reduced milk and meat yield, cost of treatment, control, disease diagnosis and surveillance. In addition to this, there are indirect losses due to the imposition of trade restrictions.

Source of Infection

By carrier or infected animals. Organisms do not live long outside of animal body.

Transmission

The disease spread through inhalation of organism present in soil and environment. The bot fly has been found to spread the infections. Experimental transmission is possible.

Host Affected

Goats are highly susceptible when exudates to sheep. Goat strain is not transmissible to cattle.

Pathogenesis

In animals with primary infection, the illness lasts for about two days and death ensues, while in other cases it may last several days. The primary clinical signs are cough with animals tending to lie down or lag behind the flock. Affected animals continue to graze for some time but eventually become anorexic, breathing becomes exudate with painful grunting and a rise in temperature up to 41°C. Gradual respiratory signs progress and accelerated, painful, and is followed by severe cough. In the terminal cases, the animals are unable to move. Affected animals have abducted legs, the stiff neck and extended downward. Saliva drools from mouth and nose is obstructed by mucopurulent discharge. The tongue protrudes and bleats distressingly. In fully susceptible flocks that encounter an outbreak, morbidity is usually 100 per cent and mortality is up to 70 per cent. The organism is reported to affect majorly the respiratory tract of goats. In endemic areas subacute and chronic cases are common and the symptoms are milder, dominated by intermittent coughing.

Clinical Signs

Acute Form

It is a highly fatal disease in sheep and goats. Mortality varies from 60-100 per cent. Incubation period is about 6-10 days. Anorexia, dullness, depression, nasal discharge, abodominal respiration, fever and dry painful cough are seen. Animal may die but no pathoglogical changes in lungs. Nasal discharge is watery in early stage and turns to thick mucopurulent to white in later stage.

Chronic Form Clinical signs are mostly similar to cattle, CCPP restricted to the respiratory tract, Cough, dyspnoea, lagging behind; lying down a lot but the animal can stand and walk. Fever 40.5°C to 41.5°C (104-106), is seen Terminal stage: Mouth breathing, tongue protrusion and frothy salivation with death in two or more days. In adverse climatic conditions disease occurs as septicemic with little signs or with evidence of pneumonia.

Necropsy Findings

Usual findings are similar to bovine but in caprine sequestra are not formed in the lungs. Lesions are restricted to lungs and pleura with hepatization of part of the lung and increase in pleural fluid with a fibrinous pleuritis. The lesions may be confined with lung.

Diagnosis

Based on clinical signs and necropsy findings. Interstitial intralobular septa are seen. More effective detection is by PCR performed on samples of pleural fluid dried on filter paper. Detection of antigen from lung tissues. Pleural fluid has to be examined by PCR. Antibody detection by CFT, ELISA and Latex agglutination test. A blocking ELISA using monoclonal antibody is highly specific for detection of CCPP.

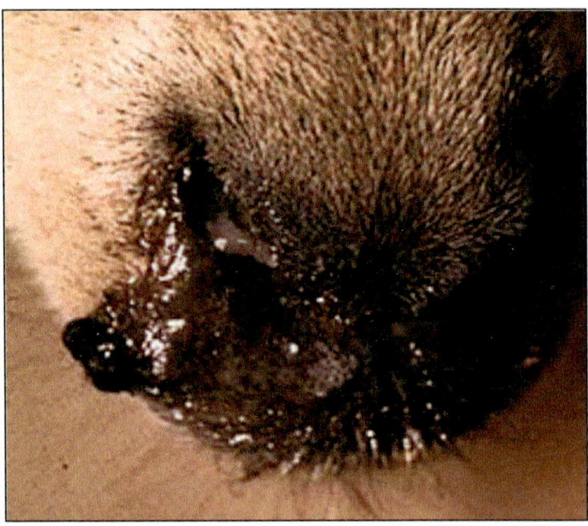

Figure 2.9. Contagious caprine pleuropneumonia.

Sample Collection

Mycoplasma is fragile and should be freeze dried and has to be a transported in time. Serum, lung tissues, pleural fluid, nasal discharges.

Differential Diagnosis

Other pulmonary mycoplasmoses and chronic respiratory diseases.

Treatment

Oxytetracycline, rolitetracycline, chlortetracycline and tylosin. The organism is highly sensitive to Oxytetracycline 15mg/kg bw/day. Tiamutin 36mg/kg bw is satisfactory. Tylosin tartrate @ 10mg/kg bw i/m along with cotrimaxazole tablet for 5-7days for the treatment with alincomycin gave satisfactory result. The macrolides (erythromycin, spiramysin, and tylosin), tetracyclines and quinolones are active against *M. capricolum* subsp. *capripneumoniae*.

2.10. Fowl Typhoid

The causal agent is *Salmonella gallinarum*. The incidence of fowl typhoid is low in the USA, Canada, and some European countries but is much higher in other countries. Although *S. gallinarum* is egg-transmitted and produces lesions in chicks and poults similar to those produced by *S. pullorum*, there is a much greater tendency to spread among growing or mature flocks. Mortality in young birds is similar to that seen in *S. pullorum* infection but may be higher in older birds. It is an infectious, enteric disease of adult and layer birds. The disease develops a more acute septicaemic condition mainly in mature birds and more severe condition in commercial laying flocks. It is often exudated by rapid spread with high morbidity and mortality.

Etiology

S. gallinarum causing fowl typhoid is a gram negative, non-capsulated, non-sporogenic, non-motile, rods shaped and flagellated organism. It survives outside the host's body for many months.

Epidemiology

Prevalence of Infection

The bacterium is fairly resistant to normal climate, surviving months, but is susceptible to normal disinfectants.

Source of the Infection

Red mites persists in poultry houses contribute the spread of infection. The organism is excreted in droppings. The organism persists in faeces for months but survive long time in the infected carcasses. Rats, dogs, foxes and wild birds may carry infection. Recovered birds act as carriers for long periods.

Transmission

It is mainly a hatchery borne infection. The lateral spread through ingestion of contaminated food and water occurs. Chronic birds remain as carrier even after treatment and may lead to re-infection. Infection also spread through eggs laid by vaccinated birds but egg transmission is not a regular feature of the disease.

Host Affected

Adult and growing birds are mostly affected with serious problems and heavy mortality. The organism also affects turkey, ducks, pheasants, guinea fowl, peafowl, grouse, quail, game birds, sparrows, parrots, canaries and bullfinches.

Pathogenesis

Infection occurs by horizontal and vertical transmission. Horizontal transmission occurs via the respiratory and oral routes. Birds ingest the organism from the contaminated environment. Infection also occurs by cannibalism. Wound infections are also possible. *Salmonella gallinarum* is transmitted by fomites which includes contaminated feed, water and litter; they may survive in a favorable environment for many months and up to several years. Wild birds, mammals, and insects can act as mechanical or biological vectors. Red mites, in particular, are involved in spreading of fowl typhoid. Rodents act as biological vectors. In growing birds and adults, *Salmonella* Pullorum infections are likely to be inapparent. Fowl typhoid can occur in older as well as young birds. Occasionally, *Salmonella pullorum* may cause a disease similar to fowl typhoid in older birds; The route of infection is oral or via the navel/yolk. Morbidity is 10-100 per cent; mortality is increased in stressed or immunocompromised flocks and may be up to 100. In young birds it cause septicemia which leads to systemic illness. Mainly affects, heart, kidney, liver and spleen. They become enlarged, congested and haemorrhagic. In adult birds it causes intestinal and kidney exudates. Reproductive system is most prominently affected.

Clinical Signs

(a) **Acute:** Affected birds shows decreased food intake, depression, ruffled feathers, closed eyes, respiratory distress, rapid breathing, watery to mucoid, yellow color exudates, pasty feathers around the vent followed by drop in production. Birds surviving 2-3 days after the onset of acute disease may follow the chronic stage. In this stage higher mortality is noticed in young chicks.

(b) **Chronic phase**: There is progressive loss of condition, pronounced anaemia, shrunken, pale combs and wattles. Incubation period 4-6 days, the disease spread rapidly through the flocks and cause 50 per cent loss.

(c) **Subacute:** Grumbling, increased dead in shell embryos, small, weak, moribund dead and chicks may be found on the hatching trays. Mortality may occur seldom but follows for a long period. In young birds signs may be non-specific.

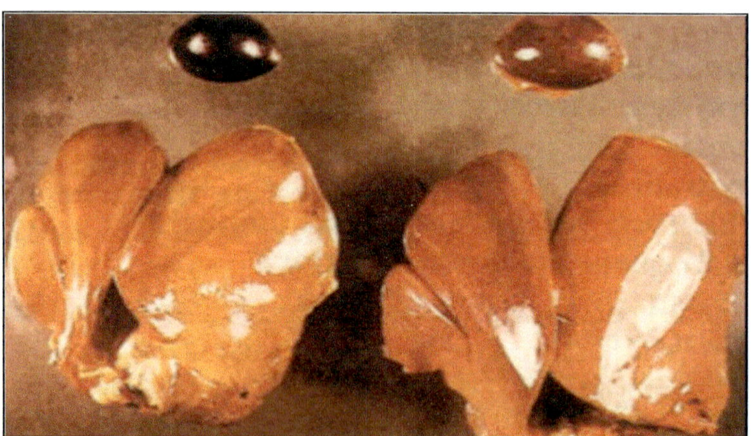

Figure 2.10. Fowl typhoid – Enlarged, bronzed to mahagony liver, mottled and brittled spleen in turkey – left one is normal.

Necropsy Findings

(a) **Acute:** Septicaemic and jaundice appearance of the carcasses, injected and prominent sub-cutaneous blood vessels and dark congested skeletal muscle seen. Swollen, friable, dark red or black colored liver is observed as a constant features of the fowl typhoid and the cut surface of the liver may shows a distinct coppery bronze sheen. Spleen may also be enlarged. Catarrhal enteritis and the affected intestine may contain viscous, slimy, bile stained material. Bone marrow may become dark.

(b) Chronic: Emaciation, intense pale carcass, xudate white focal necrosis of the myocardium, mucosa and submucosa of the initial part of the intestine, pancreas and liver may be seen. Pericarditis, accumulation of turbid yellow fluid in the pericardial sac, fibrin attachment at the surface of the heart is characterisitic for chronic fowl typhoid. Young birds have discrete, necrotic foci in the lung and gizzard and in the testicles exudates is noticed. In laying birds, retained yolk with subsequent rupture may be noticed.

In Turkeys

Liver exhibits bronze to mahogany color streak, necrosis of heart, xudate lungs are pathgnomonic lesions of this disease. Crop usually contains food which suggests paralysis of digestive tract. Mucous membrane of proventriculus sloughs off readily. Heamorrhagic enteritis (duodenum) intestinal ulceration is remarkable.

Diagnosis

Based on clinical signs and necropsy findings. Caecal tonsils and spleen from infected birds is given priority. Swabs from infected tissues, intestinal and cloacal contents should be collected aseptically. Eggs, embryos, fecal droppings and hatchery debris, fluff, dust, broken eggshells and chick box linings also be collected for the diagnosis. Tissue samples can be cultured into selective and non - selective enrichement liquid media or into agar based media (brilliant green agar) immediately following collection of samples or else, samples can be stored if there is any delay in diagnosis.

Blood Testing

Using *S. pullorum* antigen in RBPT or whole blood test (WBT) can detects carriers of *S. gallinarum*. Positive birds based on the test should be culled. RBPT is not a reliable test in turkeys and ducks. Antiglobulin indirect haemagglutination test detected serum antibodies in days after oral infection.

Sample Collection

Blood, serum, fecal sample, tissues.

Differential Diagnosis

Typhoid, Pasteurellosis, Colibacillosis, Viral exudates, Parasitic infection, Mycoplasmosis.

Treatment

Furazolidone in feed for 10 days at the level of 0.04 per cent. Use of enrofloxacin unable to completely eliminate the infection. A moxycillin, potentiated sulponamide, tetracylines, fluoroquinolones is effictive.

2.11. Glanders

Synonyms

Farcy.

Glanders is a contagious, acute or chronic, usually fatal disease of Equidae caused by *Burkholderia mallei* and characterized by serial development of ulcerating nodules that are most commonly found in the upper respiratory tract, lungs, and skin. Felidae and other species are susceptible and infections are usually fatal. The organism is infectious for people, with a 95 per cent fatality rate in untreated septicemia cases, and is considered a potential bioterrorism agent. Glanders is one of the oldest diseases known and once was prevalent worldwide. It has now been eradicated or effectively controlled in many countries, including the USA. In recent years, the disease has been reported in the Middle East, Pakistan, India, Mongolia, China, Brazil, and Africa. It is a highly contagious and chronic disease of solipedes and is characterized by the development of nodules, ulcers in upper respiratory tract, lungs, and cutaneous tissues. The disease is transmissible to human beings.

Etiology

Glanders is caused by *Burkholderia mallei* – (*Pseudomonas mallei*). *Burkholderia pseudomallei* cause Melioidiosis. *Pseudomonas* is a medium sized 0.5-1.0 x 1.5-5.0 μm in lengh. It is a gram negative, rod shaped, strict aerobic organism. Motile by one or more polar flagella. *B. malleus* is a non-motile organism. Some species produce soluble pigments. Most will grow on Mac Conkey Agar. It is an opportunistic pathogen.

Epidemiology

Prevalence of Infection

The disease is prevalent in horse rearing countries. Glanders has been reported from Eastern Europe, India and Africa. North America and Thailand are almostly free from glanders. Through strict isolation, adequate sanitation and exudate test, the disease problem has been reduced.

Sources of Infection

Soil, infected secretions, carrier animals.

Transmission

Ingestion through oral, inoculation through skin invasion, inhalation air ways, direct contact, man *via* broken skin contact with eexudates.

Host Affected

It causes glanders or farcy (the skin form) in equines. Occasional infection in dogs, goats, sheep and camels occurs. Cattle, pigs, rats infected through contaminated food and water, less commonly by aerosols and through wounds, human susceptible, *etc.*

Pathogenesis

The organism gains access through intestinal mucosa leads to septicemia in acute and bacterimia in chronic phase. It invades the regional lymphnodes through pharyngeal mucosa and undergoes proliferation. From the skin wound the organism reaches the blood stream and localized in various organs and forms nodules and ulcers in the skin. Involvement of lungs *via* inhalation leads to severe broncho-pneumonia. *P. aeurugenosa* produces a number of proteins exotoxins, entero toxins causes exudates during initial infections. Endotoxin and numerous extracellular products such as proteases and haemolysin play an important role in pathogenesis. This organism possesses pile which facilitates adherence to epithelial cells. Some strains have a capsule that is antigphagocytic in characters. Bacteriosins (pyocins) and pigments exhibit antimicrobial actions. Blue green pigment is pyocyanin can stain wool greenish blue. It is an opportunistic organism involves in primary disease very rarely.

Clinical Signs

Incubation period varies few days to several months. Chronic nasal discharge in or both nostrils grey in colour and catarrhal in nature. Formation of small, grey or yellowish nodules about the millet seed size on the mucosa of the upper repiratory tract. Submaxillary lymphnodes are edematous in nature. Nodules and ulcers formed along the lymphatic channels of the skin. Skin of the lower limbs and abdomen are mostly affected. The skin affection is ascribed as Farcy.

(a) **Acute form:** High temperature with ocular and nasal discharge, dyspnoea due to swelling of nasal mucosa and edema of glottis. Ulcers formed due to the infection is little resistant to healing.

(b) **Chronic form:** Persists for few months or even a year. Intermittent fever, cough, respiratory distress, lymphnode of the mandible turn firm and nodular. Edema of the hind limbs down upto hock region accompanied with discharges from lymphnodes. Ulcers gradually heal up leaving irregular star shaped scars.

Zoonosis

High temperature, swelling and pain usually on the hands, lips, eyes, accompanies with swelling of neighbouring lymphnodes. Ulcers develop on nose, mouth in some cases. Abscess development and pustules in the skin are the important features of the disease.

Necropsy Findings

Nodules and ulcers in nasal septum turbinate bones. Small nodules are observed throughout the lips varying in size from millet to pea size. Catarrahal bronchopneumonia and purulent lymph adenitis are also noticed.

Diagnosis

It is done on the basis of based on clinical signs and necropsy findings. Identification of organism: Gram negative, rod shaped organism can be seen in Gram staining of pus smears. Isolation of organism. Fluorescent Antibody Technique: May be useful for detection antibody, Both cell mediated and antibody mediated complement fixation test, agglutination test, haemagglutination test and counter immune electrophoresis. False positive reaction of glanders occurs where melioidosis is endemic as serological tests may detect antibodies that cross react with those of *P. pseudomallei*. Mallein test: Demonstrate hypersensitivity reaction with *P.mallei.* Mallein is a glycoprotein extracted from bacteria and injected s/c route in infected animal's results in swelling at the injection site. Conjunctival Mallein Test: (ophthalmic) in 6-12 hours an inflammatory and purulent reaction in eye develops.

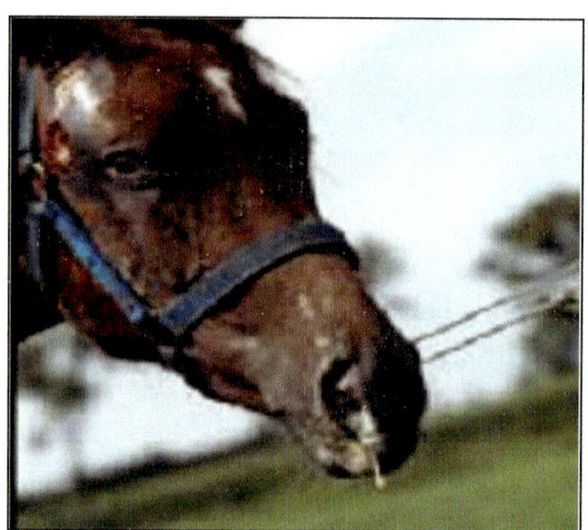

Figure 2.11. Glanders – Yellow green nasal discharge.

Intrapalpebral Test

In lower eyelid exudate is injected and produce localized edematous swelling, purulent conjunctivitis.

Strauss Reaction

Male guinea pigs are injected intra peritoneally with xudate antigen 0.5ml shows peritonitis, purulent inflammation of testicular tunica vaginalis in 2-3 days followed by orchitis.

Sample Collection

Pus material, lymphnode discharge and swabs.

Differential Diagnosis

Epizootic lymphangitis, Ulcerative lymphangitis, Sporotrichosis, Melioidosis and pneumonia.

Treatment

However, treatment with Sodium sulphadiazine has been found to be effective in experimental cases. It is highly effective. Combination of formalized preparation of exudate and sulfadiazine or exudate and sufadimidine can be given.

2.12. Listeriosis

Synonyms

Silage disease and Circling diseases.

Listeriosis is a sporadic bacterial infection that affects a wide range of animals, including people and birds. It is seen worldwide, more frequently in temperate and colder climates. There is a high incidence of intestinal carriers. Encephalitis or meningoencephalitis in adult ruminants is the most frequently recognized form. Listeriosis is primarily a disease of ruminants, particularly seen in sheep with characteristic septicemia, encephalitis, spinal myelitis, abortion, uveitis, gastroenteritis and mastitis. Occasionally septicemic form affects horses and pigs.

Etiology

Currently, six species have been identified in the genus *Listeria*. Of them *L. monocytogenes*, serotype-5 is pathogenic and *L. ivanovii* is mildly pathogenic. Based on somatic (O) and flagellar (H) antigens *L. monocytogenes* is divided into 16 serovars. Many serovars have been isolated from animals. Virulent strains multiply in macrophages and monocytes and produce haemolysin and listeriolysin O toxins. *Listeria* spp. can grow and reproduce at temperature from 4°C to 45°C. At low pH and low temperature reduces the growth rate of the organism. Grow at pH ranges from 4.5- 9.6. The organism is resistant to -20°C for 2 years even repeated freezing and thawing unable to destroy the organism. *L. monocytogenes* able to survive and grow in a wide variety of environments and has a wide range of strain variations.

Epidemiology

Prevalence of Infection

Disease is more common in temperate countries as compared to tropical and subtropical countries. It is a very important disease in North America, Europe, UK, New Zealand and Australia.

Predisposing Factors

Reduced host animal's resistance. Poor nutrition, sudden changes of weather such as very cold and wet weather. Stress due to late pregnancy, parturition and transport. Long periods of flooding and silage feeding.

Transmission

The highest prevalence of the disease due to feeding of silage has been recorded. Ingestion of contaminated food, water, milk, silage feeds, *etc.* develops listeriosis.

Host Affected

It is primarily a disease of ruminants, particularly seen in sheep and occasionally in horses and pigs. Introduction of virulent strains through migratory carrier animals, birds, sea gulls is possible. Organism persist for more than 3 months in sheep faeces and survive in soil for 1-2years. The organism has been isolated from 42 species of mammals and 22 species of birds, fish, crustaceans and insects.

Pathogenesis

Listeria is a facultative intracellular organism; infect intestinal cells by direct endocytosis. The organism is taken up by macrophages and monocytes but the phagocytic activity is prevented by bacterial superoxide dismutase. Listeriolysin which disrupts lysosomal membranes and permit organism to grow in cytoplasm. Upon ingestion, organism reaches the intestine by penetration and develops, in-apparent/sub-clinical bacteremia which may be cleared by development of immunity. Bacteremia is frequently sub-clinical and may be accompanied with excretion in milk. Septicemic listeriosis develops with or without meningitis, most commonly in neonatal ruminants and in adult sheep and goats. In pregnant animals, invasion into placenta and foetus occurs in 24 hours of onset of infection. Edema and necrosis of placenta leads to abortion. Infection in late pregnancy results in still birth or birth of young ones that quickly develop a fatal septicaemia.

Encephalitis

Acute inflammation of brain stem is unilateral. Portal of entry is by ascending infection of the trigeminal or cranial nerve following loss of the integrity of buccal mucosa resulting from trauma, shedding of teeth or from periodontitis. Asymmetric cranial nerve function, trigeminal, facial, vestibular, glosso-pharyngeal nerve leads to ipsilateral facial hypalgesia and paralysis. Involvement of vestibular nucleus leads to ataxia, circling and head tilting to the affected side. Dullness, head pressing, delirium spread along optic nerve leads to endophthalmitis in sheep and cattle. Encephalitis is the most prevalent manifestation in sheep and septicaemia in lamb in association with abortion. Mastitis: *L. monocytogenes* rarely cause mastitis in cattle. It is not invasive or perpetuating organism for the udder. *L. ivanovii* occasionally causing abortion and encephalitis in ruminants. Suppurative bronchopneumonia and lack of multifocal hepatocellular necrosis are common in aborted foetus. Case fatality rate is 25 per cent. In milk, *L.monogytogenes* present less than 1 per ml in raw milk and from bacteremic sub clinical animals with mastitis are higher 2000-5000 per ml.

Clinical Signs

Sheep and Goats

In early infection, affected sheep separate from flocks, show high temperature 40°C, cranial nerve dysfunction, run and fall in a flaccid motion. More acute death in 2-4 days of infection. Affected animals develops in-coordination, head deviation, head tilting, wallowing in circles, unilateral facial hypalgisia, paralysis of lips and face. Keratitis, corneal ulceration, strabismus, nystagmus, panopthalmitis with pus evident in anterior chamber of one or both eyes. Paresis of muscles of the jaw, dropped jaw which ensues difficulty in prehension and mastication. Poll-nose relationship, recumbent, death due to respiratory failure. In young ones onset is sudden and the course of the disease is short. Death occurs in 2-3 days. Abortion occurs in 3 months of pregnancy. Abortion is as high as 15 per cent with annual recurrence. Retained placental membrane, mortality in ewes in case of foetus retention. Abortion due to *L. ivanovii* is sporadic in cattle. In sheep and goats causes outbreak, still birth and birth of live infected lambs.

Cattle

Course of the disease in adult cattle is 1-2 weeks and in calves disease is more acute and death follows in 2-4 days. Fever 40.5ºC, abortion, still birth (sporadic) usually occurs in last trimester of pregnancy, retained placental membrane.Abortion is seen after silage feeding. Encephalitis signs include circling, ptosis, half chewed food in the mouth and unilateral facial paralysis.

Septicemic Listeriosis

Acute septicaemia – *L. monocytogenes* is not common in adult ruminants. No nervous signs but depression, weakness, emaciation, pyrexia, exudates, hepatic necrosis and gastroenteritis. Corneal opacity, dyspnoea, nystagamus and mild opisthotonus is noticed. Death occurs in 12 hours following infection. At necropsy, opthalmitis, serofibrinous meningitis observed. Septicaemia is also recorded in foals. Inflammation of single quarter or both quarters. Chronic mastitis show poor response to treatment, high somatic cell count in milk but milk appears normal.

Septic Myelitis

Fever, ataxia, initial knuckling of hind limbs, weakness, and paralysis. No cranial nerve involved. Animals affected appear to be alert, bright and eat well.

Opthalmitis

Iritis: Swelling of iris, constriction of pupil. Advanced cases, pannus and corneal opacity may be uni/bilateral.

Enteritis

Weaner sheep: Initially found dead. Lethargy, anorexia, pass loose green coloured faeces. Pregnant ewes may abort.

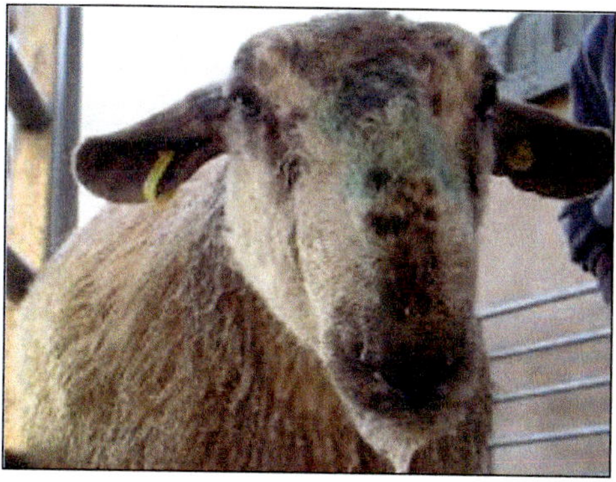

Figure 2.12. Listeriosis drooling ear, deviated muzzle.

Necropsy Findings

Encephalitis: Visual lesions occur as multiple foci of necrosis in the liver, spleen, myocardium and in septicaemic form. Enteritis, Ulcerative abomasitis, typhlo-colitis, micro-abcessess through out the intestine, infiltraton with neutrophils in mucosa or lamina muscularis of the exudates are noticed.

Diagnosis

Samples of lumbosacral CSF can be collected under local anesthesia. In cases of listeriosis, the CSF has an increased protein concentration (0.6–2 g/L [normal 0.3 g/L]) and a mild pleocytosis composed of large mononuclear cells. Listeriosis is confirmed only by isolation and identification of *L. monocytogenes*. Specimens of choice are brain from animals with CNS involvement and aborted placenta and fetus. If primary isolation attempts fail, ground brain tissue should be held at 4°C (39°F) for several weeks and recultured weekly. Occasionally, *L. monocytogenes* has been isolated from spinal fluid, nasal discharge, urine, feces, and milk of clinically ill ruminants. Serology is not used routinely for diagnosis, because many healthy animals have high *Listeria* titers. Immunofluorescence is effective for rapidly identifying *L. monocytogenes* in smears from animals dead or aborted from listeriosis and from milk, meat, and other sources.

Listeriosis can be differentiated from pregnancy exudates in ewes or ketosis in cattle by careful clinical examination, CSF changes, and 3-OH butyrate concentrations well below 3 mmol/L. Furthermore, facial and ear paralysis are absent in pregnancy exudates or ketosis. In cattle, the unilateral signs of trigeminal and facial paralysis (often subtle) help differentiate listeriosis from bovine spongiform encephalopathy, thrombotic meningoencephalitis, polioencephalomalacia, sporadic bovine encephalomyelitis, and lead poisoning. Rabies must always be considered in the differential diagnosis of listeriosis. Animals with brain abscesses and coenurosis present with circling, contralateral blindness, and proprioceptive deficits, but show no cranial nerve deficits. Vestibular disease is common in growing ruminants; these animals typically show ipsilateral spontaneous nystagmus or strabismus, and remain bright and alert without trigeminal nerve dysfunction.

Differential Diagnosis

Pregnancy toxaemia in sheep. Nervous ketosis, rabies, kid, polioencephalomalacia, middle ear disease and scrapie in cattle. Trichomoniasis, Brucellosis, Toxoplasmosis, IBRT, Salmonellosis, Contagious opthalmia. Vaginal secretions, abortion, milk, faeces, tonsils, cerebrospinal fluid, mid sagittary section of brain, brain stem (chilled or frozen), formalin fixed spinal cord segment.

Treatment

Chlortetracycline -10mg/kg BW/day for 5 days for meningo-encephalitis for Cattle Inj. Penicillin-44000 IU/kg BW, I/M daily for 7 days or 10-14 days. Supportive therapy using parenteral fluids, neurotropic vitamins and minerals.

Zoonotic Risk

Whether animals serve as a reservoir of infection for people may be questioned, because *Listeria* organisms have been isolated from feces of a significant number of apparently healthy people as well as other animals. However, despite this and the apparently low invasiveness of *L. monocytogenes*, all suspected material should be handled with caution. Aborted exudates and necropsy of septicemic animals present the greatest hazard. In cases with encephalitis, *L. monocytogenes* is usually confined to the brain and presents little risk of transmission unless the brain is removed. People have developed fatal meningitis, exudatest, and exudate exanthema on the arms after handling aborted material. Pregnant animals (including women) should be protected from infection because of danger to the fetus, with possible abortion, stillbirth, and infection of neonates. Although human listeriosis is rare (upper estimate of 12 cases per million population per yr), mortality can reach 50 per cent. Most cases involve older patients, pregnant women, or immunocompromised people.

L monocytogenes can be isolated from milk of mastitic, aborting, and apparently healthy cows. Excretion in milk is usually intermittent but may persist for many months. Infected milk is a hazard, because the organism may survive certain forms of pasteurization. *Listeria* also have been isolated from milk of sheep, goats, and women.

2.13. Paratuberculosis

Synonyms

Johne's disease.

Paratuberculosis is chronic, contagious granulomatous enteritis is also characterized in cattle by persistent diarrhea, progressive weight loss, debilitation, and eventually death. It is considered a listed disease by the OIE, meaning it is a priority disease for international trade. The etiologic agent, *Mycobacterium paratuberculosis*, also known as *Mycobacterium avium* subsp *paratuberculosis*, is believed capable of infecting and causing disease in all other ruminants (*e.g.*, sheep, goats, llamas, deer) and in captive and free-ranging wildlife. The infection has also been recognized in omnivores and carnivores such as wild rabbits, foxes, weasels, pigs, and nonhuman primates. Distribution is worldwide. National control programs include those established in Australia, Norway, Iceland, Japan, The Netherlands, Denmark, Ontario, Canada, and the USA. The highest published prevalence is in dairy cattle, with 20 per cent –80 per cent of herds infected in many of the major dairy-producing countries. Limited information is available about the prevalence in other species. The disease is of economic importance for the goat industry in Spain and the sheep industry in Australia. Paratuberculosis is mainly recognized by chronic granulomatous enteritis, emaciation and the resulting death. At very first, the disease was identified by Johnes and Frothingham in 1895.

Etiology

It is caused by *M. avium* subspecies *paratuberculosis*. It is a non-chromogenic, facultative intracellular acid fast, non-spore forming, non–motile, curved or straight or rod shaped and aerobic organisms. Map is usually identified by two forms; first is cell wall deficient (CWD) form and the second is cell wall competent (CWC) form. The species mycobacteria is broadly classified into slow growers and rapid growers. The slow growers are subdivided into pigmented and non-pigmented group.

Structure of Cell Wall of Mycobacteria

About 40 per cent of the total dry weight of the mycobacteria is made of lipid rich cell wall. It consisted of four different layers such as inner plasma membrane, immediate electron dense layer, electron transparent layer and outer membrane. The propensity of mycobacteria to clump or aggregate in culture media is attributed to the hydrophobic nature of their cell wall and the waxy material, lipoarabinomannan (LAM) present in the cell wall is associated to the acid fast property of mycobacteria.

Epidemiology

Prevalence of Infection

In Western Norway, paratuberculosis is described as endemic in goats, at the same time reported the occurrence of highest sero-prevalence in roe deer and red deer due to distribution of infection between wild and domestic animals. The disease has been reported from various parts of the world including India.

Economic Impacts

Paratuberculosis is reported to incur substantial financial losses to livestock industry. These losses have generally been estimated by calculating the reduction in milk production, lean meat production, culling and early replacement of infected cattle.

Predisposing Factors

Pregnancy, parturition and lactation are presumptive influencing factors to enhance, the development of the disease in cattle.

Source of Infection

Map survives for prolonged periods at low temperature outside the animal host and can remain viable for several months in contaminated water and soil.

Transmission

Oral ingestion of feed, water and milk contaminated with infected feces is the principal route for transmission. A single gram of infected feces can potentially infect thousands of neonates. There is interspecies transmission between cattle and sheep and goats. Infected cows, regardless of their disease status, excrete 5-8 cfu of organisms/50ml of milk. Vertical transmission of paratuberculosis is reported to occur through reproductive tract, fetus, blood, milk and colostrums of animals in advanced stages of infection.Eventually, horizontal transmission should also be considered important. Nematode larvae and nymphs of oriental cockroach acts as mechanical (passive) vectors.

Host Affected

Natural infection has been reported in cattle, sheep, goats, rabbits, antelopes and bison. Para tuberculosis in water buffaloes was detected from India. Calves younger than 4 month are highly susceptible than adult cattle.

Pathogenesis

Calves acquire infection as soon as they born, both by passive and active routes. Most of them able to eliminate the infection before they become clinically symptomatic. Due to persistence of organism in their body, which would results in a chronic disease. Persisted organism closely attached, to the glycol-proteins of the intestinal mucosa so as to escape from innate host immune mechanisms elicited by various physical, chemical and enzymatic processes. M cells, present in dome epithelium, that lack brush border, mucosal epithelium, digestive enzymes and surface mucous provide an easy access for the close attachment of the organisms and let them to cross the intestinal epithelium, through simple transcytosis process. Integrins (CR3), expressed on the apical surface of the M cells, acts as a bridge between fibronectin (FN) and fibronectin attachment protein (FAP) of map during phagocytosis process. Within the intestinal mucosal epithelium the bacteria is taken up by sub-epithelial macrophages where they can multiply and destroy macrophages. Pathogenesis and clinical signs would develop as the bacteria spread to adjacent cells. The whole process, from the time of uptake of Map by M cells and to phagocytosis by macrophages is completed in 20 hours. Secretion of pro-inflammatory cytokines and polysaccharide complexes by the infected host cells tend to produce the granulomatous enteritis especially at the terminal part of the intestine and local lymphnodes, edema and progressive thickening of both the intestines, due to infiltration of the infected tissues with a large number of inflammatory cells.

Clinical Signs

Calves are infected as young following ingestion of milk, feed and water contaminated with *M. paratuberculosis.* This causal agent is capable of living in animals for years without showing any clinical signs. Affected cattle normally appears to be healthy and bright looking without causing any changes in their appetite, nevertheless, they exhibit some of the symptoms such as decreased in milk production, loss of body conditions, and exudates in the early stage cachexia and hyporpotenemia which leads to death in the advance stage. In small ruminants, the course of the disease may vary from rapid to prolonged periods of time and the symptoms are much more similar to cattle, excepting less frequent diarrhea in the former species. Infected animals, during the clinical phase, pass as high as 10^{10}organism/gram of feces. Depending on the extensive nature of infection, the disease has been grouped into different stages;

1. **Stage I** – silent infection; includes both young and adult with no shedding of bacteria.
2. **Stage II** – subclinical excretory phase; adult carriers without clinical signs.
3. **Stage III** – clinical excretory phase; animals with characteristic signs.
4. **Stage IV** – advanced clinical disease.

Necropsy Findings

Microscopic lesions of JD is predominantly divided into two; Lepromatous and tuberculoid granulomatous lesion. Lesions are classified into four types based on the pathological features manifested by the Map infected goats.

Types	*Lesions*	*Areas Affected*	*Descriptions of Lesions*
Type 1	Focal lesions	Ileo-caecal peyers patches and lamina propria	Small granulomas
Type 2	Diffuse multi bacillary	Mainly intestines	Granulomatous enteritis (more common in goats)
Type 3	Paucibacillary	Lymphocytes (infected areas)	Diffuse lymphocytes
Type 4	Diffused mixed lesions	Macrophages and lymphocytes	Infiltrations with lymphocytes and macrophages

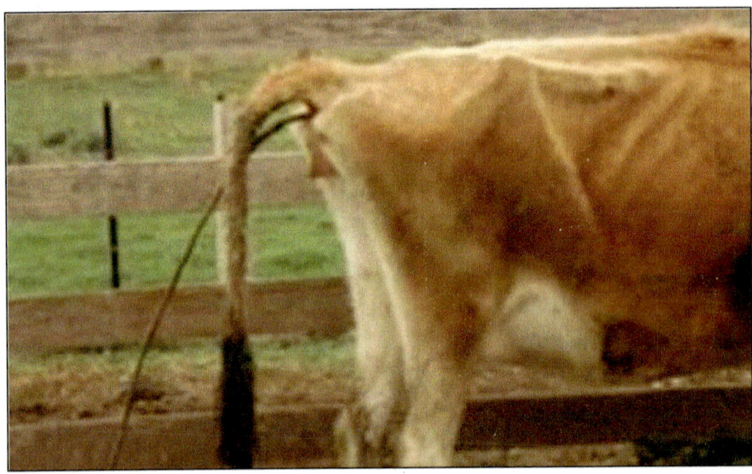

Figure 2.13. Paratuberculosis.

Diagnosis

Based on clinical signs and necropsy findings. Detection of acid fast bacilli from dung sample, intestinal mucosa and associated lymphnodes in infected animals are the most essential confirmatory diagnostic method of Para tuberculosis. Isolation of organism by culture. Solid media which includes, the egg based Lowenstein-Jensen medium (LJ) and Herold's egg yolk medium (HEYM). The culture method was described as 'gold standard'. Culture is time consuming, may require up to 3 months for incubation and labor intensive. Fecal culture test is most sensitive and could be used in herd level testing.

In BACTEC radiometric culture, the growth and recovery of colonies is observed to be greater, more sensitive and time saving than the conventional culture system. Cellular immunity is the first and strongest host response elicited during the early stages of mycobacterial diseases, is essential for the control of infection. Similarly in Para tuberculosis infected animals develops a strong CMI response in response to paucibacillary form (tuberculoid type) and a weak CMI to multibacillary form (lepromatous type). This cellular response is usually characterized by delayed type IV hypersensitivity (DTH)/intradermal test, lymphocyte transformation assay, migration inhibition test (MIT), (IFN-Y assay), and interleukin 2-R assay. *In vivo*–intradermal test is a very old technique used to measure sensitized

T-lymphocytes response to an antigen. It is a field test using 0.1-0.2ml of johnin PPD at caudal fold or the neck. The reactions of the animals are measured from a difference between the initial and the final thickness of the skin. Animal showing skin thickness of above 4mm after 72 hours of injection is considered positive. An alternative method of measuring CMI response is the gamma interferon assay, a *in vtro* test, is a sensitive test and it measures the release of interferon by exudates lymphocytes and is considered effective in screening and culling of infected herd. CMI response can also be measured by the expression of interleukin 2 receptor (IL-2R) on lymphoblasts by flow cytometry analysis. There are several methods like Complement Fixation (CFT) Test, Agar Gel Immunodiffusion (AGID) Test and Enzyme Linked Immunosorbent Assay (ELISA), used in the assessment of humoral immune response of paratuberculosis. In which CFT test has been considered a best screening test for cattle meant for international export. Molecular diagnosis by DNA probes may be of use in identifying clinically important bacteria. But for the bacteria like *M.paratuberculosis*, the use of species specific DNA probe may be essential. To date only IS900, F57 and HspX genes that are specific to this disease have been identified from its genome.

Sample Collection

Dung sample, intestinal mucosa and associated lymphnodes in infected animals are the most essential confirmatory diagnostic method of Para tuberculosis.

Differential Diagnosis

Tuberculosis, Parasitic disease, Salmonellosis, Colibacillosis, Rota viral enteritis.

Treatment

There is no treatment and antibiotics are available to control paratuberculosis. Temporarily exudates can be controlled by some antibiotics. Combined use of Streptomycin, Isoniazid and Rifambicin is suggested in some countries.

Control

No satisfactory treatment is known. Control requires good sanitation and management practices aimed at limiting the exposure of young animals to the organism. Calves, kids, or lambs should be birthed in areas free of manure, removed from the dam immediately after birth in the case of dairy cattle, bottle-fed exudates that has been pasteurized or obtained from dams that test negative, and then reared segregated as much as possible from adults and their manure until >1 yr old. Use of milk replacer is recommended instead of waste milk unless the milk has been pasteurized. A routine testing program for adults can help focus efforts in controlling the disease. Low-cost tests (*e.g.*, ELISA) have the greatest cost benefit for commercial dairy herds that are confirmed infected by culture or PCR. Animals testing positive, particularly heavy shedders or that have strong-positive ELISA results, should be sent to slaughter as soon as economically feasible. Retesting at least annually should be continued until herd tests indicate a low (<5 per cent) infection prevalence. Because intrauterine infection can occur, more aggressive control programs include culling of calves from dams that have or develop signs of the disease. Herd replacements should be obtained from herds believed to be free of the disease, and the replacements themselves should be tested before introduction to the new herd. More general procedures to minimize fecal contamination on the farm can also help, *e.g.*, elevating food and water troughs, providing piped water in preference to ponds, and harrowing frequently to disperse feces on pasture. Herd owners should be advised that paratuberculosis control takes at least 5 year.

The formulation of *M. paratuberculosis* vaccines varies by manufacturer. In many countries, their use is subject to approval by regulatory agencies and may be restricted to heavily infected herds. Vaccination of calves <1 mo old can reduce disease incidence but does not prevent shedding or new cases of infection in the herd. Vaccination thus does not eliminate the need for good management and sanitation. In the goat industry in Spain and Australia, vaccination has increased productive herd life. Cattle inoculated with an inactivated whole-cell, mineral-oil vaccine develop granulomas, one to several inches in diameter, at the site of inoculation (brisket) and may react positively on subsequent tuberculin tests. Accidental self-inoculation can result in severe acute reactions with sloughing and chronic synovitis and tendinitis.

Zoonotic Risk

There are conflicting data on the involvement of the causative organism in Crohn disease, chronic granulomatous enteritis of unknown cause in people. However, *M. paratuberculosis* is consistently detected by PCR in people with Crohn disease. This fact, coupled with its broad host range, including nonhuman primates, indicates that paratuberculosis should be considered a zoonotic risk until the situation is clarified.

2.14. Pullorum Disease

Synonyms

Bacillary White Diarrhoea.

Infections with *Salmonella* Pullorum usually cause very high mortality (potentially approaching 100 per cent) in young chickens and turkeys within the first 2–3 wks of age. In adult chickens, mortality may be high but frequently there are no clinical signs. Pullorum disease was once common but has been eradicated from most commercial chicken stock in the USA, although it may be seen in other avian species (*e.g.*, guinea fowl, quail, pheasants, sparrows, parrots, canaries, and bullfinches) and in small backyard or hobby flocks. Infection in mammals is rare, although experimental or natural infections have been reported (chimpanzees, rabbits, guinea pigs, chinchillas, pigs, kittens, foxes, dogs, swine, mink, cows, and wild rats). Transmission can be vertical (transovarian) but also occurs via direct or indirect contact with infected birds (respiratory or fecal) or contaminated feed, water, or litter. Infection transmitted via egg or hatchery contamination usually results in death during the first few days of life up to 2–3 wks of age. Transmission between farms is due to poor biosecurity. Pullorum disease is caused by *Salmonella pullorum*. It causes acute systemic infection in young chicks and localized chronic infection in adults.

Etiology

The disease is caused by *Salmonella pullorum* which belongs to the family enterobacteriaceae. It is a highly host specific organism. It is a gram negative, facultative anaerobe, non motile and rod shaped organism.

Epidemiology

Source of Infection

Parent to offspring occurs. Infected adult will become a carrier. The organism persists in the ovaries and excreted in the ova. Fluff from chicks, heavy, dry and the bacteria rapidly spread in the incubator.

Transmission

Transovarian transmission, vertical transmission from parent to chicks, rapid lateral spread from chick to hatcheries vice versa.

Host Affected

All avian species are susceptible but predominantly affects chickens, turkeys, and pheasants. All chickens less than 3 weeks are mostly susceptible.

Pathogenesis

It is a systemic infection in both domestic and wild species are affected. *S. pullorum* has tropism for reproductive tract and developing eggs following infection with particularly high numbers in the oviduct at the point of lay. Morbidity is 10-80 per cent; mortality is increased in stressed or immunocompromised flocks and may be up to 100 per cent.The development of pathogenesis is more or less similar to pathogenesis of fowl typhoid.

Clinical Signs

(a) **Acute:** Chicks of less than 3 weeks old are mostly affected. Initially there is an excessive number of dead in shell chicks or deaths shortly after hatching has been noticed. Depression, tendency to huddle, respiratory distress, loss of appetite, excretion of white viscous dropping which adhere to feathers around the vent and mortality of 100 per cent in severe condition.

(b) **Sub acute:** Grower birds are highly susceptible. Lameness, swollen hock joints in growing birds and poor growth rate is a main signs. Older birds appear listless with pale shrunken combs. Suboptimal egg production is the only sign seen in adult birds.

Necropsy Findings

(a) **Acute:** Chicks die of acute phase show no specific lesions. Chicks which die after hatching are likely to have peritonitis. Peritonitis with an inflamed un-absorbed yolk sac. Congestion of lungs, dark and swollen congested liver with haemorrhagic on the visible surface. Septicemia with liver congestion resembles dark and swollen with haemorrhage on the visible surface. Dilation of subcutaneous blood vessels is prominent. Chicks die after the development of clinical signs show typhlitis. Enlargement and distension of caeca with hard cast of dry necrotic material. Discrete, small, white, necrotic foci, often found in liver, lungs, myocardium and gizzard.

(b) **Sub-acute**: Growers and adults: Inflammation and enlargement of hock joints due to presence of excess lemon or orange colored gelatinous material around the joints. Abnormal ovary with ova, irregular cystic, misshapen, discoloured is featuristic and pedunculated with prominent thick stalks may be observed. Some infected adult birds may have small, inactive, pale ovary with underdeveloped ova. Inflammation of joints, peritoneum and pericardium is evident. Infertility, hatchability of infected eggs is very low.

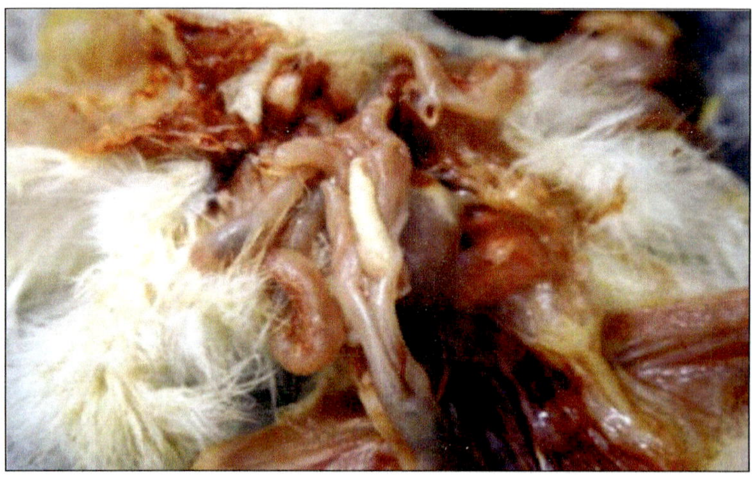

Figure 2.14. Pullorum disease.

Diagnosis

Based on clinical signs and necropsy findings. Isolation and identification of organism by culture and staining.

Sample Collection

Liver is an important specimen of choice for culture collected acute infection; whole blood and serum from chronic infection must be done by serological tests.

Test for Antibody Detection

Rapid Slide/plate agglutination test on whole blood using a stained antigen and tube agglutination test on serum can be carried out. Needle of 10 cm in length with a blunt end loop, white porcelain cavity plate, 0.02 ml of whole blood/serum drawn from the elbow joint and brachial vein 0.02 ml of antigen polyvalent crystal violet stained antigen is required for the test. Within 30 seconds after mixing the know antigen with blood/serum rapid agglutination will bee seen. If a fine, pin-point blue granules appears either through out the mixture or at the periphery in 1-2 minutes may be considered as doubtful reactions and if reactions occur in more than 2 minutes may be taken as negative. While testing the turkey, geese, guinea fowl, pheasants, partridges and quails serum result should be read in 3 minutes.

Merits

Testing of flock by RPAT is quick and easy to test. Two consecutive clean tests at an interval of one month must be done for declaring the flocks freedom from infection. Re-infection may occur through environmental contamination.

Differential Diagnosis

Fowl typhoid, Fowl cholera, New Castle disease.

Treatment

Sulfamethazine, sulfamerazine, and sulfaquinoxaline have been used successfully to reduce the death losses in chicks and poults. Furazolidone, a chemical derivative of furfural, checks losses in acute outbreaks. It may be incorporated in the feed at a low level for continuous feeding to prevent outbreaks and spread of the infection.

2.15. Q-Fever

Synonyms

Coxiellosis.

Coxiellosis is a zoonotic bacterial infection associated primarily with parturient ruminants, although domestic animals such as cats and a variety of wild animals have been identified as sources of human infection. The zoonotic infection in people associated with *Coxiella burnetii* is widely known as Q- fever. Coxiella is considered a potential agent of bioterrorism because of its low infectious dose, stability in the environment, and capability for aerosol dispersion. It is a zoonotic disease. It is a notifiable, occupational hazard of animal handlers and farm workers. Sudden onset of acute fever and liver infection followed by chronic endocarditis is observed. It is a chronic debilitating and fatal disease in animals and humans. The letter "Q" represent an abbreviated form of a query because of unknown descriptions for the disease that I before proper diagnosis had been done.

Etiology

It is caused by *Coxiella burnetii.* It is an obligate, intracellular parasite, gram negative, non-motile pleomorphic – ovoid to rod shaped organism. It exists in two antigenic phases: Phase-I – more infectious. The organism is resistant to external environmental influences. It has been divided into 6 genomic groups on the basis of restriction fragment length polymorphism.

Epidemiology

Prevalence of Infection

The disease is worldwide in distribution. The organism prevails in a wide range of wildlife species and their ecto-parasites. The rates of infection vary between farm animals, locations, regions and countries. In cattle, the prevalence of 6-82 per cent and 23-96 per cent of herds has been reported. The prevalence is significantly higher in cattle as compared to sheep and goats. Ticks and feral animals maintain the organism. Worldwide except in New Zealand the disease has been distributed.

Predisposing Factors

Those who with pre-existing valvular heart disease and vascular graft done. Transplant recipients. Patients with cancer. Those with chronic kidney disease are at risk of developing chronic Q. fever.

Source of Infection

Infection spread by contact and inhalation. In pregnant animals recrudescence of infection occurs and the organism excreted from intestine, uterus, placenta, udder during parturition. Placenta, fetal fluids, vaginal fluids, and urine consist of highly significant concentration of the organism. The organism excreted through the feces of sheep from 11-18 days post-partum.

Transmission

Parturient period may be the major period for transmission of infection. The organism present in the semen of sero-positive bulls and venereal transmission is suspected. More than 40 species of ticks infected and transmit the infection by transovarian mode. Feces contains 10^{10} infectious units/1g of of feces. The organism survives for 1 year at an ambient temperature.

Transmission in Human

Human acquires the infection by inhalation of infected airborne dust, contact with infected soil, wool, urine, feces, reproductive discharges, and other inanimate objects. Using the infected ovine manures as a garden fertilizers spread the infection in human. Sheep is a major reservoir of infection for humans. Urban population as they have close association with large dairy herds increasingly susceptible to infection due to their reservoir status. Drinking of infected milk from cattle, sheep and goats transmits the infection, however, pasteurization kills the organism. It is also an occupational hazard in human (veterinarians, livestock dealers, dairy plant, slaughter house workers, shearers), who are having close contact with infected domestic animals and their products. Several incidences in sheep attributed to parturient period in sheep and goats. In human, tick bite and human to human contact also transmits infection.

Host Affected

Sheep are at greater risk for infection. Cattle, sheep and goats are main reservoir of infection for humans. Non-pregnant animals maintained the silent infection followed by latency until the animals get pregnant.

Pathogenesis

Coxiella multiply in trophoblast of placenta. Unpasteurised milk has 10^5 organisms/ml of milk. Infective dose for human is approximately one organism as it is highly infectious. Infection ensues abortion, stillbirth, and poorly viable lambs. Lambs born to ewes excreting the organism are found to be clinically normal.

Though there is no abortion occurs in successive pregnancy in sheep but resurgence of infection occurs with excretion of organism immediately after the parturition. Goats excrete the organism in milk and feces for upto 2 weeks to 52 days following kidding. In cattle maximum shedding occurs for 2 weeks but in milk, cattle sheds for 2 years. Goats are also affected with abortion.

Clinical Signs

Animals

Infection in ruminants occurs at any time usually clinically in-apparent. Abortion in sheep and goats during later part of the lambing period in the flock and in the latter period of pregnancy in individual ewes. Correlation between herd level seroprevalence and herd infertility are clear. In pregnant animals, abortion, still birth, metritis, retained placenta, infertility and a prematurity occurs due to transplacental transmission, sometimes between 306 weeks of pregrancy. The interval between primary infection and the first signs of endocarditis last between 6 months and 10 years.

Human

(a) **Acute infection**: Mostly half of the infected human population shows clinical signs. Immuno-compromised persons are at greater risk for disease. Sudden onset of high fever (104-105°F), sweat, non productive cough, severe headache, general malaise, myalgia, confusion, sore throat, chills, nausea, vomition, diarrheoa, abdominal pain, chest pain, *etc.*, Fever last for 1-2 weeks, weight loss persists for some time. About 30-50 per cent of patients suffering from pneumonia. Liver function tests indicate the presence of hepatitis. Most of the acutely infected persons recover from infection and only 1-2 per cent dies of acute Q fever. Prevalence of infection in farm animals leads to subsequent increased infection in humans. It is considered as a potential agent of bio-terrorism.

(b) **Chronic infection**: Persists for more than 6 months and is a much more severe disease and is uncommon. Within a year, the infection in acutely infected people become chronic and persists as long as 20 years. A serious complication of Q. fever is endocarditis, generally having aortic heart valves and less in mitral valves. Less commonly pneumonitis, hepatitis, meningoencephalitis. Endocarditis, and hepatitis are highly manifested during chronic infection. About 65 per cent of the people with chronic Q. fever may die of disease. It has shorter incubation period for 2-3 weeks. If people recover from infection will develop life long immunity against re-infection.

Necropsy Findings

The liver, lungs, kidneys of the aborted fetuses shows exudatest foci of necrosis and inflammation. Placenta shows thickening and purulent exudates and large red brown foci of necrosis in its inter-cotyledonary areas.

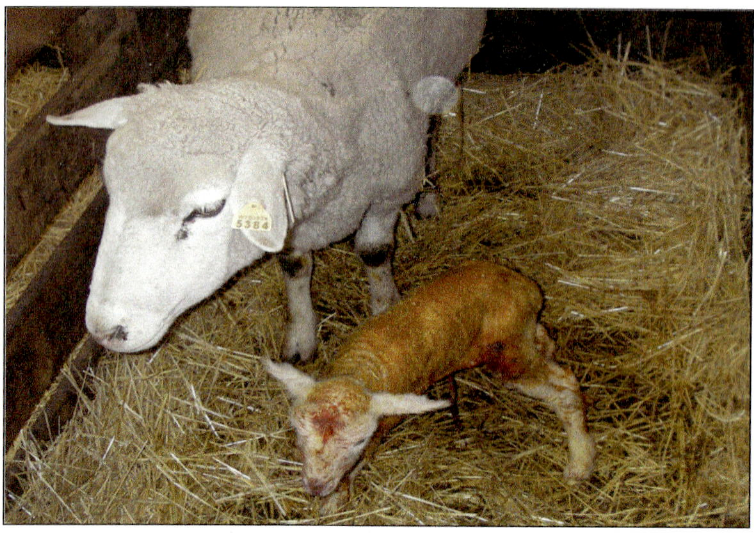

Figure 2.15. Q-Fever birthing stall.

Diagnosis

Based on clinical signs and necropsy findings. Identification of organism. Isolation of organism: Even the repeated blood culture shows negative results. Decreased platelet count and thrombocytopenia. Q. fever hepatitis is characterized by small granulomas with epitheloid cells in rosette formation. Serological detection of phase variants of antibody by Complement fixation test, micro-aggluatination test, ELISA, indirect fluorescence and indirect xudat-fluorescence test can be carried out. Phase –II antibody is associated with recent and acute infections and phase I with chronic infection. Abnormal liver function test shows the increase in bilirubin and alkaline phosphatase.

Samples for Collection

From buffy coat of blood and necrotic tissue material.

Differential Diagnosis

Ornithosis, Mycoplasmal pneumonia, Atypical pneumonias, Salmonellosis, Leptospirosis.

Treatment and Control

Q. fever in people is a notifiable disease in the USA, primarily because of its status as a possible bioterrorism agent; reporting requirements for animals vary by state. Vaccines for people and animals have been developed but are not commercially available in the USA. Vaccination has prevented infection when administered to uninfected calves and has improved fertility and reduced shedding in previously infected animals.

There is little evidence-based data to suggest that antibiotic treatment in animals provides significant benefit. Human clinical disease is typically treated with tetracyclines, but significant benefit from tetracycline treatment has not been demonstrated in controlled studies in abortion outbreaks of sheep in Europe. Despite the lack of evidence, some practitioners still advocate the use of parenteral tetracyclines during abortion storms. In known infected herds, the periparturient period represents a significant risk period for transmission because of the large amount of environmental contamination associated with abortion. Standard abortion control measures, including prompt removal of aborted materials (using zoonotic precautions), segregation of animals by pregnancy status, and diagnostic evaluation of abortions, are all warranted.

Zoonotic Risk

Q. fever occurs more frequently in persons who have occupational contact with high-risk species. The clinical presentation in people is highly variable clinically, ranging from a self-limiting, influenza-like illness to pneumonia, hepatitis, and endocarditis. *C. burnetii* is highly infectious, and a single organism can reportedly cause infection via the aerosol route in people. Individuals who have artificial heart valves are at particular risk, as well as anyone who is significantly immunocompromised. *C. burnetii* has been associated with human abortions, and pregnant women should take precautions to prevent exposure.

The majority of outbreaks in people have been associated with wind dispersion of desiccated reproductive products, contaminated with *C. burnetii*, from sites where sheep, goats, or cattle are kept. Farmers and veterinarians are at risk while assisting birthing. Slaughterhouse workers are at risk from contact with infected carcasses, hair, and wool. Transmission may also occur by consumption of unpasteurized milk. Handling of infected tissue poses a threat to laboratory personnel. Q fever has been seen in personnel and human patients in medical institutions where latently infected sheep were used for research. Medical facilities using ruminants in research should attempt to purchase animals from flocks free of coxiellosis or use male animals when possible. In addition, workers should use adequate personal protective equipment to protect against small droplet and aerosol exposure during high-risk medical procedures.

2.16. Salmonellosis

Synonyms

Paratyphoid.

Salmonella, a rod-shaped gram-negative bacterium belonging to the family Enterobacteriaceae, is the causative agent of salmonellosis. Salmonellosis in warm-blooded vertebrates is in most cases associated with serovars of *Salmonella exudate*. The most common type of infection is the carrier state, in which infected animals carry the pathogen for a variable period of time without showing any clinical signs. Clinical disease is characterized by two major syndromes: a systemic septicemia (also termed as typhoid) and enteritis. Other less common clinical presentations include abortion, arthritis, respiratory disease, necrosis of extremities, and meningitis. Only a few serotypes produce clinical salmonellosis in healthy animals and typically have a narrow range of host species, a phenomenon termed serovar-host specificity. *Salmonella enteric, Serovar typhi* (*S. typhi*) and *S. paratyphi* produce typhoid in people; *S. gallinarum* produces a similar disease in poultry, *S. abortusovis* in sheep, *S. choleraesuis* in pigs, *S. xudat* in cattle, *etc.*

The remaining serovars (serotypes) rarely produce clinical systemic disease in healthy, adult, nonpregnant animals. However, they colonize in the gut of many species of animals, enter the human food chain, and produce gastroenteritis in people (food poisoning). *S. typhimurium* and *S. enteritidis* are the most frequent causes of enteritis in people (nontyphoidal salmonellosis) but are also able to produce typical typhoid infections in mice; hence, the basis of pathogenicity is unclear. Strains from this latter group may also produce more severe disease, with systemic involvement resembling typhoid in very young animals if they have received insufficient protective antibody from their dam or when they are particularly susceptible, *e.g.*, as a result of old age, disease, or pregnancy. The host species from which a serotype is characteristically isolated is not necessarily the only species that can act as a host; thus, epidemiologic factors are important in determining prevalence.

Young calves, piglets, lambs, and foals may develop both the enteritis and septicemic form. Adult cattle, sheep, and horses commonly develop acute enteritis, and chronic enteritis may develop in growing pigs and occasionally in cattle the chapters on intestinal diseases in each of the major domestic species, Intestinal Pregnant animals may abort. The clinically normal carrier animal is a serious problem in all host species. Salmonellosis is seen infrequently in dogs and cats and is characterized by acute diarrhea with or without septicemia.

It is an acute, chronic and contagious disease of all species of animals, birds and human beings exudatestd by the development of severe dysentery and gastroenteritis. It causes the most important zoonotic problem in human beings:

Etiology

Until recent times more than 2500 salmonella serotypes have been identified and all of which may be considered potentially pathogenic. The exudates agent is a gram negative, non-sporing and rod shaped organism. It is killed by drying, sunlight and heat. But they may remain alive in soil for 7 months in water, feces and pasture. In moist soil they may remain viable for 12 months or more. The organism can be destroyed at 60°C for 20 minutes. Some of the important *Salmonella* species are as follows.

Two type of *Salmonella* species: *Salmonella exudate* – the type species. *S. bongori. S. exudate subsp. exudate* is again classified as four serotypes. *S. enteritis, S. typhimurium, S. typhi, S. cholerasuis, S. tyhphi, S.paratyphoic*- Human. *S. typhimurium*- cattle, sheep and goats, pig and horses. *S. exudat* –Cattle. *S. cholerasuis*-Pigs. *S. exudates xudat*-Horse. *S. aborus ovis* – sheep.

Epidemiology

Prevalence of Infection

The disease is world wide in distribution however; almost it has been reported from all the tropical countries. In India, many states have reported the prevalence of salmonellosis, despites various steps taken at national and international levels by the direction of the FAO and WHO human salmonellosis and has been increasing in the recent years. The disease has got economic importants as it causes high morbidity and mortality.

Sources of Infection

Animal may contract the infection from human sources. Carrier states can exist. Carrier animals excrete the causative agents through their feces. Besides domestic animals, deer, elk, raccoons, possums may remain spread the infection to cattle. Contaminated water is an important source of transmission.

Transmission

The infection is transmitted horizontally by direct exposure of the susceptible animals from the infected population. Infection is directly spread by means of ingestion. Cattle acquire infection from infected cattle or pigs or horse or sheep or dogs or poultry and pigeon.

Host Affected

Salmonellosis is prevalent in cattle, sheep, human, rodents, horse and dogs. Most animals are affected by specific salmonella species.

Pathogenesis

Infection is spread by ingestion through oral route followed by reaching the distal ileum, caecum and from there invade the mucosa, where in they replicate in submucosa and payers patches. In young animals and adults those have decreased immunity the organism spread beyond mesenteric lymphnode and establishes the infection in reticuloendothelium cells of liver followed by rapid entry into the blood circulation. Invasion of the organism in the blood stream causes pyrexia in 24-48 hours and acute infection in 5-9 days. It is a rapidly fatal condition. If invasion is sufficient to cause only a bacteremia, acute enteritis may develop and abortion is a final sequelae in sheep and cattle. Many animals may survive out of infection and the organism localized in the mesenteric lymphnode, liver, spleen, particularly in gall bladder. In chronic cases, organism shed intermittently from gall bladder and causes the foci of infection in the intestinal wall into the feces and occasionally into milk.

Enteritis

Develop at first time in carrier animals. The enteric salmonellosis much more complex than cholera, involving an increase in mucosal cell cyclic AMP content and prostaglandin concentration and inflammatory response to invading bacteria. Within a minute following infection in ileal loops in calves, salmonella can be seem to enter both M cells and enterocytes that process to over lie the domed villi associated with lymphoid follicles and absorptive villi. The organism must invade the intestinal mucosal epithelium to cause disease. *S. typhimurium* requires a function of type III secretions system encoded by salmonella pathogenecity island (SPII) to cause exudates. SPII secretions system directs the secreted effector protein into target epithelial cells. These effector proteins are virulent factor required for invasion and the induction of fluid secretion inflammatory response.

Virulent Factors

Adhesion pili, flagella, cytotoxin, enterotoxin, LPS, and inflammatory response that they initiate in the intestinal wall.

Salmonella cholerasuis: In pigs it in 36 hours causes erosion, edema of caecal mucosa. In 64 hours intestinal wall is thickened, diffuse and caseation overlying the erosions. In 96-128 hours, necrotic membrane sloughs and loses all function. In 176 hours whole intestine is inflamed and obliteration of muscular coat occurs. Colon is majorly affected in *S. typhimurium* can cause either local or diffuse colitis. Organism proliferates in intestine, invades the epithelium and reaches the mesenteric lymphnode. *S. cholerasuis* invade enterocytes by penetration of the brush border epithelium, results in local loss of microvilli and the bacteria endocytosed in to membrane bound vacuoles.

Clinical Signs

Septicemic Form

New born foals, calves, young pigs upto 4 months old are highly susceptible. Prominent depression, dullness and prostration. High fever 40.5-42°C and death occurs in 24-48hours.

(a) **Acute enteric form:** Adult animals are highly affected. High fever. Severe fetid exudates, dysentery and occasional tenesmus. Feces with putrid odor and contains mucus, blood, fibrinous casts, complete tubular casts of intestine. Intestinal mucosa in casts or sheets. Complete anorexia and increase thirst. Increase heart and respiration rate and congestion noticed. Pregnant animals abort. Severe dehydration, toxaemia, loss of weight, weakness, recumbent, and death in 2-5 days.

(b) **Chronic enteric form:** A severe outbreak. Occasional in cattle and horses. Calves intermittent or persistent exudates. Occasional spots of blood, mucus and firm fibrous casts present. Loss of weight and emaciation are seen.

Cattle

(a) **Septicemic form**: Depression, toxaemia, fever, dyspneoa and weakness. Nervous signs include incoordination, nystagamus, diarrhoea and dysentery.

(b) **Acute enteric form:** Abortion in pregnant cows and polyarthritis in calves. Dysentery with large blood clots. Complete agalactiae, abdominal pain, with kicking of abdomen, rolling, crackling, groaning and looking at the flanks are more. Rectal examination at this stage creates severe distress.

(c) **Chronic enteric form:** Inappetance, decrease weight gain, unthriftiness, acute enteritis.

Pigs

Dark purple discolouration of skin in abdomen and ear. Subcutaneous petichial hemorrhages. Nervous signs: Tremor, weakness, paralysis, convulsion and fatality 100 per cent. In four weeks old, meningitis, prostration, clonic convulsion and encephalitis. Enteritis and pneumonia.

Horses

Sporadic occurrence is common. Asymptomatic animals shed organism. Subacute enteric form in adult horses. Endemic form: Fever, depression, neutropenia –left shift, acute fulminating enteritis and exudates.

Necropsy Finding

Lesions in the brain, neuro encephalitis, polyarthritis and fatal meningo encephalitis. *S. agona* in 7 days old foals causes head tilt, seizures and exudates. In gastric mucosa develops haemorrhage and edema, In intestinal mucosa hyperaemia necrosis and ulcers. Caecum zebra markings is seen produced. Liver is enlarged with necrotic foci. Spleen is enlarged and become pulpy, Mesenteric lymphglands are haemorrhagic. In Lungs and pleura, pleural adhesion and abscess present. Pericardial and subpericardial haemorrhage occurs. Skin becomes discolored in pigs.

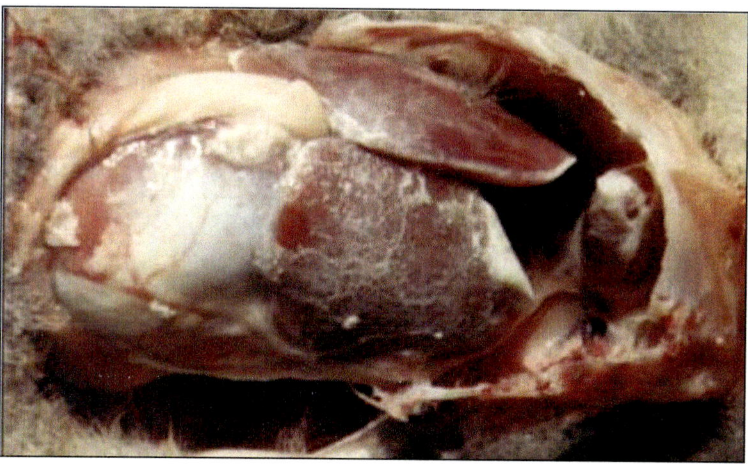

Figure 2.16. Salmonellosis pericarditis.

Diagnosis

Diagnosis of salmonellosis depends on clinical signs and isolation of the pathogen from feces, blood, or tissues of affected animals. The presence of organisms may also be sought in feed, water supplies, and feces from wild rodents and birds that may inhabit rearing premises to determine the source of the organism. Bacteria are usually identified by a range of biochemical tests. Identification to serotype may be done, followed by further subdivision on the basis of susceptibility to selected bacteriophages (phage typing).

Serologic tests are available and are increasingly used as a diagnostic tool in salmonellae surveillance and control programs. These tests are normally developed to identify a limited spectrum of salmonellae serovars and serogroups. Serologic tests are difficult to interpret in individual animals, because a seropositive animal may no longer be infected. Furthermore, specificity issues mean that in countries with low infection prevalence, many positive results are false-positive.

The clinical syndromes usually are characteristic but must be differentiated from several similar diseases in each species as follows: **cattle**—diarrhea due to enterotoxigenic *Escherichia coli*, dysentery due to verotoxigenic *E.coli*, coccidiosis, cryptosporidiosis, the alimentary tract form of infectious bovine rhinotracheitis, bovine viral diarrhea, hemorrhagic enteritis due to *Clostridium perfringens* types B and C, arsenic poisoning, secondary copper deficiency (molybdenosis), winter dysentery, paratuberculosis, ostertagiosis, and dietetic diarrhea; **sheep**—enteric colibacillosis, exudatest due to *Haemophilus* sp or *pasteurellae*, and *coccidiosis;* **pigs**—enteric colibacillosis and *Clostridium difficile* of newborn pigs and weanlings, swine dysentery (*Brachyspira hyodysenteriae*), campylobacteriosis, and the exudatest of growing pigs (which include erysipelas, *Lawsonia intracellularis*, classical swine fever, and pasteurellosis); **horses**—exudatest (due to *E.coli*, *Actinobacillus equuli*, or streptococci); **poultry**—coliform enteritis and *Yersinia pseudotuberculosis*.

Sample Collection

Feces, blood, serum, milk, body fluid and tissues.

Differential Diagnosis

Coccidiosis, Pasteurellosis, Liver fluke infestation, Poisoning, Colibacillosis, Paratuberculosis.

Treatment

Ruminants

Ceftiofur 5mg/kg 1/m 24 hours is effective. Concentration should be maintained above MICs. Amoxicillin, ampicllin, Trimethoprim, sulphadiazine, sulfadimidine and Framycetin and Nitrofurazone can be used.

Horses

Genetamycin 3mg/kg. combined with ampicillin 20mg/kg bw I/V 8-12 hours intervals in given. Trimethoprim and sulfonamide twice daily i/v combine dose 30mg/kg bw id effective. Combined sulfadoxin, sulfadiazine and sulfamethaxazole can be used in combined dose. Foals: Trimethoprim and sulfadoxine.

Supportive Therapy

Five per cent Sodium bicarbonate solution 5-8 L/400 kg bw I/V over a 2 hours period. Potassium chloride 30g in 8 L water id given twice daily.

Zoonotic Risk

Infections with *Salmonella* in food-producing animals present a serious public health concern, because food products of animal origin are considered to be a significant source of human infection. Most common sources of infection are eggs and related products, and meat from poultry and other food animal species. Milk and dairy products have also been associated with outbreaks of salmonellosis in people. In addition, contamination of fruit and vegetables by infected water may also be a source of infection. In Europe, *S. enteritidis* and *S. typhimurium*, and in the USA, *S. typhimurium* are the most prevalent serovars associated with human disease.

2.17. Strangles

Synonyms

Equine Distemper and Infectious adenitis.

Strangles is an infectious, contagious disease of Equidae characterized by abscessation of the lymphoid tissue of the upper respiratory tract. The causative organism, *Streptococcus equi equi*, is highly host-adapted and produces clinical disease only in horses, donkeys, and mules. It is a gram-positive, capsulated dippa-hemolytic Lancefield group C coccus, which are an obligate parasite and a primary pathogen. It is an extremely contagious disease of horses, most commonly affecting foals. The marked swelling of the retropharyngeal lymphnodes in throat causes "strangled breathe sounds" the disease is named "Strangles". Prolonged carrier status noticed in asymptomatic animals. The guttural pouches empyema causing respiratory distress in severely affected horses followed by death attributable to aspiration pneumonia.

Etiology

Strangles is caused by *Streptococcus equi* subspecies *equi.* It is an obligate, gram positive and cocco-bacillus organism. The organism expresses beta haemolysin around the colonies in blood agar. Similarities exist between the genome of *S. equi* and *S. zooepidemicus.* High virulent nature of the organism is due to the presence of M protein, hyaluronic acid capsule and leukocidine toxin. The mild atypical form of the disease is associated with non-capsulated variant of *S. equi.*

Epidemiology

Prevalence of Infection

The disease has been widely distributed around the world. It is also recorded from Punjab and other places in India and Pakistan. The occurrence is highest in foals during February to the start of May compared to winter and summer seasons.

Predisposing Factors

Sudden exposure to cold, high humidity, poor ventilation and severe stress are considered most important.

Source of Infection

10-40 per cent of recovered horses are carriers and hold the the organism in pharynx, guttural pouches for a long time. Discharges from nostrils, abscesses, contaminated grazing land, tracks, stalls, feed and water troughs, grooming kits, clothes of horses are sources of infection. Horses with guttural pouch empyema may excrete the organism for more than 3 years. About 25 per cent of the recovered horses not immune and are susceptible to second cycle of infection. Overpopulated farms are at high risk.

Economic Impact

Death of infected horses, time required and expenses incurred for treatment, aesthetic unpleasantness due to running noses and draining abscesses are responsible for economic losses.

Trasmission

Direct and indirect contacts with fomites are important for infection. Inhalation also possible. Through skin wound from external environment.

Host Affected

Horses, donkeys and mules around the world are susceptible. Morbidity rate is (20-100 per cent) usually more in foals and yearlings than in adults. Age specific attack rates in foals 20-40 per cent and brood mares 20 per cent. Case fatality rate is 10 per cent in untreated and 1-2 per cent in treated horses has been recorded. Outbreaks occurs frequently in breeding farms, polo and race horses.

Pathogenesis

The virulence of the *S. equi* is due to the presence of surface M protein, a hyaluronic acid capsule and production of a leukocidine toxin.

Surface M Protein

It is mainly known for three functions. Attachment to oral, nasal and pharyngeal tissues. Entry into pharyngeal tonsils and associated lymphoid structures. Prevention of host phagocytic activity by evading host immune response. There are two surface M proteins namely, SeM and Szpse. Of the two M protein, SeM is considered unique to *S. equi* which interfere with the action of c3b complements and therefore enhances the attachment of fibrinogen binding protein (Fbp) of the bacteria to host pharyngeal cells. M protein avoids the phagocytic process by host neutrophils. Hyaluronic acid capsules resist against phagocytosis and increases pathogenesis. Non-capsulated *S. equi* does not produce disease. On exposure the bacteria lodged in pharyngeal and tonsillar lymphoid tissues undergo rapid multiplication. The release of streptolysin O and streptokinase enzymes causes damage to tissues by directly injuring cell membranes and indirectly activating plasminogen leading to bacteraemia. Infiltration of neutrophils in lymphoid structures develops swelling and abscessation which causes disruption of lymph drainage and interfere with deglutition and respiration. Death due to pneumonia caused by aspiration, asphyxiation due to swelling secondary to upper airways and metastatic infection are seen. Rarely death occurs due to purpura hemorrhagica in horses as sequlae to *S. equi* and is associated with high serum antibody titre to SeM.

Metastatic Infection or Bastard Strangles

It is a chronic illness eventually leading to death. Arise due to bacteraemia or extension of infection in lymphnodes. Heart valves, brain, eyes, joints, tendons, sheath are affected. Meningitis, hyperaesthesia, rigidity of the neck and terminal paralysis. Abscess in brain leads to depression, head pressing, abdominal gait, circling and seizures.

Purpura Haemorrhagica

It is a sequlae to *S. equi* infection. Two myopathic syndromes occur in horses.

Muscle Infarction

Due to immune mediated vasculitis, associated with purpura haemorrhagica with infarction in the gastrointestinal tract, skin and lungs. Rhabdomyolysis and subsequent muscle atrophy, stilted gait, elevated serum creatinin kinase, muscle derived enzymes due to cross reactivity of anti-SeM antibody with myosin.

Clinical Signs

(a) **Acute form**: Incubation period is 1-3 weeks. Fever 103-105°F, sudden onset of anorexia, serous, copious and mucopurulent nasal discharge, abscessation of sub-mandibular, retropharyngeal lymphnode and guttural pouch develop. Severe pharyngitis, laryngitis and mild conjunctivitis noticed. Distinct enlargement of sub-mandibular lymphnode is seen. Pain in throat due to abscess, dysphagia, soft moist cough, extension of head. Hot, painful swelling of retropharyngeal lymphnode causes obstruction of oro-nasopharynx with respiratory distress which leads to death due to asphyxiation. Affected nodes rupture and discharge thick creamy, white to yellow pus in 10 days. The course of the disease may be from 3 weeks to 3 months in severe cases. Retropharyngeal lymphnode rupture and drain into guttural pouches leads to empyema and chondroids formation. In severe cases, pharyngeal, sub-maxillary, parotid and retrobulbar nodes have abscess and spread to local lymphatic vessels develops obstructive edema.

(b) **Atypical form**: It is characterized by widespread sub-clinical infection. In which animals have transient fever, profuse nasal discharge.

Strangles in Burros

Slow developing debilitated disease and have caseation and calcification of abdominal lymphnodes.

Chronic Form (Metastatic infection or Bastard strangles)

It is a chronic illness eventually leading to death. Arise due to bacteraemia or extension of infection in lymphnodes. Heart valves, brain, eyes, joints, tendons, sheath are affected. Abscess in brain leads to depression, head pressing, abdominal gait, circling and seizures.

Complications

Suppurative necrotic bronchopneumonia occur due to aspiration of pus from ruptured abscess in the upper airways/metastatic infection of lungs. Spreading of infection from RLN into guttural pouches is seen due to rupture-uni/bilarteral nasal discharge.

Necropsy Findings

Suppuration of liver, spleen, lungs, pleura and peritoneum. Meningitis, hyperaesthesia, rigidity of the neck are seen. Lesions occur in guttural pouch and in various lymphnodes.

Diagnosis

Based on clinical signs. Lsolation and identification organism is done. Using nasal swab collected and stained by a special Gram stain reveals *S. equi* as fluorescent purple color. A commercial test, measures the serum IgM antibody titer to SeM used to identify vaccination immunity. The test is not suitable in diagnosis of acute diseases. Serum antibody titre to SeM are very high (>1:12800) in horse with metastatic infection or purpura haemorrhagica. Detection of shedding S.equi DNA. It is more specific than culture. Acute form: Leucocytosis with neutrophilia reaches the peak.

Hyper-fibrinogenaemia is a characteristic of both acute and chronic disease.

Lucocytosis with a Hyperproteinemia

Polyclonal gammaglobinemia is an important change of metastatic and chronic abscessation. Hypoalbuminaemia is seen. Affected animals may or may not have anaemia, it depends on haemolytic effect of streptolysin O and immune mediated hemolysis.

Sample Collection

Nasal, pharyngeal, guttural pouch exudates and abscess swabs from animals with active diseases and carrier state.

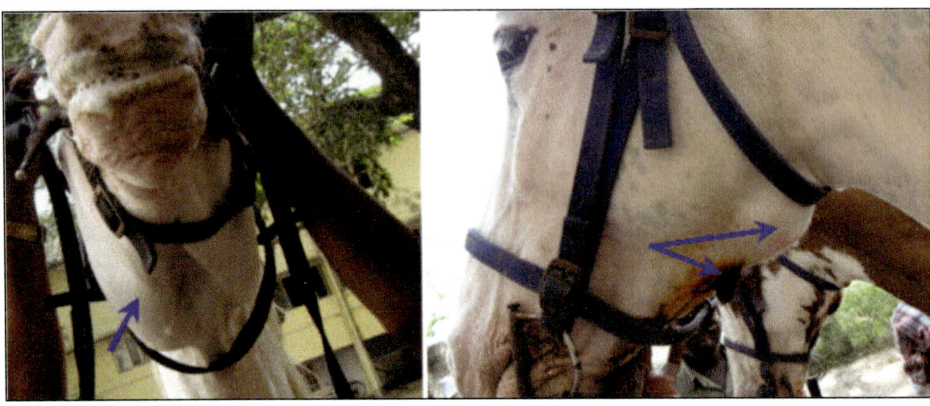

Figure 2.17. Strangles.

Differential Diagnosis

Strangles. Equine viral arteritis, equine viral rhinopneumonitis, equine influenza, equine rhinitis virus and equine adeno virus.

Treatment

Provide horses more comfort by feeding and watering. Perfect monitoring in order to avoid the development of secondary bacterial infection. Penicillin prevent recurrent and metastatic infection. For fever, anorexia, depression, purulent discharge, Procaine penicillin G 22,000IU/kg bw by I/m for every 12 hours for 5 days is given. Tetracycline 6-7.5 mg/kg bw i/v for every 12-24 hours. Sulphonamide-trimethoprim combination 15-30 mg/kg orally or i/v every 12 hours may be effective but only be used if procaine penicillin administration is not possible. Guttural pouch empyema is flushed with sterile isotonic electrolyte solution (0.9 per cent NaCl). Non-steroidal, anti-inflammatory drugs (NASAIDS) and hot poultices to reduce swelling relieve pain and rupture of abscess.

Control

Clinically affected horses should be physically separated from the herd and cared for by separate caretakers wearing protective clothing. The rectal temperature of all horses exposed to strangles should be obtained twice daily, and horses developing fever should be isolated (and potentially treated with penicillin). Contaminated equipment should be cleaned with detergent and disinfected using chlorhexidine gluconate or glutaraldehyde. Flies can transmit infection mechanically; therefore, efforts should be made to control the fly population during an outbreak. Farriers, trainers, and veterinarians should wear protective clothing or change clothes before exudates to the next equine facility. Additions to the herd should be carefully scrutinized for evidence of disease or shedding (nasopharyngeal culture) and quarantined for 14–21 days. Two negative nasal swab cultures should be obtained during the quarantine period.

Most horses continue to shed *S.equi* for ~1 mo after recovery. Three negative nasopharyngeal swabs, at intervals of 4–7 days, should be obtained before release from quarantine, and the minimal isolation period should be 1 mo. Prolonged bacterial shedding (as long as 18 mo) has been identified in a small number of horses. Guttural pouch empyema is the source of infection in most prolonged carrier states. Bacterial culture of nasopharyngeal swab and/or guttural pouch lavage is used to identify persistent carriers.

2.18. Tetanus

Synonyms

Lockjaw.

Tetanus toxemia is caused by a specific neurotoxin produced by *Clostridium tetani* in necrotic tissue. Almost all mammals are susceptible, although dogs and cats are relatively more resistant than any other domestic or laboratory mammal. Birds are quite resistant; the lethal dose for pigeons and chickens is 10,000–300,000 times greater (on a body woght basis) than that for horses. Horses and lambs seem to be the most sensitive of all species, with the possible exception of people. Although tetanus is worldwide in distribution, there are some areas, such as the northern Rocky Mountain section of the USA, where the organism is rarely found in the soil and where tetanus is almost unknown. In general, the occurrence of *C tetani* in the soil, especially in cultivated soil, and the incidence of tetanus in people, horses, and lambs are higher in the warmer parts of the various continents. It is a noncontagious, non-febrile, infectious disease of mammals affected by toxins released by *Clostridium tetani.* It is characterized by spasmodic contractions of skeletal muscles.

Etiology

Clostridium tetani is a gram positive, a long, slender, rod shaped anaerobe with rounded ends. The organism develops terminal spores and has a drumstic appearance. It lives in the intestine of herbivores as a normal inhabitant. The organism grows mainly under strict anaerobic condition. Spores are resistant and persists in soil for many years. The organism releases three types of toxins under anaerobic condition which are Tetanospasmin, Tetanolysin and Fibrinolysin.

Epidemiology

Prevalence of Infection

The disease is more common in tropical countries than in temperate. It is a sporadic disease in India. Case fatality rate in young cattle may be over 80 per cent. Mortality rate may be 50 per cent in animals die of acute infection.

Predisposing Factors

Infected nature of soil, climatic conditions and environment influences the infection. Wound or break in the skin, and accidental injury. Shearing, docking, parturition period, favors the infection.

Sources of Infection

Infected soil, discharges and exudatest.

Transmission

The organism present in soil gain access into animals during parturition, shearing, docking, castration, spaying and any other unprotected surgical and accidental injury. Spread can also occurs through ingestion.

Host Affected

Farm animals are probably most affected. Horses and mules are highly susceptible. Cattle are relatively less susceptible than man and horses. Sheep, goats and pigs are more susceptible compared to cattle.

Pathogenesis

The organism enters through any broken skin or injury does not cause tetanus. For the tetanus to develop need some favourable conditions such as; access of spores in to body tissues. Tissue damage causes localized impairment in blood supply oxygen creates anaerobic condition. Anaerobiosis leads to germination of spores. Following germination of spores vegetative growth occurs rapidly and releases toxins; tenospasmin, (neurotoxin), tetanolysin (haemolysin), and fibrinolysin (muscle and tissue cell lysis). All these toxins are released by cellular autolysis and get absorbed from site of production and spread into blood stream, exert neuro-toxic effect in peripheral nervous system by retrograde intra axonal transport, via motor nerves to central nervous system via brain and spinal cord, along the nerve route. Among these toxins tetanospasmin is considered very important and potent toxin. Through axonal terminal and intra axonal transport mechanism the toxin gains the central nervous system. From the CNS toxins reach dendrites and transferred to neurons that synops with cells. Generally, toxin can not cross the blood brain barrier. The released toxin binds with a "protogon", which is made of cerebrocide and oligosaccharides like N-Acetyl galactosamine and galactose. The toxin acting on the inhibitory synapses interfere with action of the inhibitory transmitter thus cause hyperirritability and there by leads to spasm. As the toxins enter the blood stream causes spastic paralysis, and invasion into nerve endings develops flaccid paralysis. Death usually occurs due to asphyxiation as a result of fixation of respiratory muscles. Mortality in horse is 50 per cent and cattle 80 per cent.

Clinical Signs

Horses

Initially affected animals are very hypersensitive to the external stimuli. Inability to open the mouth is seen. Animals continue to be with spasm for several days with mild muscle spasm. Saw horse stance, exudates of the third eye lid, erection of ears, immobility of the ears seen as predominant signs. Head, neck, and leg are in extended position. Spasm of facial muscle, masseter muscle leads to trismus. Mastication impairment, drooling of saliva because of spasm and swallowing difficulty. It is very sensitive to light and noise. Trembling and profuse sweating occur. At the end, affected animals unable to stand and die due to asphyxia in 3-10 days.

Cattle and Buffaloes

Affected animals exhibits mild problems and identified at the initial level recover from the infection. Affected animals restrict its movement, exhibits muscle stiffness, difficulty in walking and decrease milk yield. Lock Jaw, hyper irritability, exudates of the 3rd eyelid, pump handled position of the tail are more common and unique sign of tetanus in these cattle. Lateral recumbency, extend rigidity and opisthotonus. Suspension of rumination, drum like appearance of the rumen and left abomasal displacement. Animal dies due to asphyxiation.

Sheep and Goats

Dullness, head is drawn on one side or backward, opisthotonus, hypersensitivity to noise and bending of neck. Kids and lambs fail to suck milk due to tonic contraction of masseter muscle. Death occurs by asphyxiation.

Dogs

Localised: Rigidity of one leg, hypersensitivity, erection of ears, wrinkling of forehead, hypertonicity, opisthotonus, masseter muscle spasm, caudal retraction of the lips are noted.

Generalized: Clinical signs may be prominent in 10 days of infection. Dyspnoea, laryngeal spasms, mitosis and stiff gait. Out stretched tail, difficulty in rising or lying is the most common. Constipation, retention of urine due to spasm of the sphincter. Affected animals die of respiratory muscle failure, muscle spasm, laryngeal dysphagia, decrease secretion from respiratory tract and death occurs in 5 days.

Human: Rigidity of muscles, painful paroxysmal spasms of voluntary muscles, (masseter), the facial muscle paralysis and the muscles of back.

Necropsy Findings

Rigor mortis develop very quickly. Congestion of spinal cord and medulla. Hyperaemia of lungs is seen due to asphyxia. Skeletal muscles reveal haemorrhages, loss of cross striation and atrophy of the myofibrils.

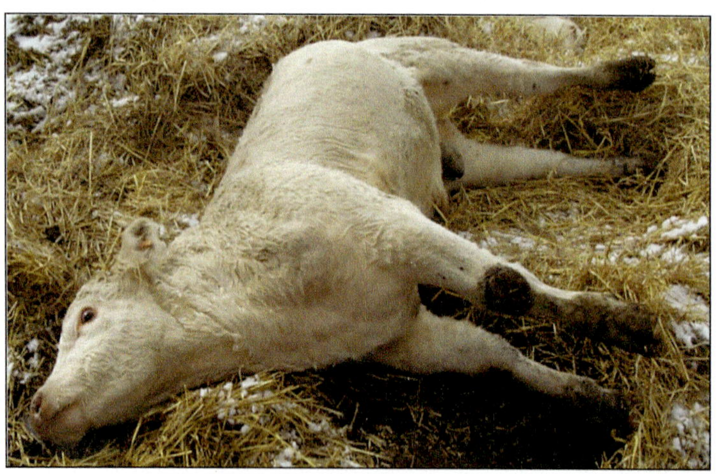

Figure 2.18. Tetanus.

Diagonsis

It is done on the baris of clinical signs and necropsy findings. Biological Inoculation: Challenging of mice, rabbit and guinea pig with cultured *C. tetani*. Demonstration of toxin. In acute case elevation of serum creatinine Phosphokinase (CRK) is give.

Differential Diagnosis

Strychnine poisoning, Grass tetany, Milk fever, Rabies, Epilepsy.

Principles of Treatment

These are neutralization of free toxin, destruction of tetanus organism, relaxation of muscle to prevent asphyxiation and supportive care.

Neutralization of Free Toxin by Tetanus Anti Toxin (TAT or ATS)

TAT may be mixed in saline and administered through I/V over a period of 30 min. It can be given in mares following, foaling and new born foals. It is given during last week of pregnancy. It can be administered following castration, docking and other operations. For prophylaxis (1500IU) is given which provides transient immunity, *i.e.*, only for 21 days but elicits quicker action.

Neutralization of Toxin by Tetanus Toxoid (TT)

It is a toxoid which establishes active immunity. Vaccination with tetanus toxoid is recommended for healthy domestic animals as preventive measures. Tetanus toxoid can be given at the same time with anti toxin provided in different sites.

Destruction of Organism

Early tetanus in cattle responds to the treatment. In very early cases high doses of Penicillin may be helpful, particularly if combined with local treatment of the infected site. Penicillin G 22,000 IU/kg bw 3-4 times I/M. De-bridement in used, Wound is cleaned, debrided with H_2O_2 followed by administration of antitoxin/antibiotics at the site of wound. Topical hydrogen peroxide infiltration increases the local oxygen tension and prevents bacterial growth.

Relaxation of Muscle

Affected animals should be kept in dark place and muscle relaxant must be given.

Treatment and Control

When administered in the early stages of the disease, curariform agents, tranquilizers, or barbiturate sedatives, in conjunction with 300,000 IU of tetanus antitoxin IV, bid, have been effective in the treatment of horses. Good results have been obtained in horses by injecting 50,000 IU of tetanus antitoxin directly into the subarachnoid space through the xudate magna. Such therapy should be supported by draining and cleaning the wounds and administering penicillin or broad-spectrum antibiotics. Good nursing is invaluable during the acute period of spasms. The horse should be placed in a quiet, darkened box stall with feeding and watering devices high enough to allow use without lowering the head. Slings may be useful for horses having difficulty standing or rising.

The same approach as described for horses is used in treatment of dogs and cats, except that caution must be exercised in the IV administration of antitoxin, because the equine antitoxin may induce anaphylaxis. In one study, antitoxin was given to dogs with tetanus only after an intradermal test to detect hypersensitivity reactions. In addition, all dogs received IV penicillin and some also received metronidazole orally. A combination of chlorpromazine and exudatestd or diazepam may be used to reduce hyperesthetic reactions and convulsions.

Active immunization can be accomplished with tetanus toxoid. If a dangerous wound occurs after immunization, another injection of toxoid to increase the circulating antibody should be given. If the animal has not been immunized previously, it should be treated with 1,500–3,000 IU or more of tetanus antitoxin, which usually provides passive protection for as long as 2 weeks. Toxoid should be given simultaneously with the antitoxin and repeated in 30 days. Even though it is not scientifically based, yearly booster injections of toxoid in animals are advised; in people the toxoid is given every 10 year. The toxoid vaccination interval is currently debated among vaccine recommendations for sport horses. Mares should be vaccinated during the last 6 wk of pregnancy and foals vaccinated at 5–8 wk of age. In high-risk areas, foals may be given tetanus antitoxin immediately after birth and every 2–3 wk until they are 3 months old, at which time they can be given toxoid. The decision to vaccinate lambs or calves depends on the prevalence of the disease in the area. All animals that have recovered from tetanus should be regularly vaccinated. Animals surviving tetanus do not build a good immunity and should be vaccinated with tetanus toxoid.

All surgical procedures should be conducted with the best possible aseptic techniques. After surgery, animals should be turned out on clean ground, preferably grass pastures. Only oxidizing disinfectants such as iodine or chlorine dependably kill the spores.

Large Animals

- Chlorpromazine 0.04-0.1mg/kg bw.
- Promazine 0.5-1mg/kg bw.
- Acetyl Promazine 0.03mg/lb bw.
- Sodium pentobarbital 5 per cent solution 2-4ml/kg bw I/V.
- Diazepam 0.01-0.4mg through I/V.

Dogs

- Acepromazine 0.25-0.5mg/kg bw 3-8 hours intervals I/V or I/m or S/C.
- Chlorpromazine 0.25 – 1.0mg/kg bw 4-8 hours intervals I/V or I/M.
- Diazepam 1.0mg/kg bw 1-4 hours intervals I/V.
- Phenobarbitone 2-6mg/kg bw 6-12 hours I/V or I/M.

Horse and Dog

- Nasogastric tube feeding can be given.
- Enema and use of catheter to remove stagnant urine and faecal matters.
- Tympany is relieved by rumenotomy.
- Use of indwelling tube should be done to avoid disturbances caused during repeated passing of stomach tube.
- Moist and soft feed should be given.
- Animals should be provided clean water, feed and bedding material to avoid injury.

2.19. Tuberculosis

Synonyms

Consumption, Pthisis, Pearl's disease and Scrofula.

Most of the general discussion above applies to bovine TB. The introduction of milk pasteurization was a major step in the fight against *Mycobacterium bovis* TB and continues to be an important control procedure in many nonindustrialized countries. Tuberculosis is a chronic, contagious, granulomatous disease characterized by development of tubercle nodules followed by caseation and calcification, debility and muscle wasting. The disease is transmissible between animal and human beings.

Etiology

As based on species of genus mycobacterium, affecting animals, human and birds, it is classified majorly into four types: **Bovine type:** Animals and human. **Human type:** Human and animals. **Avian type:** Fowls, pigs, horses and dogs. **Volebacillus:** Murrines species.

Different species of mycobacterium affecting different animals and human beings. **Cattle**: *M. bovis and M. tuberculosis.* **Human** – *M. tuberculosis* and *M. bovis.* **Horses**: *M. bovis* (majorly), *M. tuberculosis* and *M. avium.* **Dogs**: *M. bovis, M. tuberculosis* and *M. avium.* **Pigs**: Bovine, human and avian type. **Birds**: *M. avium.*

Mycobacterium is a slender, rod shaped organism, appears as single or pair or in group, resembles bundle of faggots. The cell wall of the organism is rich in mycolic acid (waxy coat) and sulphur rich glycolipids, which facilitate the bacteria to take up certain dyes such as Aniline and Ziehl Nielsen stain. During heating due to relaxation of the cell wall, the stain taken up inside the cell is retained in itself and thereby help resisting acid alcohol decolourisation. It is a characteristic phenomenon of mycobacterium hence why it is ascribed as acid fast organism.

Physical and Chemical Features

The organism is a slow grower in laboratory media. It is sensitive to heat. The organism is killed by creosote and sodium orthopheno phenoate. Resistant to chlorine and 6 per cent NaOH. It remains viable in organic materials.

Epidemiology

Prevalence of Infection

Tuberculosis is prevalent worldwide both in animals and human beings. TB is endemic in India both in animals and human beings.

Economic Impact

Apart from the mortality and productive loss, disease is relatively benign in pigs. Discarding and condemning of infected carcasses at slaughter.

Predisposing Factors

Some predisposing factors are overpopulation in small area, purely intensive rearing, and intercurrent infection. Poor sanitation, inadequate ventilation, Vitamin A and C deficiency, young age groups and malnourishment. are also included in it.

Source of Infection

Exhaled air, feces and infected meat, nasal discharge, sputum and tracheal mucus, contaminated inanimate and animate objects, reproductive discharges, feed, water and soil arer some souras of it in faction.

Reservoirs and Carriers of Infection

South West England: Badgers (*Meles meles*) – During their nocturnal visits in the farm buildings, excrete organism through urine and cattle in the same premises pick up the infection. New Zealand: Brush tailed possum (*Trichosarus vulpecula*)- Cattle infected when get along with possums in pasture. North America: Mule deer (*Odocoileus hemianus*), whilte tailed deer, elk, (*O. viriginianus* and *Cervus elaphus Canadensis*), Bison (*Bison Bison*). Great Britain: Red deer is playing very important role. South Africa: Buffaloes (*Syncrus caffer*) and water buffaloes (*Bubalis bubalis*) acts as maintenance hosts. India: Infected animals and human being acts as source of infection.

Transmission

It occwrs nasal discharge and tracheal mucus, communal use of feed and water troughs. Ingestion of tuberculosis infected animals milk and their products, direct contact with infected animals are alos sourus ginfection. Inhalation of droplet nuclei from aerosol, congenital infection by vertical transmission.

Host Affected

Cattle are the primary host highly susceptible for the infection. Pure bred and cross bred are highly affected as compared to zebu cattle. Sheep and goats more or less resistant to infection. Badgers, possums, pigs, dogs, primates, large cats and elephants other than cattle are affected and acts as maintenance host. Infected cattle are the main source for human infection.

Pathogenesis

Mechanism to Develop Infection

The cells wall of the mycobacteria is constituted by 40 per cent of the lipid which is of trehalos-6, 6′dimycolate and sulphur containing glycolipids. Virulent tubercle bacilli destroy the phagosome and causes failure of phagolysosomal fusion and so there is survival of mycobacteria within the phagocytic cells.

Primary Tubercle Complex or Ghon's Focus

The mycobacteria which gain entry in the host by inhalation get lodged in the alveolar surface of the lung and its bronchial and thoracic lymphnodes. By ingestion the organism reaches pharyngeal and mesenteric lymphnodes get locked up there. Within the corresponding lymphnodes the mycobacteria undergoes multiplication and develop small tubercles. The focus of such infection in the lymphnodes in "Primary complex of infection" or "Ghon's focus" condition.

Post Primary Dissemination and Stage of Late Generalization

Through draining of lymphnodes, bacteria reach the blood circulation and spread into other body cavities due to drop in immune response. As a result the bacteria overcome the killing effect by host immune mechanism and causes infiltration and necrosis of neutrophils. Together, the bacteria and the dead immune cells are surrounded by multi epitheloid cell layers which are called as Langhan's giant cells or granulomas and further this is surrounded by lymphocytes and fibrous connective tissues.

Clinical Signs

(a) **General form**: Affected animals become docile, lethargic but seem to be bright and alert. Cows with prominent exudates tubercle lesions are clinically normal. Progressive emaciation, capricious appetite, fluctuating body temperature and rough/sleek hair coat. In spite of good appetite animal does not put up weight. All these general signs are pronounced following calving.

(b) **Respiratory form**: Silent or paroxysmal cough especially during early morning and chilled weather. Chronic cough due to bronchial pneumonia. Rapid respiration with dyspnoea revealed by auscultation and percussion of the chest due to enlargement of bronchial lymphnode and obstruction of air ways. Squeaking crackles are audible but noise audible over the caudal lobes. Enlargement of retropharyngeal lymphnode causes dysphagia and noisy breathing due to pharyngeal obstruction.

(c) **Reproductive form**: Metritis and inflammation of placenta leads to infertility, abortion and failure in conception. A nervous sign in horse painful cervical osteomyelitis causes stiffness of neck and difficulty to eat.

Sheep and Goats

Lesions caused by *Mycobacterium bovis* in the lungs and lymph nodes of sheep and goats are similar to those seen in cattle, and the organism may sometimes disseminate to other organs. Sheep and goats are quite resistant to *M. tuberculosis* infection. The intradermal skin test is commonly used for diagnosis. The comparative tuberculin skin test conducted in the cervical region using biologically balanced purified protein derivative tuberculins of *M. bovis* and *M. avium* can be used to differentiate sensitization to other mycobacteria. The responses should be observed at 48 and 72 hr for induration and swelling. are seen. Intestinal ulceration with diarrhea is rare in cattle. Enlarged lymphnode of alimentary tract. Kids more progressive to early death.

Pigs

Pigs are susceptible to *M. tuberculosis*, *M. bovis*, and *M. avium* complex. *M. avium avium* and *M. avium hominissuis* are most frequently isolated; serologic identification of isolates is useful in epidemiologic investigations. Granulomatous lesions are most often found in the cervical, submandibular, and mesenteric lymph nodes, but in advanced disease lesions may also be found in the liver and spleen. Typically, enlarged nodes contain small, white or yellow, caseous foci, usually without any evidence of mineralization. Pigs with disease due to *M. tuberculosis* may have similar regionalized lesions. Pigs are particularly susceptible to *M. bovis*, which is usually acquired from shared grazing or ingestion of contaminated dairy products. This can cause a rapidly progressive, disseminated disease with caseation and liquefaction of lesions. The single intradermal test conducted on the dorsal surface of the ear or in skin of the vulva is often useful for diagnosis. Test responses should be observed at 48 hr after injection of tuberculin. TB lesion is seen cervical lymphnodes.

Horses

Horses are relatively resistant to tuberculosis caused by *Mycobacterium tuberculosis*; however, they are susceptible to *M bovis*. When tuberculosis does develop, tuberculous, noncalcified lesions are often found in the liver, mesenteric lymph nodes, lungs, and other sites. Tuberculin test results are rather erratic. Cervical vertebrae show osteomyelitis, and causes stiffness of neck.

Zoonosis

It is an important zoonotic disease. There is an increase incidence with an increase spread from animal to human. *M. bovis* is responsible for 5-10 per cent of human tuberculosis. Children getting infected via drinking of infected breast milk.

Necropsy Findings

Cattle, Sheep, Goats

Granulomatous lesion in bronchial, retropharyngeal AND mediastinal lymphnodesn is seen. Firm and enlarged pharyngeal lymphnode, swelling in dorsum of the pharynx occur. Miliary abscesses in lung. Pus is characteristic creamy and cheesy. TB nodule present in pleura and peritoneum. TB lesions are covered with fibrous capsule. Lesions in placenta with chronic purulent material is seen. Enlargement of supramammary lymphnode – TB lymphomatosis occur.

Chronic Lesions

Discrete, nodular, thick yellow to orange caseous material followed by calcification covered by a thick fibrous capsule is seen.

Pigs

Enlarged exudates TB localized in tonsils, submaxillary, cervical, hepatic, bronchial, mediastinal, exudates lymphnode with white caseous calcified material surrounded by a strong fibrous capsule.

Horses

TB lesion is seen in intestinal wall, mesenteric lymphnode and spleen. Cut surface of the LNs appears fleshy and resemble neoplastic tissue. Mineralisation and tissue necrosis is noticed.

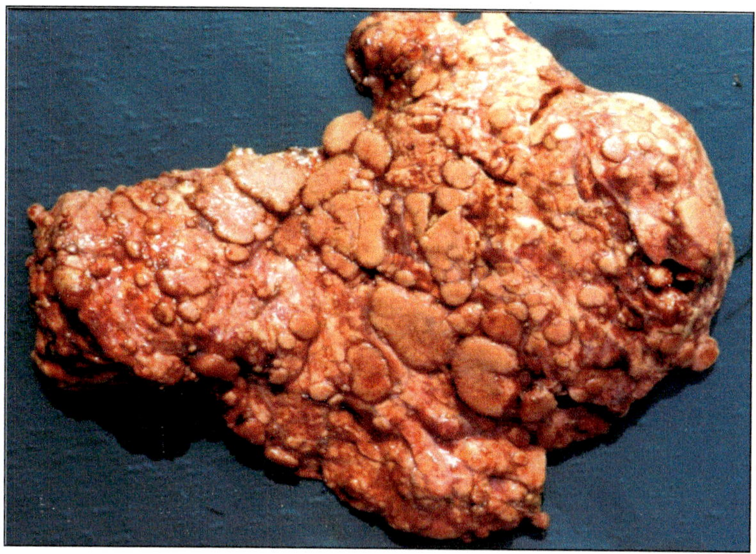

Figure 2.19. Tuberculosis of lung.

Diagnosis

It is based on clinical signs and necropsy findings. Palpation of supramammary lymphnode essential for suspected TB mastitis cases. Isolation and identification of organism is done by culture or acid fast staining.

The following are the tests for detection of cell mediated immunity.

Single Intradermal Test

PPD injection is given at caudal fold at base of the tail in sheep and goats/lateral center portion of the neck in cattle is highly sensitive. Initial skin thickness measured with a Vernier Caliper. DOSE: 0.1 ml herds with unknown status of sensitivity. 0.2 ml herds with known infected herds. Final skin thickness and inflammatory changes at 72 hours post injection should be taken. Increasing skin thickness more than 4mm is taken as positive.

Demerits

Lack of specificity. Nonvisible lesions reactors (NVLs).

Short Thermal Test

Intradermal tuberculin 4ml injected s/c in the mid neck of cattle. Initial rectal temperature 39°C (102° F) at the time of injection. If the temperature increases in 4, 6, 8 hrs to above 40°C animal is classed as positive reactor.

Stormont Test

First intradermal injection of 0.1 PPD at middle of the neck followed second injection should be given 0.1 after 7 days at the same site. Increase in skin thickness of 5 mm or more at 24 hrs. after this second injection is considered positive. Cattle with *M. avium* does not give positive reaction but skin TB cases do. It is more accurate than SID.

Comparative Test

For testing the animals for TB, along the side of PPD tuberculin injection, 12 cm apart, *M. avium* PPD should be given and the test result should be compared. Test results read after 72 hrs. This test is not used for initial screening but can be used as a primary test when there is a high incidence of Avian TB and JD.

False Positive

No gross lesions reactors. Nonpathogenic mycobacteria, Nocardia.

False Negative Reaction

Advance case of TB. Anergic animals are those with visible lesions of TB. But do not react to intradermal DTH test. Early cases until 6 wks after injection. Cows which have calved within preceding 6 weeks.

Gamma Interferon Assay

This test measures the amount of gamma interferon released from the antigen stimulated whole blood cells. Elisa test is done for detection of antibody. Molecular diagnosis is done by PCR. Sputum, feces, milk, blood and tracheal secretions must be collected for the diagnosis.

Differential Diagnosis

Lung abscess. Pleurisy, Pericarditis, Traumatic reticulitis, chronic contagious bovine pleuropnemonia, Upper respiratory tract infection, Actinobacillosis, Bovine leukosis, Lymphadenopathy, Mastitis.

Treatment

There is no antibiotic treatment successful in control tuberculosis. Supportive treatment to enhance the immune response can be done.

Prevention

All animals over six months and above should be tested by tuberculin test. Positive reactors disposed of according to local legislation. Suspicious cases must be retested by comparative test. Retesting: If incidence is higher, retesting should be done in 45-60 days after desensitization of intradermal injected animals. Annual testing of all cattle, quarantine, test positive herds should be slaughtered. Identification of individuals and wild life reservoir. BCG vaccination is available for calf hood vaccination. But vaccinated animals react positive to the skin test. Immunity is not strong and long lasting. Most probably cell mediated immunity is predominant. Accredited areas set up: All cattle in this area are tested and reactors removed and monitored until next generation off-springs become free from infection by tests.

Control

The main reservoir of *M. bovis* infection is cattle. However, other animals have been found to be reservoirs in some countries, including badgers and red deer (England, Ireland); red deer, possums, and ferrets (New Zealand); mule deer, white-tailed deer, elk, and American bison (North America); African buffalo (South Africa); and water buffalo (Australia). The prevalence of disease in such reservoirs influences the incidence of disease in other species. Carnivores and scavengers can acquire *M. bovis* by consumption of infected carcasses. These species include lion, coyote, wolf, hyena, cheetah, black bear, bobcat, and leopard. Warthogs, ferrets, raccoon, European wild boar, opossums, and feral pigs have also been found to be infected with *M. bovis*.

The three principal approaches to the control of TB are test and slaughter, test and segregation, and chemotherapy. The test and slaughter policy is the only one assured of eradicating TB and relies on the slaughter of reactors to the tuberculin test. In an affected herd, testing every 2 mo is recommended to rid the herd of individuals that can disseminate infection. Routine hygienic measures aimed at cleaning and disinfecting contaminated food, water troughs, *etc.*, are also useful. Test and slaughter has been used widely in the UK, USA, Canada, Germany, New Zealand, and Australia. In some European countries, where test and slaughter would have been impractical, varying forms of test and segregation have been used, with test and slaughter used only in the final stages of eradication.

The BCG (exudate Calmette-Guérin) vaccine, sometimes used to control TB in people, has proved to provide little protection against virulent *M. bovis* in most animal species, and inoculation often provokes a severe local granulomatous reaction. Moreover, BCG-vaccinated animals usually respond on the tuberculin skin test. Disinfection of utensils with 5 per cent hot phenol and cresol. Feeding of calves with milk free from infection should be done. Test and introduce new stock. Educate public about the significance of the disease.

2.20. Clamydiosis

Synonyms

Psittacosis/Chlamydiosis: *It is a term used to indicate the disease in psittacine birds, humans and animals.*

Bacteria of the order Chlamydiales are ubiquitous, obligate intracellular gram-negative bacteria. Within the host cell, they replicate via a unique developmental cycle competing with the host for intracellular nutrient pools. Virtually any chlamydial organism can infect any eukaryotic host cell, resulting in various infections. Chlamydial taxonomy with two genera, *Chlamydia* and *Chlamydophila*, was proposed in 1999 but is no longer valid. A single genus, *Chlamydia*, is now used, as well as nine species (*abortus, caviae, felis, muridarum, pecorum, exudates, psittaci, suis*, and *trachomatis*). Genome comparison revealed a high level of sequence conservation and synteny across taxa with the major exception of the human pathogen *C. trachomatis*. Two additional new species have been discovered recently, *i.e., C. avium* and *C. exudatest*.

Ornithosis

Disease affecting birds other than psittacines.

Etiology

C. trachomotis – mainly humans and other mammals. *C. psittaci*- humans, mammals and poultry. *C. exudates*- humans. *C. pecorum*- ruminants and other mammals. *Chlamydia psittaci* is a gram negative, coccoid organism and has a distinct life cycle. The organism has obligatory type of replication intracellularly within the cytoplasmic vacuoles of eukaryotic cells.

Epidemiology

Prevalence of Infection

C. psittaci prevails in psittacine birds and is endemic in tropical and subtropical region especially South America, Australia and in feral pigeons in many parts around the world. World wide in distribution. In poultry it is exudatest epidemic in nature. Sporadic occurrence of the disease noticed in flocks. Mortality rate is 0-30 per cent.

Predisposing Factors

Stress due to migration, transportation, changes in diet/environment, concurrent infection with other organisms such as Salmonella or *Pasteurella multocida*.

Sources of Infection

The infectious elementary body is highly resistant outside the host and so able to survive in dried excreta and in manure for longer periods. The organism is destroyed in putrified carcasses. Elementary bodies found in feces and respiratory secretion.

Transmission and Zoonotic Risk

Recent studies indicate that host specificity of different species is not as clear as previously thought. Most members of the genus *Chlamydia* have shown to be transmissible among species, including people. Zoonotic transmission from animals to people is well known for *C. psittaci*, *C. abortus*, and *C. felis*. Conversely, chlamydial species of people have been detected in numerous animal species.

Transmission of avian *C. psittaci* strains to people may result in atypical pneumonia or even life-threatening acute illness (*i.e.*, psittacosis in people). Transmission between companion parrots and dogs or cats, respectively, has also been associated with clinical cases. Furthermore, *C. psittaci* has been found in numerous other mammalian species (*e.g.*, cattle, swine, horses, small ruminants, rodents, wildlife). An association between *C. psittaci* genotypes with host species has recently been detected, but the pathogenetic relevance as well as the zoonotic potential of non-avian *C. psittaci* strains have yet to be defined. *C. abortus* may cause abortion and fetal death in pregnant women after transmission from goats or sheep. It has also been found in other animals (cattle, swine, wild suidae, horses, and birds). Zoonotic risks resulting from these hosts and the role of this pathogen in these hosts are unknown. Natural transmission of *C. felis* mostly occurs through close contact with other infected cats, their aerosol, and fomites, but the pathogen has also been found in dogs. With respect to people, there is clear evidence that *C. felis* acquired from cats may occasionally cause keratoconjunctivitis. Reports are rare, attributing this pathogen to serious systemic disease or atypical pneumonia. The known human pathogen *C. exudates* was detected in cats with conjunctivitis and also infects koalas, horses, and frogs. *C. trachomatis*, the other human pathogen, was found in pigs and birds so far. The risk of zoonotic transmission of other chlamydial species found in numerous animal species beside their main hosts, including the two new species *C. avium* and *C. exudatest*, has yet to be defined.

Host Affected

Turkeys are highly susceptible. Ducks, pigeons and chickens are rarely affected. Wild birds are affected by less virulent strains. Young birds are more susceptible than older birds. Psittacine birds, ducks and turkeys cause severe infection in human beings

Pathogenesis

During multiplication of the organism within the eukaryotic cells two inclusion bodies are produced. Elementary body: A small, infectious form, measures 250- 300 nm diameter which is surrounded by a rigid walled. Reticulate body: A larger, non-infectious form, measures 400- 600 nm diameter, flexible walled, develops from a small elementary body. Reticulate body divides by binary fission and produce daughter elementary bodies. These daughters elementary bodies attaching to the cell membrane of the host and undergo maturity before they rupture. On rupture the inclusion bodies libearated from the host. Inclusions able to survive outside of the host for long time until they acquire another host. The entire process of life cycle is being completed in 28-32 hours. The organism gain entry through inhalation reaches various organs, such as lungs, air sacs and under obligatory mode of replication within the cytoplasmic vacuoles in the exudates cells. Via the haematogenous route spread into pericardium, liver, spleen and kidney where in the organism undergo further multiplication and produce elementary bodies and exudates body. Incubation period varies upon factors such as virulence, the host species affected, age of the host and it may be 5- 60 days.

Clinical Signs

Mild to severe form of disease occurs in turkeys, ducks, pigeon. Depression, ruffled feathers, anorexia, purulent nasal exudates and conjunctivitis. Tracheitis, rales, grey-green exudates, exudatest droppings may be gelatinous with blood.

Nervous signs: In ducklings, trembling and an unsteady gait noticed. Pigeon affected by temporary ataxia. Chickens are rarely affected.

Necropsy Findings

The development of lesions varies depends on the severity and acute nature of the disease. Serosal surfaces covered by serofibrinous exudates. Pericarditis, congestion of lungs and cloudiness of wall of the air sac. Enlargement and softening of liver, spleen with small necrotic foci and petechiation noticed. In pigeons spleen may rupture.

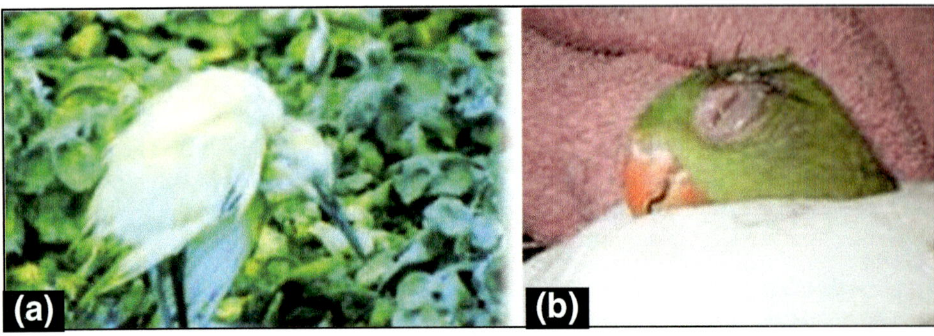

Figure 2.20

(a) Psittacosis affected birds, (b) Parrot affected with Psittacosis.

Diagnosis

Clinical signs and gross lesions. Confirmation by demonstration of causal organism or its isolation, identification and serological examination of paired sera. Wrap carcass for laboratory. Examination should be made in biohazard cabinet.

Demonstration of Casual Organism

Direct smear examination, Demonstration of chlamydial antigen and sera, Demonstration of chlamydial DNA, Culture and identification of organism.

Direct Smear Examination

Smear from exudates, lesion on the surface of liver or spleen, cloacal, tracheal, conjunctival swabs stained by modified Ziehl-Neelsen stain. Elementary bodies stain red while the back ground is blue-green, Giemsa, Machiavello, Castanada and an Iodine technique also used. Direct smear examination identifies only elementary bodies and so they lack sensitivity. Demonstration of inclusion bodies by inoculation into embryonated eggs, tissue cultures and mice inoculation.

Demonstration of Chlamydial Antigen

Verification of specific Antigen. Fixed infected tissue processed for FAT or IPT. Identification of Chlamydia after growth in eggs or cell culture.

Sample Collection

Tissues, eexudates and feces collected in exudates containing antibiotics, which reduce contaminants but have no adverse effect on Chlamydia.

Differential Diagnosis

Borreliosis, Pasteurellosis, Salmonellosis, Infectious laryngotracheitis.

Treatment

Chlortetracycline, in turkeys- 200-800g/ton of feed or 0.2-0.4gm in one liter of drinking water. Doxycycline by oral route for complete elimination of infection. Medicated corn, mash diets with 1 per cent chlortetracycline (CTC) and 0.7 per cent calcium. White millet seed with 0.5 mg CTC/g of seed, for budgerigars, parakeets and finches only for 30 days. A special diet is necessary for Lories and lorikeets, which feed on nectar and fruit in the wild. Doxycycline 40-50mg/kg body weight by oral once a day for cockatiels, cockatoods and parrots. Doxycycline 75-100mg/kg body weight IM for every 5-7 days for the first 4 weeks.

2.21. Collibacillosis

Synonyms

Scour in ruminants.

Colibacillosis occurs as an acute fatal septicemia or subacute pericarditis, airsacculitis, salpingitis, and peritonitis. It is a common disease of economic importance in poultry and is seen worldwide. *Escherichia coli* is a normal inhabitant of the digestive tract of mammals and birds. Many strains of the *E. coli* are non-pathogenic but some strains causes different disease conditions. In poultry, it causes Yolk sac infection, coligranuloma (Hjarre's disease), egg peritonitis and coli septicemia. Colisepticemia is a common disease of calves and lambs below one week old and chronic bacteremia with localization of organism occurs. The disease is usually sporadic and is more common in dairy than beef calves.

Etiology

E. coli is a gram negative, flagellated and rod shaped organism. It measures 2-3um in length 0.6um in width. Serotypes are mainly identified by their somatic antigen (O), capsular antigen (K) and flagellar antigen (H). The capsular antigen can be identified by Rapid Slide Agglutination test.

Epidemiology

Predisposing factors - Poultry

Colispeticemia

The disease occurs due to poor ventilation in houses. Inter current infections such as Mycoplasmosis, Colispeticemia, coccidosis, New Castle disease, infectious bronchitis, infectious bursal disease, viral tracheitis, Haemorrhagic enteritis, Aspergillosis and nutritional deficiency.

Egg Peritonitis

Flock peritonitis outbreak associated with cannibalism or vent pecking. Overcrowding and huddling leads to vent pecking.

Yolk Sac Infection

Intercurrent infection caused by *Bacillus cereus, Staphylococcus, Pseudomonas proteus, Clostridia* and yolk sac infection. Humid environment in poultry houses favors the incidence of yolk sac infection.

Source of Infection

E. coli involves either as a primary source of infection or as a secondary opportunistic pathogen.

Transmission

Poultry

Yolk sac infection occurs through unhealed navel. Sometimes, following fecal contamination of egg shell occurs. Ingestion of contaminated materials feeds and water.

Animals

In groups of calves, transmission occurs by direct nose-to-nose contact, urinary and aerosols, through navel, and feco-oral route.

Host Affected

All poultry and avian species are susceptible for infection. *E. coli* affecting, chicken, turkeys, ducks, pheasants but most commonly chicken are affected. Yolk sac infection mainly in chicks in the first week of age. All animals are susceptible and young age groups are highly susceptible.

Pathogenesis

Calves

Invasion occurs mainly via nasal and oral route. The organism crosses the intestine or via the umbilicus and umbilical veins. Septicemic phase is followed by death due to endotoxemic shock. In a prolonged course of the disease localization of infection occurs resulting in polyarthritis, meningitis, less commonly uveitis and nephritis. In chronic phase in calves marginal levels of circulating immunoglobulin present. The organism is excreted in nasal and oral secretions such as urine and feces. Excretion starts during the preclinical bacteremic phase.

Poultry

Collisepticemia

E. coli found in large numbers in digestive tract especially in lower part of small intestine and caeca. The organism enters the body through respiratory tract to develop characteristic lesions.

Yolk Sac Infection

The organism multiply in the intestines of newly hatched chicks, and spread rapidly to other chicks in hatchery and brooders. It causes 100 per cent mortality in a batch of chicks in first week of life. After first week the mortality may be 5 per cent to 10 per cent. The infection is associated with thick exudates navel.

Pigs

Neonatal exudates or scour in piglets occur. *E. coli* normally present in the gut of pigs and in other mammals. Haemolytic *E. coli* are highly pathogenic. This is a harmful bacteria attached to the wall of the intestine and produce toxins. It affects the function of the intestine and causes loss of fluid in to gut and produces scour and dehydration.

Clinical Signs

Calves

In acute disease, the clinical course is short (3-8 hr), and signs are related to the development of septicemic shock. Rectal temperature is subnormal. Calves show listlessness, loss of interest in sucking, depression, poor response to external stimuli, recumbency and collapse. Tachycardia, a poor pulse rate and a prolonged capillary refill time is observed. The feces are loose and mucoid. Mortality approaches 100 per cent. In prolonged clinical course, the infection localizes and develops polyarthritis and meningitis. In such calves, tremor, hyperesthesia, ophisthotonus, and convulsions are seen occasionally, but stupor and coma are more common.

Poultry

Colisepticemia

Very young birds are affected. Inappetance leads to listlessness, dejection, dry and ruffled feathers. Rapid xudate breathing, occasionally gasping with snicking. Mortality <5 per cent and morbidity >50 per cent. Following recovery unsatisfactory performances of the birds are noticed.

Yolk Sac Infection

Affected birds appear distressed with distended abdomen. Tendency to huddle, visibly thick navel which is prominent and necrotic.

Coligranuloma

This disease causes a sporadic death in adult. There are no specific signs but the affected birds die of infection a fter depression and loss of bodily condition.

Necropsy Findings

Colisepticemia

Lesions are very featuristic. Air sacculitis, peritonitis, perihepatitis, pericarditis and fibrinous pericarditis seen. Pericardial sac appears to be thick with white membrane adhering to the surface of heart is a characteristic finding. In septicaemic carcasses, liver, spleen, lungs and kidneys appears dark. Liver surface is covered by a thin fibrinous material. Air sacs are thickened, opaque and with white deposits adhere to this.

Egg Peritonitis

Egg peritonitis is indicated with salphingitis, peritonitis, impaction of the oviduct. Inspissated yolk mass, yolk debris and caseous materials are the important signs under post mortem examination. Milky fluid present in the abdominal cavity. Inflammation and distortion of ovaries, salphingitis, seen. Obstruction of oviduct by a core of inspissated and exudatest debris due to rupture of oviduct wall may be observed. A whole or partly developed egg found in the oviduct. Immediately after death organism should be isolated. The percentage of death in layers is less that 1 per cent.

Yolk Sac Infection

In septicemic carcasses, the blood vessels supplying to the yolk sac and sub-cutaneous route is engorged and dilated. Congested liver and dark swollen kidneys are observed. Inflammed unabsorbed yolk sac with abnormal colour and consistency of the yolk is a striking feature. Yolk is yellow/brown in color, watery and often fetid. Peritonitis and haemorrhagic lesion in serosal surfaces of intestines is a regular picture.

Coligranuloma

Hard yellow, nodular granulomas in mesenteric wall of intestine and particularly in caeca. Affected liver exhibits hard, blotchy, swollen and discoloured liver. In addition, synovitis, arthritis, tracheitis, air sacculitis, panophthalmia and localized abscesses are caused by *E. coli* in poultry. Presence of severe purulent peritonitis is characteristic feature of this disease.

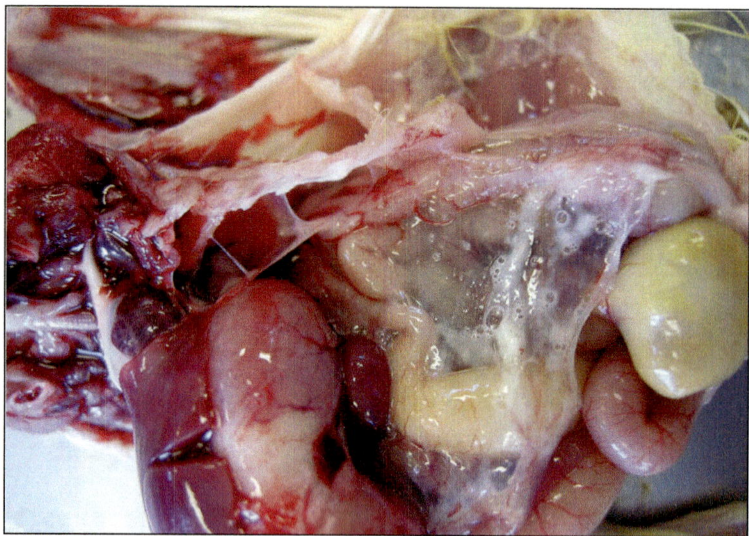

Figure 2.21. Colibacillosis.

Diagnosis

Unlike pathogenic *E. coli* associated with illnesses in other animal species, avian isolates are generally nonhemolytic on sheep (5 per cent) blood agar. Isolation of a pure culture of *E. coli* from heart blood, liver, or typical visceral lesions in a fresh carcass indicates primary or secondary colibacillosis. Consideration should be given to predisposing infections and environmental factors. Pathogenicity of isolates is established using multiplex PCR panels for plasmid-mediated virulence genes or when parenteral inoculation of young chicks or poults results in fatal septicemia or typical lesions within 3 days. Pathogenicity can also be detected by inoculation of the allantoic sac of 12-day-old chicken embryos. Resulting gross lesions include cranial and skin hemorrhages in addition to encephalomalacia in embryos inoculated with virulent isolates.

Calves

A moderate level of leukocytosis and neutrophilia in early stages followed by exudates in terminal stage. The joint fluid contains increased inflammatory cells and protein. CSF shows pleocytosis and an increased protein concentration. Organism is visible by microscopic examination. Culturing and characterization of organism is necessary for confirmation. Demonstration of deficiency of circulating IgG in the affected calves can be done using Zinc sulfate turbidity test or total protein estimation.

Differential Diagnosis

Pullorum disease, Fowl typhoid, Fowl cholera, Salmonellosis.

Treatment

Antimicorbials such as Furazolidone 0.04 per cent in feed for 10 days, Chlortetracyclin 600mg/5 liters of water for 5 days usually is effective. Other antibiotics, vitamins and minerals should be added in water or feed materials.

Calves

Initially bactericidal antibiotics having efficacy against gram-negative organisms. Antibacterial therapy combined with aggressive fluid, drug, and other supportive therapy.

2.22. Dermatophilosis

Synonyms

Mycotic dermatitis, cutaneous streptothricosis, Lumpy wool of sheep and cutaneous actinomycosis.

This infection of the epidermis, seen worldwide but more prevalent in the tropics, is also erroneously called mycotic dermatitis. The lesions are characterized by exudative dermatitis with scab formation. *Dermatophilus congolensis* has a wide host range. Among domestic animals, cattle, sheep, goats, and horses are affected most frequently, and pigs, dogs, and cats rarely. It is commonly called cutaneous streptothricosis in cattle, goats, and horses; in sheep, it is termed lumpy wool when the wooled areas of the body are affected. Infection in camel herds has been related to drought and poverty. Recent isolates from chelonids may represent a new species of *Dermatophilus*. It is also a common disease in farmed crocodiles. The few human cases reported usually have been associated with handling diseased animals. It is a disease of superficial skin of animals and man, manifested by exudation with matting of hairs, wools and formation of crusts and scab.

Etiology, Transmission, and Epidemiology

D. congolensis is a gram-positive, non-acid-fast, facultative anaerobic actinomycete. It is the only currently accepted species in the genus, but a variety of strains can be present within a group of animals during an outbreak. It has two characteristic morphologic forms: filamentous hyphae and motile zoospores. The hyphae are characterized by branching filaments (1–5 μm in diameter) that ultimately fragment by both transverse and longitudinal septation into packets of coccoid cells. The coccoid cells mature into flagellated ovoid zoospores (0.6–1 μm in diameter). The natural habitat of *D. congolensis* is unknown. Attempts to isolate it from soil have been unsuccessful, although it is probably a saprophyte in the soil. It is believed to be spread by direct contact between animals, through contaminated environments, or possibly via biting insects. It has been isolated only from the integument of various animals and is restricted to the living layers of the epidermis. Asymptomatic chronically infected animals are considered the primary reservoir.

Factors such as prolonged wetting by rain, high humidity, high temperature, and various ectoparasites that reduce or permeate the natural barriers of the integument influence the development, prevalence, seasonal incidence, and transmission of dermatophilosis. Ticks and lice are major predisposing factors in cattle and sheep, respectively.

The organism can exist in a quiescent form within the epidermis until infection is exacerbated by climatic conditions. Epidemics usually occur during the rainy season. Moisture facilitates release of zoospores from exudatest lesions and their subsequent penetration of the epidermis and establishment of new foci of infection. High humidity also contributes indirectly to the spread of lesions by allowing increases in the number of biting insects, particularly flies and ticks that act as mechanical vectors. Shearing, dipping, or introducing an infected animal into a herd or flock can spread infection. Dermatophilosis is contagious only in that any reduction in systemic or local skin resistance favors establishment of infection and subsequent disease.

Prevalence of Infection

Disease is prevalent through out tropical and temperate region of the world.

Economic Impact

Causes major economic losses in Africa, Australia, NewZealand, Europe, Middle east N, C, South America, India and Bangladesh.

Predisposing Factors

Moist and cold weather conducive for spread of the diseases and most of the outbreaks occur during rainfall. Concurrent infection like contagious ecthyma in sheep. Humidity and warm temperature, abundance of biting arthropods (*Amblyomma variegatum, Boophilus microplus, Hyalomma*), Sarcoptes, Demodex, mosquitoes, stinging and bloodsucking flies are some other predisposing factors.

Source of Infection

Exposure of surface of the body to water retention area.

Transmission

Direct contact with infected materials and infected animals. Mechanical transmission through instruments, brushes, harnesses, bedding materials are possible. Transmission occurs through anthropod vectors like flies, *Musca domestica, Lucilia cuprina, Stomoxys calcitrans and Calliphora* spp. Ticks and sheep keds acts as a mechanical vector. The disease also spread from one animal to other while dipping. Infection spread through abrasion.

Host Affected

Most commonly seen in cattle, sheep and horse. Reported also in goats, donkeys, dogs, fox, cat, deer, antelope, zebra, pig, monkey, exudates and wide variety of wild animals. Experimentally transmitted in camel and rabbit. Man is readily infected with dermatophilosis therefore, may be considered as zoonotic disease.

Pathogenesis

The organism invades hair follicles, sweat glands and other epidermal layer. The organism is highly proteolytic and liberates urease, increased exudatest casein, exudates gelatin and coagulates serum.

Three stages of development have been observed.

Hairs of the infected animals mats with eexudates and form crust. The hairs adhere strictly and difficulty to remove. The greasy scabs removed and there is a formation of dry scabs, Scars turn hard and confluent which make alopecia. Mild cases disappear spontaneously. Histological studies show filaments and mature multiple organisms in the cornified epithelial cells, leucocytes and dermis of animal. Pathogenic changes are exudates to epidermis and to some extent in the underlying dermal suface.

Clinical Signs

Cattle

Purulent eexudates below the crust and removal of crust will reveal moist and inflamed areas of granulation tissues. Systematic signs are not apparent except the febrile reaction. Milk yield reduced. Acute cases with extensive lesions complicated by secondary bacterial infection may lead to death due to endotoxemia. A chronic form of disease with deep encrustation is common.

Horse

Itching is absent, skin is thickened and dried up eexudates mat together form scab and plague. Removal of scab will exhibit a bleeding surface.

Sheep

Disease may appear in mild form, which may so unnoticed except loss of wool. In sheep it is ascribed as mycotic dermatitis. Eexudates mat the fibres together at the base and form crust. Crust spread in a pyramidal fashion, affect flank, rump occasionally sides and outer sides of legs. Heavy mortality in young lambs. Sore mouth are in sheep and goats. Lesions prominently present on scrotum, coronet, mouth and nose.

Dogs and Cats

Exhibits the feature of exudative dermatitis manifested as discrete, multiple focal raised lesions. The incidence is extremely rare in cat.

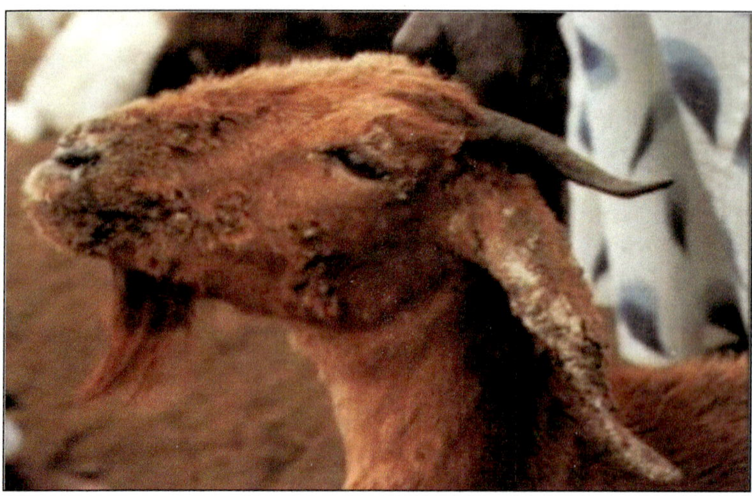

Figure 2.22. Dermatophilosis – Crusty, scaly lesions involve this goats head, ears and neck.

Necropsy Findings

Lesions on neck, body of the udder and extend down to the legs and assume a mosaic pattern with diameter 2.5 cm. It is common in back, sides and on rump. Lesion in muzzle, face, eyes, produces lacrymation and nasal discharge. Lesion also observed in all parts of body, abdomen and thorax. Proliferative dermatitis, known as strawberry foot rot is noted where scabs on removal would exhibit bleeding points. On fleshy mass resembling fresh strawberry and this condition is ulcerative dermatitis which affects the skin of legs from the coronet to above the knee or hock. Individual lesions coalesce, enlarge produce wart like masses and cover the entire legs. The lesions may appear tumor like in mouth is known as oral dermatophilosis. It is characterized by granuloma affecting tongue and crypts of tonsil.

Diagnosis

Presumptive diagnosis depends largely on the appearance of lesions in clinically diseased animals and demonstration of *D. congolensis* in stained smears or histologic sections from scabs. A definitive diagnosis is made by demonstrating the organism in cytologic preparations, isolation via culture, and/or via skin biopsy. An indirect fluorescent antibody technique and a single dilution ELISA test have been developed for large serologic and epidemiologic surveys. The most practical diagnostic test is cytologic examination of fresh crusts and/or impression smears of the underside of freshly avulsed lesions. Fresh crusts are minced on a glass microscope slide with a sterile scalpel blade in several drops of sterile saline. The slide is allowed to air dry and is then stained with a fast Giemsa or Romanowski stain. The organisms are seen under oil immersion as 2–6 parallel rows of gram-positive cocci that look like railroad tracks. Differential diagnoses include dermatomycoses in most species, warts and lumpy skin disease in cattle, contagious ecthyma and ulcerative dermatosis in sheep, and dermatophytosis and immune-mediated scaling diseases of horses (*e.g., pemphigus foliaceus*).

Differential Diagnosis

FMD, Scabby mouth, Photosensitization.

Treatment and Control

It was previously thought that because acutely infected animals usually heal rapidly and spontaneously, treatment was indicated only for cosmetic reasons in food-producing animals. However, in certain parts of the world, the disease is associated with significant morbidity and mortality, loss of body condition, decreased milk production, and increased somatic cell counts in milk. Treatment is recommended in horses because the lesions interfere with use and are painful. Organisms are susceptible to a wide range of antimicrobials: erythromycin, spiramycin, penicillin G, ampicillin, chloramphenicol, streptomycin, amoxicillin, tetracyclines, and novobiocin. Two doses of long-acting oxytetracycline (20 mg/kg) 1 day apart have shown to be curative in 85 per cent of cattle and 100 per cent of sheep, compared with cure rates of 71 per cent in cattle and 80 per cent in sheep for a single dose. In food-producing animals, topical applications of lime xudate are a cost-effective adjuvant to antibacterial therapy. Insecticides applied externally are frequently used to control biting insects.

In horses, the lesions should be gently soaked and removed. Topical antibacterial shampoo therapy is effective as adjuvant therapy. Chlorhexidine is recommended. Topical treatment with povidone-iodine is superior to parenteral oxytetracycline alone (100 per cent and 66 per cent effective, respectively). Isolating clinically affected animals, culling affected animals, and controlling ectoparasites are methods used to break the infective cycle. Preventing chronic maceration of the skin and keeping the animals dry are important. Zinc levels should be checked in the feed of cattle, because outbreaks have been associated with zinc deficiencies.

Zoonotic Risk

Dermatophilosis can be transmitted to people. Direct contact with an infected animal can lead to infections on the hands and arms. Affected animals should be handled with gloves, and thorough handwashing with an antibacterial soap is recommended after contact with an infected animal.

2.23. Enterotoxaemia – Type A

Synonyms

Yellow lamb disease.

Type A strains of *Clostridium perfringens* are commonly found as part of the normal intestinal microflora of animals and lack some of the powerful toxins produced by strains of other types. *C. perfringens* enterotoxin (CPE) is the principal toxin involved in *C. perfringens* foodborne illness and is associated with nonfoodborne diarrheal disease in different animals. *C. perfringens* also produces a necrotizing toxin associated with necrotic enteritis in poultry and dogs, colitis in horses, and diarrhea in pigs. *C. perfringens* type A is implicated in a rarely occurring hemorrhagic diarrhea in dogs and has been associated with nosocomial and acquired acute and chronic diarrhea in dogs. The acute form is characterized by necrotic enteritis in which there is massive destruction of the villi and coagulation necrosis of the small intestine. Many large, gram-positive rods are visible in fecal smears, and large numbers of *C. perfringens* type A are recovered on anaerobic culture of feces of dogs with acute diarrhea. Fecal tests are not useful in determining the cause of diarrhea, however, because of a high number of false-positive results. A commercial ELISA for CPE in dogs is quite specific. PCR for CPE gene expression in dogs is being evaluated. Type A strains from pigs with diarrhea have produced enterotoxin *in vitro,* and anti-enterotoxin antibodies in sows indicate that enterotoxin is produced *in vivo.* E nterotoxin has also been demonstrated in the feces of pigs with diarrhea but not in feces of healthy animals. *C. perfringens* isolated from pigs with diarrhea are typically nonenterotoxigenic but produce the cytotoxic dippa2 toxin, which possibly plays a role in disease. Experimental disease has been produced in pigs challenged orally with *C. perfringens* type A.

It is a sporadic disease affecting all groups of animals. *Clostridium perfringens* Type A –It is a major cause for abomasal inflammation, which may result in abdominal distension, abomasal ulcers in young calves. Varying degrees of exudates, and occasionally sudden onset of weakness and coma. It affects calve 2 weeks to 4 weeks old. Haemolytic enterotoxaemia in foals and in goats developed by alpha toxin, which possess phospholipase C and sphingomyelinase acitivity.

Etiology

Clostridium perfringens isolates are categorized in to type A-E as based on their ability to produce alpha, beta, epsilon, and Iota toxins. These toxins are important to exert their effect in developing pathogenesis. It is caused by *Clostridum perfringens* Type – A alpha toxin. *Clostridium perfringen is a* gram-positive, spore-forming, anaerobic bacteria.

***Clostridium perfringens* types, major toxins, and associated syndromes**

Toxin Type	*Major Toxin*	*Syndromes*
A	Alpha	1. Abomastitis (stomach inflammation) in calves 2. Bloating in calves 3. Mild diarrhea in calves 4. May be associated with hemorrhagic bowel syndrome (HBS) in dairy cattle
B	Beta, Alpha, Epsilon	1. Hemorrhagic enteritis
C	Beta, Alpha	1. Sudden death in very young calves 2. Hemorrhagic enteritis (bloody scours)
D	Epsilon, Alpha	1. Enterotoxemia resulting in sudden death, usually in calves on feed (finishing cattle)
E	Iota, Alpha	1. Fatal enterotoxemia in newborn calves

Epidemiology

Prevalence of Infection

Clostridium perfringens type A has been suggested as a cause of xudat hemorrhage syndrome in beef and dairy cattle and calves in most of the temperate countries predominantly in Canada, Belgium, in the western United States including in India.

Predisposing Factors

It is also occasionally associated with wound contamination and gas gangrene.

Sources of Infection

Organisms found in many environments, including soil, water, poorly preserved feeds, contaminated or improperly thawed exudates or milk, Calf sheds and the normal bovine intestinal tract.

Transmission

Contact with infected group of animals. Ingestion of contaminated feed and water materials with organism. Inhalation of spores.

Host Affected

All animals such as cattle, sheep and goats, horses, pigs are affected. Young one of the above species is highly susceptible to the disease.

Pathogenesis

C. perfringens type-A produce alpha toxin. It possess phospholipase C and sphingomyelinase activity and consequently, haemolytic action. The presence of Beta 2 toxin in these strains may contribute to the pathogenecity leading to high temperature, jaundiced mucous membrane, haemoglobinuria. Affected animals die in 12 hours. Cattle develops xudat haemorrhagic syndrome.

Clinical Signs

Horse

Acute profuse exudates with high mortality in adult. Affected animal die following strenuous exercises.

Pigs

Enteritis, watery yellow exudates, in piglets less than 5 days of age. High morbidity and low fatality.

Cattle, Sheep and Goats

Haemorrhagic enteritis in calf and adult cattle. Haemolytic disease in goats. An acute increase in body temperature, severe depression, pale mucous membrane, jaundice, hamoglobinuria, dyspnoea and severe abdominal pain. Affected animals collapse and die in 12 hours.

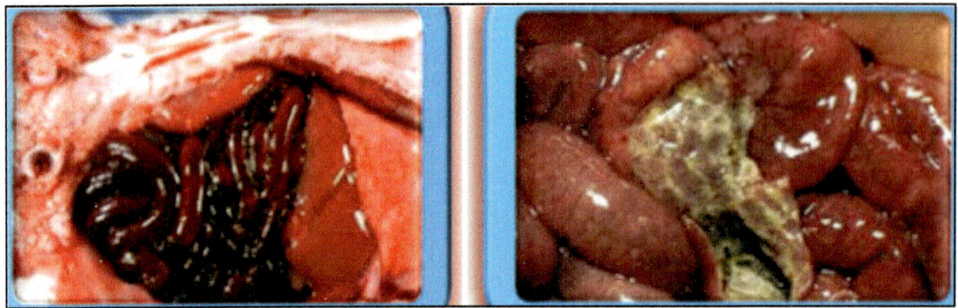

Figure 2.23. ***Clostridium perfringens*-Type-A, Haemorrhagic, necrotizing enteritis, with a abundant fibrin in a week old pig**

Necropsy Findings

Horse

Cecitis and colitis.

Pigs

Mild enterocolitis and villous atrophy.

Cattle, Sheep and Goats

The disease is highly fatal. Haemolytic disease and haemorrhagic enterotoxaemia. Jaundiced mucous membrane, swollen kidney, dark brown in colour and contains infarcts. Liver is pale and enlaged. Hydropericardium and pulmonary edema are noted. Extensive necrosis of the intestine occure.

Diagnosis

Isolation of organism from young and adult animals feces with enterocolitis. The organism can be isolated from young one even when they are 3 days old. Identification of Beta 2 toxin in feces (enterotoxin gene). Beta toxin detection in gut contents. It may cause protease degradation. Cytotoxic assays and immunoassays. The organism present in the intestine of normal calves. Culture of the organism from the calf is not sufficient to confirm a diagnosis of disease due to *C. perfringens*. So culture results should be confirmed with clinical signs, lesions in the tissues, and, in some cases, toxin identification, to obtain a true diagnosis. Tissue samples from calves should be collected soon after death and preserved.

Differential Diagnosis

Chronic copper poisoning.

Treatment

In subacute and chronic cases, antitoxin along with Tetracycline orally at the rate of 11 to 22 mg/kg bodyweight will usually effective. Supha group of drugs as injection or tablets may be given. Sometimes sulpha drugs in combination with trimethoprim can be tried.

2.24. Enterotoxaemia – Type B

Synonyms

Lamb exudates and Pine (Older lambs).

Infection with *C perfringens* types B and C causes severe enteritis, dysentery, toxemia, and high mortality in young lambs, calves, pigs, and foals (Enterotoxemia Caused by *Clostridium perfringens* Types B and C). Types B and C both produce the highly necrotizing and lethal beta toxin responsible for severe intestinal damage. This toxin is sensitive to proteolytic enzymes, and disease is associated with inhibition of proteolysis in the intestine. Sow exudates, which contains a trypsin inhibitor, has been suggested as a factor increasing the susceptibility of young piglets. Type C also causes enterotoxemia in adult cattle, sheep, and goats. Focal areas of necrosis produced in the small intestine.

Epidemiology

Prevalence of Infection

The organism prevalils in animal housing environment and as normal inhabitant in the alimentary tract of healthy animals. It is widely prevalent in other countries and lesser extent in India.

Predisposing Factors

Poor management factors exudatest the disease, well nourished animals are affected more.

Sources of Infection

Infected soil, environment, infected animals, and aerosol infection.

Transmission

By contact with infected animals, inhalation of spores, ingestion of contaminated materials.

Host Affected

Cattle, sheep and goat is highly susceptible for infection.

Pathogenesis

Type B organism produces beta toxin and a trypsin sensitive toxin. Dormant spores in tissue and dissemination of alpha toxin yields systemic effects with acute or per acute death. Cardio, necrotic, histo and hepatotoxic effects produce edema, serosal effusion and focal hepatic necrosis. Darkening of inside skin due to venous congestion. This venous congestion leads to death in cattle and sheep.

Clinical Signs

Lambs

(a) **Per acute**: Sudden death without any signs.

(b) **Acute**: More common. Loss of suckling, severe abdominal pain, bleating, stretching and looking at the abdomen. Lambs pass brown colored feces and sometimes with blood. Defecation is often accompanied with painful straining. Death usually occurs after a period of recumbency and coma and within 24 hours of onset of illness.

(c) **Chronic**: In older lambs causes abdominal pain, reluctance to suck, and without exudates.

Pigs

Rapid death in young ones. More prolonged disease in older piglets. Dull, depressed, exhibit, exudates, reddening of mucous membrane. Watery yellow feces initially, and sometimes haemorrhagic and red brown in color. Feces contain necrotic debris. In old pigs yellow colored exudates without any evidence of blood in feces. Rapid dehydration, hypoglycemia, hypothermic and comatose. Clinical course is less tha 24 hours.

Foals

Depression, prononunced toxaemia, marked abdominal pain and bloody feces. Subnormal body temperature, rapid pulse and respiratory rate. Death within a few hours after colic. In subacute cases, recovery is slow and requires 10-14 days.

Necropsy Findings

Pigs

Less commonly cause necrotic enteritis. Acute outbreak is followed by necrotizing enteritis. Localised areas of necrosis more evident in ileum. Intestinal mucosa is dark and red ulcers are large up to 2-5cm in diameter. Transmural intestinal contents are bloody with blood clots. Peritonitis, subendocardial and subepicardial haemorrhage.

Diagnosis

Isolation of organism from feces. Stained intestinal content shown large numbers of clostridium organism. Demonstration of toxin in feces. ELISA and Rapid Passive Latex Agglutination Test. Multiplex PCR for detecting gene encoding major toxin. Samples 20-30 ml intestinal contents frozen in glass or plastic leak proof container.

Differential Diagnosis

Salmonellosis, Enteric colibacillosis, Cryptosporidiosis, Isospora suis infection, Transmissible gastro enteritis, Strongyloides, Actinobacillus.

Treatment

Fluid and supportive therapy. Hyper immune serum is a specific therapy. Oral and parenteral administration of penicillin prevents the further proliferation of organisms.

2.25. Enterotoxaemia – Type C

Synonyms

Struck.

It is a sporadic disease occurs in orphan lambs especially reared on milk replacer. Type- C one of the more commonly encountered types of C. perfringens. It is virulent in calves less than 10 days old. The disease is exudatestd by bloody exudates but calves even die before this stage.

Etiology

C. perfringens isolates are categorized in to type A-E as based on their ability to produce alpha, beta, epsilon, and Iota toxins. These toxins are important to exert their effect in developing pathogenesis. It is caused by *Clostridum perfringens* Type-C produces beta and alpha toxin. *Clostridium perfringen* is a Gram-positive, spore-forming, anaerobic bacteria.

Epidemiology

Prevalence of Infection

Prevalent in cold weather. Lamb dysentery reaches 20-30 per cent. In an outbreak disease initially affects 1-4 days old lambs and the clinical course is very short. During the lambing period disease incidence increase. The cases fatality rate approaches 100 per cent

Predisposing Factors

Gross contamination. In lambs, goats due to close stocking in shed.

Sources of Infection

Poor quality feed facilitate infection. Feeding of milk in excess.

Transmission

Ingestion of infected feed and water. Close contact with infected animals.

Host Affected

Upto 2-3 weeks age groups of lambs and calves are affected. Sporadic disease occurs in orphan lambs reared on milk replacer. Necrotic enteritis of pigs: Important disease in piglets, particularily in intensive pig units. Organism is recoverable from the skin of sows and faces. Piglets up to 7 days are most commonly affected. Foals and calves are susceptible for type C and B.

Pathogenesis

Organism occurs as normal intestinal flora or any dietary changes significantly cause pathogenesis. Poor quality of feed facilitates abomasal and small intestinal multiplication of organism with resulting mucosal necrosis. Fluid accumulation in peritoneum and thoracic cavity and leading to toxaemia, enteric lesions, dysentery, exudates, often absent. Beta toxin affects central nervous system. Organism proliferates and attaches to the epithelial cells of the intestinal villi but toxin production and mucosal damage precede the attachment.

(a) **Alpha toxin**: It is a lethal toxin, produced in varying amounts by isolates. It is a phospholipase which hydrolysis the membrane phospholipids in RBC, platelets, leucocytes and endothelial cells, results in cell lysis or often develops cytotoxicity.

(b) **Beta toxin**: It causes increased vascular permeability and may facilitate the uptake of toxins from intestine. It is a exudatest toxin, initially produces damage to microvilli, degeneration of mitochondria with external distinction and desquamation of the intestinal epithelial cells. Which also develops haemorrhagic enteritis and ulceration of the intestinal mucous membrane. Beta toxin is highly sensitive to inactivation by trypsin which is a component of normal pancreatic proteases. Colostrum contains trypsin which inhibits organism in affected young animals. In the absence of trypsin the organism multiply within the intestine and exudatest of organism in the intestine of young animals.

Clinical Signs

Haemorrhagic enteritis, ulceration of intestinal mucosa, exudates, dysentery in young sheep, lambs, goats, calves, pigs, foals along with beta 2 toxin. High fatality rate, rapid course, haemorrhagic exudates, abdominal pain, and toxaemia.

Necrosy Findings

Areas of necrosis, extensive involvement of entire segments of small intestine, peritonitis, often, subendocardial, and sub pericardial haemorrhage, malignant edema, yellow fibrinous depositis in the intestinal mucosa, accompanied with large quantity of watery, mildly blood stained ingesta in the lumen.

C. perfringens type-C –	*C. perfringens* type-C –	*C. perfringens* type-C –
Small intestine mucosa in lamb with haemorrhagic enteritis.Dark red necrotic mucosa and the large amount of fibrin present in the lumen	Small intestine serosa in lamb with haemorrhagic enteritis. Distended intestine with gsa produced by alpha toxin and with haemorrhagic fluid	Small intestine in lamb with haemorrhagic enteritis. Complete necrosis of the epithelium and bacilli mixed with fibrin, desquamated cells and leukocytes in the lumen

Diagnosis

Frequently the organism is isolated from systemic faeces of newborn lambs and kids with haemorrhagic enteritis. Identification of organism.

Sample Collection

20-30 ml frozen intestinal contents. Air dried smears of mucosal surface from several levels of small intestine, ileum, jejunum, segments of several organs. Demonstration of toxin.

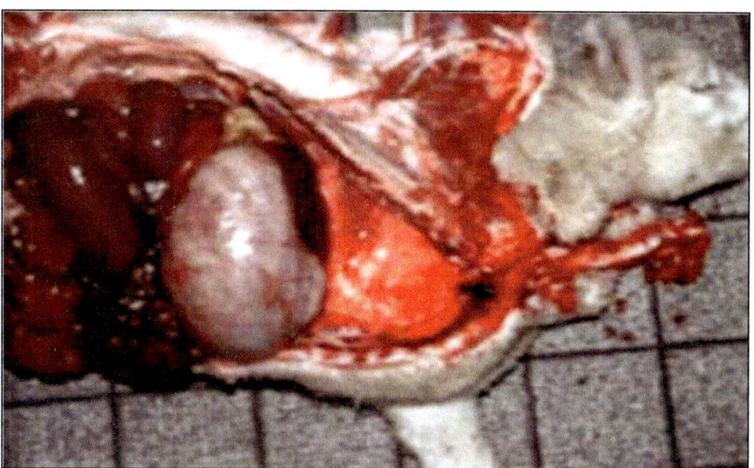

Figure 2.24. ***C. perfringens*** **type-C, Blood filled small intestine in sheep.**

Differential Diagnosis

Rota viral enteritis, Coronal viral enteritis, Parvo viral enteritis, Oother enterotoxaemic infection.

Treatment

Fluid therapy and supportive treatment are preferred. Hyper immune serum is a specific therapy. Oral and parenteral administration of penicillin prevent further proliferation of organism. In the subacute and chronic case, antitoxin along with Tetracycline orally at the rate of 11 to 22 mg/kg bodyweight will usually effective. Supha group of drugs as injection or tablets may be given. Sometimes sulpha drugs in combination with trimethoprim can be tried.

2.26. Enterotoxaemia – Type D

Synonyms

Overeating disease, and Pulpy kidney.

This classic enterotoxemia of sheep is seen less frequently in goats and rarely in cattle. It has a worldwide distribution and affects animals of any age. It is most common in lambs either <2 wk old or weaned in feedlots and on a high-carbohydrate diet or, less often, on lush green pastures. The disease has been suspected in well-nourished beef calves nursing high-producing cows grazing lush pasture and in sudden death syndrome in feedlot cattle; however, supportive laboratory evidence in the latter is lacking. Enterotoxemia due to *C. perfringens* Type D is sometimes associated with sudden death in cattle due to proliferation of organism in the presence of high amount of carbohydrates in diet.

Etiology

C. perfringens isolates are categorized in to type A-E as based on their ability to produce alpha, beta, epsilon, and Iota toxins. These toxins are important to exert their effect in developing pathogenesis. It is caused by *Clostridum perfringens* Type-D produces alpha and epsilon toxin. *Clostridium perfringen is a* Gram-positive, spore-forming, anaerobic bacteria.

Epidemiology

Prevalence of Infection

The disease prevails mostly in sheep and goats reared on young grass routes and shoots. The disease has been widely recorded from many countries.

Predisposing Factors

Upset in gut flora. Sudden changes to a rich diet. Continuous feeding of concentrates. Presence of excess dietary starch in the small intestine. Enterotoxemia may also seem to occur spontaneously due to sudden or dramatic changes in weather or other stressors.

Source of Infection

Infected materials, fomites, excesss rich diets containing organism, soil infection and environmental infection, *etc.*

Transmission

By contact, ingestion of excess diet and inhalation.

Host Affected

All age group of sheep affected except new born. Lambs 3 weeks to 10 weeks old, suckling lambs and lactating ewes are commonly affected.

Pathogenesis

Degenerative necrosis in the central nervous system is typical and focal encephalomyelitis is a chronic neurological manifestation of non-fatal disease. In normal course ingested organism are destroyed in large numbers in the rumen and exudates, where in the organism multiply and produce toxin. Toxaemia does not occur because the movement of ingesta keeps the bacterial population and toxin content down to a low level. Sometimes if stocked produce toxaemia. Passage of large quantities of starch granules in to the duodenum when a sheep overeat grain diet or/are change suddenly from a ration consisting largely of roughage to a consisting mainly of grain. Heavy milk feeding. Slowing of intestinal movement permit the accumulation of toxin and intestinal stasis predisposes the disease. The epsilon toxin of the *C. perfringens* type D increases the permeability of the intestinal mucosa to this and other toxins, thereby facilitating its own absorption. A receptor for epsilon toxin has been identified on vascular endothelial cells. Clinical signs and pathology develops due to widespread vascular damage and increase in vascular permeability.

Acute

In brain, degeneration of vascular endothelium, Perivascular and intracellular edema, and microscopic foci of necorsis in the basal ganglia, thalamus, internal capsule, substantia nigra, subcortical white matter, and cerebellum. Vascular endothelial damage leads accumulation of prolin rich fluid effusions in heart, brain and lung. Post mortem autolysis of kidney tissue rapidly and is the characteristic of pulpy kidney. Pronounced hyperglycemia due to mobilization of hepatic glycogen due to mobilization of hepatic glycogen, severe haemoconcentration and elevation of blood concentration of pyruvate, lactate, alpha-ketoglutarate. In goats, (in contrast to sheep), develop haemorrhagic enterocolitis. A degree of natural immunity may be attained by non lethal exposure to the toxin, as a proportion of lambs and calves appear to be exposed to subclinical but antigenic levels of *C. perfringens* toxin so that they become immune chanism. The extent of in co-ordination and convusion is directly related to the severity of lesions. Peritoneal and pericardial effusions typical in sheep. Glycosuria is Common characteristic.

Clinical Signs

Toxin facilitates its own absorption, toxaemia with no enteritis, dullness, retraction of the head, opisthotonus, convulsions and sudden death.

Lambs

Course of the illness is very short. Less than 2 hours and never more than 12 hours. Many lambs found dead with no signs.dullness, depression, yawning, facial movements and loss of interest in feed.

Acute

Severe chronic convulsion is higher with frothing at the mouth and rapid death. Cases susrvive for a few hours show a green, pasty exudates, staggering, recumbency, ophisthotonous, and severe, clonic convulsion. With normal temperature and increase in the case of severe convulsion. Death occurs due to convulsion after a period of coma.

Adult Sheep

Survive for a long periods upto 24 hours, Lagging behind the flock staggering and knuckling, Champing of the jaw, salivation, rapid shallow, irregular respiration. There may be bloat in the terminal stages, Irritation-convulsion, muscle tremor, grinding of teeth and salivation, Less common than in lambs.

Calves

Similar to that of adult sheep, Nervous signs predominating, Peracute cases found dead no, no struggling.

(a) **Acute**: Common-sudden onset of bellowing, mania, convulsion persists until death 1-2 hours later.

(b) **Subacute**: Many recover do not drink guiet and docile and appear to be blind. Eyes Preservation reflex persists. They may continue to be in this state for 2-3 days and recover quickly and completely. In an outbreak of the disease in calves all three forms of the disease may be seen.

Goats

Diarrhoea is a prominent signs

(a) **Peracute**: Young kids-convulsions, after initial attack of fever 40.5 degree centigrade, severe abdominal pain, dysentry, death in 4-36 hours occur.

(b) **Acute***:* More common in adults, there is usually no fever, abdominal pain, exudates, prominent with death or recovery in 2-4 days.

(c) **Chronic***:* goat may be ill for several weeks, anorexia, intermittent severe exudates, xudates with epithelial shreds in the feces. Chronic wasting, anemia, eventual emaciation, in chronic cases.

Necropsy Findings

Pericardial and peritoneal effusion is typical in sheep, acute lysis, hyperaemic, toxin damaged tissues and pulpy kidney.

Goats: Catarrahal, fibrinous haemorrhageic enterocolitis.

Chronic: Pulpy kidney absent.

Diagnosis

Based on clinical signs, and post moretem examinations. Bacteriological examination by culture (isolation and identification). Definitive diagnosis, can be made in the laboratory. Affected sheep is positive for glycosuria.

Sample Colletion

Intestinal contents should be preserved by adding 1 ml of chloroform to 10 ml of contents which have been collected in glass within 12 hours of death.

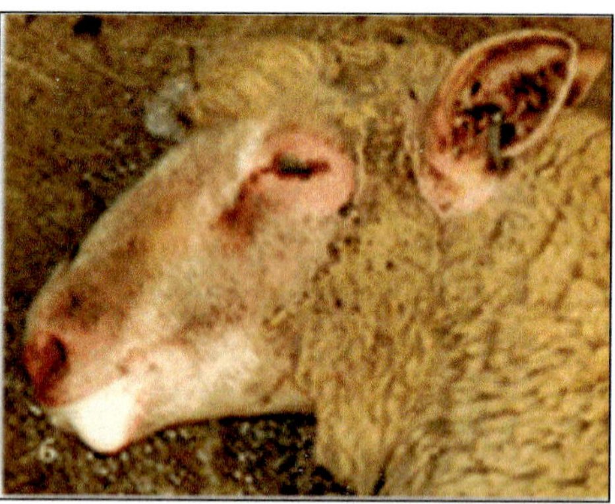

Figure 2.25. C. perfrigens type-D – Recumbent lamb with acute anterotoxaemia frothing by the mouth.

Differential Diagnosis

Coccidiosis, Salmonellosis, Rumen impaction.

Treatment

Benzathine penicillin and amoxicillin are given at birth. Bacitracin 300 mg/kg feed and Salinomycin 60 mg/kg feed are give. Treatment is ineffective against the peracute and acute cases. However, if ante mortem diagnosis is made one should attempt the use of 50 ml. of specific hyperimmune serum intravenously every 4 to 8 hours in the valuable animal.

2.27. Leptospirosis

Synonyms

Weil's disease, Canicola fever, Canfield fever, Seven day fever and Rat scratch yellow fever and Paddy field fever.

Leptospirosis is a zoonotic disease with a worldwide distribution caused by infection with any of several pathogenic serovars of *Leptospira*. The disease affects virtually all mammals and has a broad range of clinical effects, from mild, subclinical infection to multiple-organ failure and death. Leptopsirosis is a potentially re-emerging, epidemic disease creates public health problems. It causes an acute, severe, septicemic infection leading to death following multi-organ failure.

Etiology

Leptospira are aerobic, gram-negative spirochetes that are fastidious, slow growing, and have characteristic corkscrew-like motility. The taxonomy of *Leptospira* is complex and can be confusing. Traditionally, *Leptospira* were divided into two groups; the pathogenic *Leptospira* were all classified as members of *L interrogans*, and the saprophytic *Leptospira* were classified as *L biflexa*. Within each of these species, leptospiral serovars were recognized, with >250 different serovars of pathogenic *Leptospira* identified (based on surface antigens) throughout the world. The serovars are often grouped into antigenically related serogroups. With the increased use of genomic information for the classification of bacteria, the genus *Leptospira* was reorganized. There are currently 21 recognized genomospecies of leptospires, including pathogenic, intermediate, and nonpathogenic organisms. Pathogenic leptospires are now identified in 9 species of *Leptospira*, with 6 species being regarded as intermediate in pathogenicity, and 6 being nonpathogenic. Some of the common leptospiral pathogens of domestic animals now have different species names. For example, *L. interrogans* serovar Grippotyphosa is now *L. kirschneri* serovar Grippotyphosa. The two types of serovar Hardjo have been formally split into two species: serovar Hardjo type hardjo-bovis (found in the USA and much of the world) is now *L. borgpetersenii* serovar Hardjo and the less common serovar Hardjo type hardjo-prajitno (found primarily in the UK) is now *L. interrogans* serovar Hardjo. The revised nomenclature is now reflected in the scientific literature but not on labels for vaccines and pharmaceutical products. Fortunately for clinicians, the serovar and serogroup names remain in common use and are useful when discussing the epidemiology, serology, clinical features, treatment, and prevention of leptospirosis.

Cattle

L. hardjo, L. xudat, L. icterohaemorrhagiae, L. canicola, L. grippotyphosa, L. exudates, L. hardjoprajitna, hardjobovis and *L. autumnalis.*

Dogs

L. icterohaemorrhagiae, L. canicola, L. xudat, L. grippotyphosa and *L. exudates.*

Sheep

L. xudat, grippotyphosa, hardjo and *L. exudates.*

Horses

L. serovar L. xudat type kennewickii and *L. exudates.*

Pigs

Serovar, L. exudates is widely prevalent. *L. xudat, L. grippotyphosa, L. canicola* and *L. tarassovi.*

Human

L. hardjo and *L. xudat.*

Epidemiology

Prevalence of Infection

It is worldwide in distribution. The disease is highly prevalent in India in animals and human beings.

Economic Impact

Sub-clinical infection – abortion storm, still births and birth of weak calves, infertility, increased culling rate, agalactia, milk drop syndrome (*L. hardjo*) and death rate in – cattle, sheep, horses and pigs causes heavy economic losses.

Predisposing Factors

Organism is susceptible to dryness and pH <6 or >8 inhibits the survival. Temperature < 7-10 °C/>34-36 °C is sensitive to inactivate the organism. Moisture and dampness increase the incidence of leptsopirosis. In high rainfall area *L. hardjo* and in low rainfall areas *L. pomona* is prevalent. There is a direct correlation exists between incidence and rainfall. Stagnant water preserves more organism than the flowing water.

Transmission

Rat is peri-domiciliary mammals excrete leptospires in urine. Fox is a sylvatic carrier. Human contact with contaminated soil and infected materials able to contract the infection. Through licking of urine, penetration via abraded/injured skin, mucous membrane and eyes infection mostly occurs in dogs. Natural and artificial insemination would spread the infection. Venereal transmission is possible.

Host Affected

All animals including human beings are susceptible.

Pathogenesis

Upon entry through skin leptopsires soften skin, cross the mucosal surface and bind to the epithelial cells. And get attached with exudatestd matrix components by an active process initiated by expressed surface proteins. Pathogenic leptospira is found extracellularly between cells of liver and kidney and release lymphokines, TNF-α from monocytes through the endotoxic activity. TNF-dinna damage the endothelial cells and produce hemorrhage in severe leptospirosis. Vascular lesion is aggrevated by lipopolysaccharide and endotoxin of leptopspires. Intravascular hemolysis and interstitial nephritis, septicemia, abortion and mastitis. In acute severe septicemic leptospirosis, endotoxaemia, haemorrhages, hepatitis, nephritis and meningitis. Subacute leptopsirosis is a moderately severe disease manifested by nephritis, hepatitis, agalactia and meningitis. Chronic leptospirosis is exudatestd by abortion, stillbirth and infertility. In occult form no clinical illness seen.

Clinical Signs

Per acute leptospirosis: Young calves below one month age is exudatestd by high fever, rapid respiration, haemoglobinuria and death. Acute Leptospirosis: Sudden onset of agalactiae in adult dairy cattle and sheep, Icterus and haemoglobinuria in young animals, meningitis, acute renal failure and jaundice in dogs. Chronic leptospirosis: Abortion, still birth, retained placenta, weak offspring, infertility, chronic renal failure in cattle, jaundice in dogs and periodic ophthalmia and conjunctival suffusion in horses. Persistence: In chronically infected animals the organism persists in the kideney and genital tract. Chronically infected animals carrying the infection for life and become reservoir.

Dogs

Incubation period is 2-20 days. Decrease urine output, anuria proteinuria. Jaundiced sclera indicates hepatitis. Vomition, fever, dysuria and dark or brown urine. Cough, haemoptysis, dyspnoea and exudates respiratory rate. Meningitis, fatigue, hearing impairment, respiratory distress, azotemia, renal interstitial tubular necrosis, renal and liver failure in severe form of Weil's disease.

Cattle

Acute Cases

Cattle is a reservoir for serovar *L. hardjo* and type *L. hardjo* bovis and it causes nephritis. Leptospirosis is septicaemic in calves and lambs. Dyspnoea, pulmonary congestion, icterus, haemoglobinaemia, haemoglobinuria last for 48 to 72 hours. Haemolytic anaemia leading to death and sometimes recovered animals become normal in 7-10 days. Enzootic infection in adult cattle. Abnormal haemorrhagic milk in dairy cattle. No haemolysis noticed. Mortality rate is 10-30 per cent and CFR – 5 per cent. Abortion 30 per cent. Flabby bag syndrome – (Sudden drop milk syndrome) – Somatic cell counts are 10-75 per cent. Udder uniformly affected and resume milk production in 10-14 days. Leptospiruria is present in upto 30 per cent of affected cows.

Chronic Cases

Abortion and still births is more common in 6-12 weeks of gestation. Abortion storm – In midterm to lastterm pregnancy.

Pigs

Abortion occurs in 2-4 weeks of pregnancy.

Clinical Signs

Human

Incubation period is 4-14 days. Disease is biphasic in nature.

First Phase: Flu like fever, chills, myalgia, intense headache and become asymptomatic.

Second phase: Flu like signs with muscle pain, abdominal pain, vomition, exudates, rash, red eyes, renal failure, meningitis, liver damage, jaundice and highly lethal pulmonary haemorrahge.

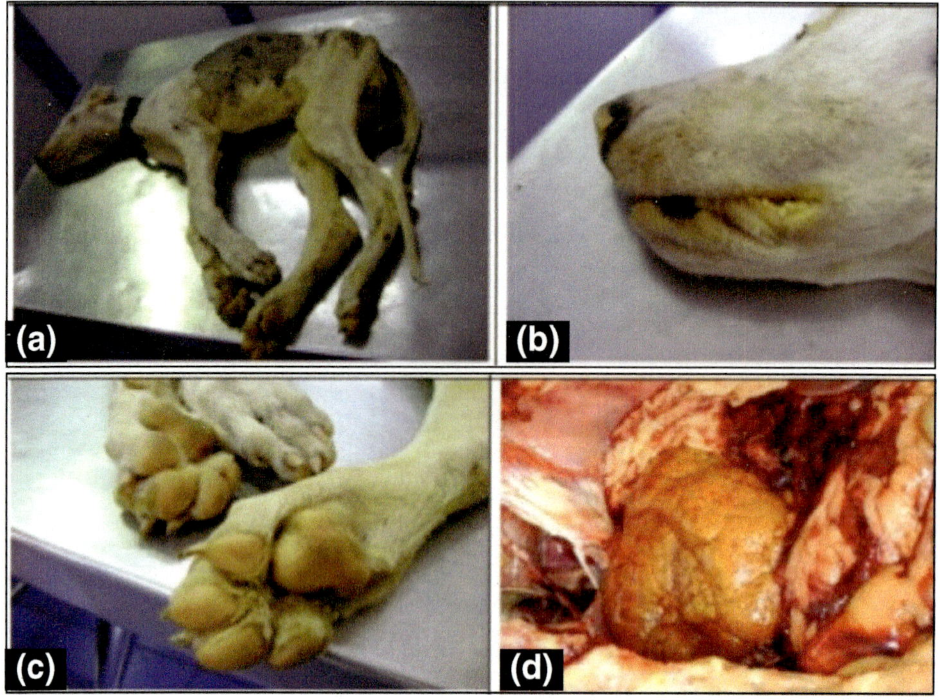

Figure 2.26

(a) Icteric dog with acute leptospirosis infection, (b) Icteric condition of the mucous membrane, (c) Icteric of the foot pad, (d) Liver after postmortem appears as icteric mottled.

Hypotension, irregular pulse-ECG reveals the type of arrythymia. Bleeding of vascular tubules and decreased platelets. Increased neck rigidity and cells in cerebrospinal fluid.

Necropsy Findings

Generalised pale and icteric carcass, enlargement of liver, Hepatitis, nephritis, placentitis and leathery placenta are seen.

Diagnosis

Diagnosis of leptospirosis depends on a good clinical and vaccination history and laboratory testing. Diagnostic tests for leptospirosis include those designed to detect antibodies against the organism and those designed to detect the organism in tissues or body fluids. Serologic testing is recommended in each case, combined with one or more techniques to identify the organism in tissue or body fluids.

Serologic assays are the most commonly used technique to diagnose leptospirosis in animals. The microscopic agglutination test (MAT) is most frequently used. It involves mixing appropriate dilutions of serum with live leptospires of serovars prevalent within the region. The presence of antibodies is indicated by the agglutination of the leptospires, with the reported titer being the highest dilution of serum that results in 50 per cent agglutination. The MAT is a complex test to perform and interpret, and it requires the maintenance of live leptospiral cultures. An ELISA test to diagnose canine leptospirosis is offered by a commercial laboratory in the USA. This test detects antibodies to LipL32, a membrane protein found on pathogenic leptospires. The currently available assay provides a qualitative negative or positive result and will also detect antibodies induced by vaccination. A comparison of this test to the MAT has not been reported, and it is likely that the numerical titers provided by the MAT will provide more diagnostically useful information than a qualitative ELISA.

Interpretation of serologic results from the MAT is complicated by a number of factors, including cross-reactivity of antibodies, antibody titers induced by vaccination, and lack of consensus about the level of antibody titer that indicates infection. Antibodies produced in an animal in response to infection with a given serovar of *Leptospira* often cross-react with other serovars. In some cases, these patterns of cross-reactivity are predictable based on the antigenic relatedness of the various serovars of *Leptospira*, but the patterns of cross-reactive antibodies vary between host species. Paradoxical reactions may occur with the MAT early in the course of an acute infection, with a marked agglutinating antibody response to a serovar other than the infecting serovar. In addition, there is evidence of lack of consistency between diagnostic laboratories. For these reasons, the infecting serovar in an individual animal cannot be reliably identified as the serovar to which the animal develops the highest titer. The real value of the MAT is in providing a numerical titer to allow comparison of acute and convalescent values.

Widespread vaccination of dogs and livestock with leptospiral vaccines also complicates interpretation of leptospiral serology. In general, vaccinated animals develop relatively low agglutinating antibody titers (1 : 100 to 1 : 400) in response to vaccination, and these titers persist for 1–4 mo after vaccination. However, some animals develop high titers after vaccination which persists for dikhuaaa 6 mo.

Consensus is lacking as to what constitutes a diagnostic titer for leptospiral infection. A low antibody titer does not necessarily exclude a diagnosis of leptospirosis, because titers are often low in acute disease and in maintenance host infections. In cases of acute leptospirosis, a 4-fold rise in antibody titer is often observed in paired serum samples collected 7–10 days apart. Diagnosis of leptospirosis based on a single serum sample should be made with caution and with full consideration of the clinical picture and vaccination history of the animal. In general, with a compatible clinical history and vaccination >3 mo ago, a titer of 1 : 800 to 1 : 1,600 is good presumptive evidence of leptospiral infection. The use of paired acute and convalescent titers is strongly recommended whenever possible. Antibody titers can persist for several months after infection and recovery, although there is usually a gradual decline with time.

Immunofluorescence can be used to identify leptospires in tissues, blood, or urine sediment. The test is rapid and has reasonable sensitivity, but interpretation requires a skilled laboratory technician. Immunohistochemistry is useful to identify leptospires in formalin-fixed tissue but, because there may be small numbers of organisms present in some tissues, the sensitivity of this technique is variable. A number of PCR procedures are available, and each laboratory may select a slightly different procedure. Unfortunately, few publications have confirmed the validity of all the commercially available PCRs, which likely vary considerably in their performance. PCR techniques allow detection of pathogenic leptospires in blood, urine, or tissue samples but do not determine the infecting serovar. Culture of blood, urine, or tissue specimens is the only method to definitively identify the infecting serovar. Blood may be cultured early in the clinical course; urine is more likely to be positive 7–10 days after clinical signs appear. Culture is rarely positive after antibiotic therapy has begun. Culture of leptospires requires specialized culture medium, the organisms are fastidious and slow-growing, and diagnostic laboratories rarely culture specimens for the presence of leptospires. Thus, culture is of little value to clinicians.

Kidney

Increased serum creatinine and blood urea nitrogen.

Liver

Serum bilirubin, with normal or mildly elevated SGPT, SGOT and CPK.

Lung

Chest X-ray shows lower and mid zone opacities. Molecular diagnosis by PCR.

Samples Collection

Acute phase: Liver, lung, brain, kidney, body fluids, blood, milk, cerebrospinal fluid, thoracic and peritoneal fluids.

Chronic phase: Urine, kidney, fetal fluid, uterine and other reproductive discharges.

Differential Diagnosis

Dengue fever, Haemorrhagice fever and Hepatitis. Viral meningitis, Malaria, Typhoid fever, Influenza and Parvo. Brucellosis, SMEDI, (Still birth, mummification, early embryonic death, and inferitility, *etc.*).

Prevention

Avoidance of exposure to free-ranging wildlife and domestic animals that may be maintenance hosts for *Leptospira* is difficult because rodents, raccoons, opossums, and skunks are frequently found in rural and urban environments. The cornerstone of leptospirosis prevention is vaccination with polyvalent inactivated vaccines. Immunity to leptospirosis is believed to be serovar specific and, therefore, vaccines are formulated for various species to include the relevant serovars. There are currently no leptospiral vaccines for horses. Leptospiral vaccines are generally designed and evaluated for the ability to prevent clinical signs of disease, although some vaccines have also been shown to significantly reduce renal colonization and urine shedding.

Treatment

Doxycycline 100mg/oral/every 12 hours period for one week. Penicillin 20,000 IU/kg bw for every 4 hours for one week. Doxycycline 200-250mg once a week in adult as a prophylaxis per oral. Dogs – penicillin- leptospiraemic phase and doxycycline eliminate the carrier status. Detoxification, hydro-electrolyte balance with glucose and salt solutions. Dialysis in serious cases must be done. K and P may be increased due to renal failure. Corticosteroid (eg.prednisolone 30-60 mg for 7-10 days).

Zoonotic Risk

People are susceptible to infection with most of the pathogenic serovars of *Leptospira* but are incidental hosts and, therefore, not important reservoirs of infection. Occupational exposure is a rick factor, and veterinarians, veterinary staff, livestock producers, and dairy workers are at increased risk. In addition, recreational exposure to waters contaminated with urine of domestic animals or wildlife presents a risk. Animal owners have contracted leptospirosis via contact with infected companion animals and livestock. The principal route of infection is contact with infectious body fluids (blood in acute cases or urine) via mucous membranes. In people, the disease varies from subclinical to severe and can be fatal when renal or hepatic failure occurs. The most common signs are fever, headaches, rash, ocular pain, myalgia, and malaise. Transplacental infection, abortion, and infection of infants via breast feeding have been described, making exposure of pregnant women of particular concern. Laboratory techniques are necessary for a definitive diagnosis. Because diagnosis of leptospirosis in animals is difficult based on clinical signs, veterinarians may wish to implement an infection control program in which animal body fluids are handled only with gloved hands and hand washing is routine. It is also essential for staff to take precautions when handling or nursing animals suspected or confirmed to have leptospirosis. Appropriate precautions include wearing gowns, shoe covers, and gloves to avoid contaminating exposed skin or spreading organisms. Face shields should be worn when handling wet bedding or cleaning cages, stalls, or runs to avoid contact of aerosolized organisms with mucous membranes.

2.28. Mastits

Synonyms

Mammitis, Inflammation de la ubre.

Almost any microbe that can opportunistically invade tissue and cause infection can cause mastitis. However, most infections are caused by various species of streptococci, staphylococci, and gram-negative rods, especially lactose-fermenting organisms of enteric origin, commonly termed coliforms. From an epidemiologic standpoint, the primary sources of infection for most pathogens may be regarded as contagious or environmental.

Except for *Mycoplasma* spp, which may spread from cow to cow through aerosol transmission and invade the udder subsequent to bacteremia, contagious pathogens are spread during milking by milkers' hands or the liners of the milking unit. Species that use this mode of transmission include *Staphylococcus aureus, Streptococcus agalactiae,* and *Corynebacterium bovis*. Most other species are opportunistic invaders from the cow's environment, although some other streptococci and staphylococci may also have a contagious component. Additionally, contagious transmission infrequently occurs for pathogens typically associated with environmental reservoirs, *e.g.*, through the development of host-adapted virulence factors (*Escherichia coli*) or by shedding of overwhelming numbers of bacteria from infected udders (*Trueperella* [formerly *Arcanobacterium*] *pyogenes*). Mastitis is an inflammation of the mammary gland. In which the milk undergo physical, chemical and microbiological changes where as mammary glandular tissue under go physical and pathological changes. In which infected milk colour, consistency change and contains more amount of leucocytes.

Etiology

Mastitis is caused majorly by *Staphylococcus, Streptococcus* and coliform bacteria and less importantly by other organism such as other bacteria, viruses, and fungus.

Epidemiology

Prevalence of Infection

Mastitis due to staphylococcus, streptococcus infection is more prevalent in India. Mastitis is prevailing in dairy animals. Greater risk occurs in 10-12 per cent of individuals herds. Clinical mastitis increases with increasing parity.

Economic Impact

It is one of the most economically important diseases of dairy cows. The economic loss occurs due to reduction in milk, changes in quality milk and milk products. In addition, disqualification of dairy cow due to chronic mastitis.

Predisposing Factors

Stages of lactation, Milking condition, Genetic factors, Poor hygiene, Hybrid animals.

Source of Infection

S. agalactiae and *S. aureus* resides primarily in the udder of infected cows. Exposure to uninfected quarters is limited to milking process. *Strepoccus uberis, S. dysgalactiae* and coliforms are normal inhabitants of the cows environment.

Transmission

Invasion through teat canal pore. Through milkers hands. Through ingestion of infected material from environment. Fly biting influences the entry of organism. Contact occur at any time during the life of the cows including milking time between milking dry period prior to first calving in heifers.

Host Affected

Cows, buffaloes, sheep, goats, pigs, horses are highly susceptible for mastitis. Heavily producing cows are mostly susceptible than less producers.

Pathogenesis

Infection occurs mainly through teat canal pore. The set up of infection occurs in two stages: 1. Invasion stage and 2. Infective stage. Invasive stage: In which, organism enter through teat canal and reaches the mammary tissue. *Streptococci* enters the epithelium of the ducts develops inflammation and promotes in turn the development of many folds of granulation tissue under the epithelium and become polypoid swelling. In the epithelium some of the organisms are destroyed by immune cells, neutrophils and all other remaining organism causes oedema in the interstitial tissues and leads to infiltration in the lymphatics. The epithelial acini vacuolated and desquamated and forms fibrosis due to accumulation of eexudates. In advance and severe cases of mastitis, secretion through teats ceases. Udder become hard indurated due to inflammation of interalveolar tissues and retention of secretion which results in collapse of acini and granulation of tissues followed by filling of interstitial space with large number of lymphocytes. Finally, udder is small, hard and is called shrunken udder. There is no regeneration of glandular tissue occurs in severe cases of mastitis. Infective stages: At this stage, bacteria undergo multiplication and causes damage to udder tissues. In acute cases, infection set up toxaemia and leads to death. Affected udder is hard, swollen, and painful in surviving animals. Milk becomes scanty with blood. The diffusion of bacterial toxins in to other unaffected quarters leads to infection. Gangrene develops as the infection progress in to blood vessel and causes thrombosis. At this time, the udder become cold, and becomes greenish or bluish in color. Pits on pressure and edema are noticed at the side of the flank. The accumulation of gas in the affected area produces crackling sound on palpation. In mild cases, necrotic foci appear and are surrounded by fibrotic tissues. Granulomatous lesions develop. Summer mastitis is caused by Corynebacterium pyogenes. More pus produced in abscess. Fistula develops and discharges pus to the exterior which leads to necrosis and sloughing.

Clinical Signs

Per acute form: Pyrexia, anorexia, respiratory distress, swollen, hot and painful udder. Cessation od milk production. Exudate is often blood stained. Mostly, *Staph. aureus, Str. dysgalactiae, Cory. pyogenes, E. coli,* and *P. aerugenosa.*

(a) **Acute form**: Swollen udder, changes in quality of milk. Milk becomes curd like, yellow, brown fluid with flakes and clots.

(b) **Subacute form**: No changes in the udder tissue.

(c) **Chronic form**: Udder is haemorrhagic, and fibrotic. Swollen and palpable supra mammary lymphnode. Udder is thick, firm, nodular and atrophic, yellowish or white fluid with clots and flakes.

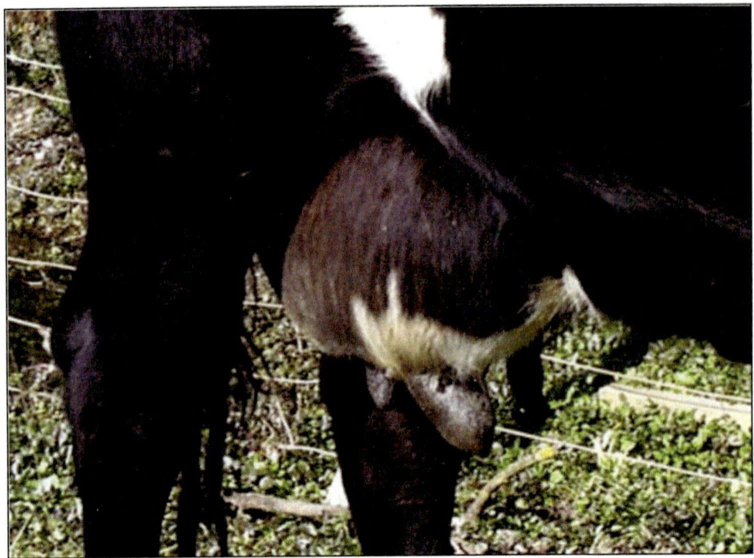

Figure 1.27. Mastitis swollen udder.

Zoonosis

Mastitis milk is unsuitable for public consumption because many diseases such as tuberculosis, brucellosis, staphylococcal infection, streptococcal sore throat, scarlet fever and gastroenteritis are spread through milk to human beings.

Necropsy Findings

In severely affected dead animals necrotic foci appears which is surrounded by fibrous tissues. Granulomatous lesion is seen. In summer mastitis, abscess, fistula and discharged pus to the exterior and sloughing leads to loss of quarters are observed.

Diagnosis

Physical examination of the udder. Tests done for the milk abnormalities: Strip cup test. Bromothymol Blue Test (BTB). Bromocresol purple test. Chloride test. California mastitis test. White side test. Catalase test.

Direct Test

Isolation and identification of the organisms. Cultural examinations. Biochemical test. Animal inoculation test. Serological test. Miscellaneous tests. Electrical conductivity test. Radial immune diffusion test. Milk antitrypsin assay.

Differential Diagnosis

Various types of mastitis:*Staphylococcal mastitis, Coliform mastitis, Summer mastitis, Mycoplsmal mastitis,Nocardial mastitis, Pseudomonas mastitis, Anaerobic mastitis.*

Treatment

Stripping out the milk from the infected quarters. Cleaning of infected quarters with normal saline and distilled water. Infusion of antibiotic therapies immediately after the infection. Contineuos use for antibiotics as per the antibiogram. Combination of drugs may be used for better remedy. The following combination of drugs can be used as based on the stages of mastitis with antibiogram results. Penicillin and its derivatives, Streptopenicillin, Oxtetracycline, Gentamycin, Cloxacillin, Lincomycin, Neomycin, Cotrimoxazole and Enroflaxacin. Antipyretics and anti-inflammatory drugs can be used as per the exudatest. Antihistamin can be used. Application of astringents over udder tissues to reduce the swelling. Intravenous therapy using normal saline or dextrose saline solutions to reduce the toxic level in the blood. In non-responsive cases animal should be dried out. It is done by infusing 30-60 ml of 3 per cent silver nitrate solution, or 20 ml of 5 per cent copper sulphate.

Prevention and Control

Use of inactivated vaccine containing *Str. agalactiae, Str. uberis, Staph. pyogenes, Staph. aureus* and *E. coli* in some countries. Reduction of time of infection. Treatment and drying off quarters. Immediate treatment of affected animals. Culling of non-responding animals. Control of development of new infection. Dipping of quarter with disinfectant. Personal hygiene of the milk man before milking. Seggregation of infected animals and proper treatment based on the antibiogram. Routine disposal of the soiled exudates and thorough cleaning of shed using disinfectants.

2.29. Ulcerative Lymphangitis

Synonyms

Big leg.

In horses, *Corynebacterium pseudotuberculosis* causes ulcerative lymphangitis (an infection of the lower limbs) and chronic abscesses in the pectoral region and ventral abdomen. It is one of the most common and economically important infectious diseases of horses in California and Texas and is increasing in prevalence in other western and Midwestern states of the USA. In cattle, the bacteria most commonly cause cutaneous excoriated granulomas. Large, ulcerative skin lesions resembling infected granulation tissue and lymphangitis may occur in 2 per cent –5 per cent of cows. Location on the animal is variable but is often associated with skin trauma.

Healing often occurs without treatment or with limited topical treatment in 2–4 weeks. Abortion and mastitis may also occur. Rarely, visceral involvement has been reported.

It is characterized by the development of cutaneous form of pyo-granulomatous abscess in sub-cutis, mastitis, and internal abscessation, a necrotic and ulcerative dermatitis on the heel of the foot. Lesions are restricted to limbs. Edema and lameness of the affected limb noticed.

Etiology

The disease is caused by *Corynebacterium pseudotuberculosis* biotype-2. It is a saprophytic and intracellular organism. Biotypes causing ulcerative lymphangitis in cattle and horses are not the same biotype that causing caseous lymphadenitis in sheep and goats. They are gram-positive and catalase positive, non-spore forming, non-motile, rod-shaped bacteria that are straight or slightly curved. The bacteria group together in a characteristic way, which has been described as the form of a "V", "palisades", or "Chinese letters". They may also appear elliptical. They are aerobic or facultative anaerobic, chemo-organotrophs, with a 51–65 per cent genomic G:C content. They are pleomorphic through out their life cycle. They come in various lengths and frequently have thickenings at either end, depending on the surrounding conditions. Their size falls between 2-6 micrometers in length and 0.5 micrometers in diameter.

Epidemiology

Prevelence of Infection

The disease affects the ability of the horses. It is the most important disease of North Africa, Israel and Asia. Generally, the morbidity rate is 5 per cent but during epidemic period the morbidity recorded was found as 5-35 per cent and culling mortality rate is 16 per cent.

Economic Impact

The loss usually associated with a increased culling rates, a decrease in milk production and changes in quality of the bulk tank milk due to increase in somatic cell count.

Predispoing Factors

Unhygienic and wet conditions predispose animals to infection, particularly of the lower legs and ventral region.

Sources of Infection

Arthropod vectors such as *Habronema* spp. larva and stable flies and contact with fomites such as contaminated soil and grooming equipment.

Transmission

Sporadic form of cutaneous ulcerative lymphangitis and outbreak form occurs during the summer months of the year and is correlated to the prevalence of house flies. The bacteria probably enter via skin wounds including IM injections, arthropod

Source of Infection

Aspergillus has been isolated from placenta of aborted cows, uterine discharge of repeat breeder and semen of bull. Mouldy, damp food and moist grains are conducive for growth of *Aspergillus*. Spores liberated in large numbers from infected eggs opened at incubation or hatching. Contaminated feed or poultry house litter acts as source of infection. Wet litters favour the growth of spores and present in aerosol when litters are dried. Spores liberated in large numbers from infected eggs opened at incubator hatchery. Contaminated feed or poultry house litter acts as source of infection. Wet litters favour the growth of spores and present in aerosol when litters are dried.

Transmission

Human, animals and birds contract infection through inhalation and ingestion of *Aspergillus* spores present in the aerosol. Infection occurs by inhalation of spores. Infection may also spread through abraded skin, mucous membrane and set up lesions in the embedded organs and systems. Direct transmission from animal to animal and to human is not reported.

Host Affected

Cattle, buffaloes, sheep, goats, birds, and human beings are affected. All birds are susceptible for infection. Chicken, turkeys, ducks, quails are mainly affected.

Pathogenesis

Aspergillus species are responsible for respiratory infection. In birds, acute Aspergillosis is known as "Brooder pneumonia" and causes heavy mortality in them. *Aspergillus* is incapable of utilizing keratin, normally they do not establish infection on skin but able to penetrate the skin through epithelial defects and thus capable of establishing infection on subcutaneous tissue to develops chronic suppurative granulomas. Fungi may disseminate to other organs and systems through haematogeonus route. Even the fungi infects placenta and leading to placentitis and mycotic abortion, skin of some cases may also show gramulomatous changes. *Aspergillus* are not highly pathogenic and may not produce clinical signs, however, due to some predisposing factors such as prolonged use of antibiotics and corticosteroids, exposure to radiation, neoplastic diseases, malnutrition and tuberculosis makes the animals more prone for infection.

Brooder Pneumonia

Conidia present in aerosol or environment spread through conjunctival, nasal, tracheal, para bronchial and air sac epithelium and form discrete, granulomas of 1-15 mm diameter, containing white plaques or nodules at these sites. It may have necrotic centre with dichotomous branching septate of 4-7 µm diameter hyphae. Older lesions contain pleomorphic hyphae upto 12 µm in diameter but are confused with zygomycotic infections. Older lesions in air filled centres appear as green to black due to development of pigmented fungal conidiophores. Fungi tend to proliferate with in the granuloma and rarely invade adjacent tissues in umiga competent birds.

Chronic

In turkeys often pulmonary blood flow impeded by enlarging pulmonary granulomas and this cause right ventricular dilatation or ascites. In chronically infected bird's accumulation of umigate in the trachea or syrinx producing acute respiratory embarrassment. After inhalation, spores are disseminated rapidly through haematogenous route to other tissues and cause lesions in brain, pericardium, bone marrow and kidneys, *etc.* Lesions in m eninges, leading to large superficial white plaques over the caudal cerebral cortex and in umiga and iris leading to fungal ophthalmitis and iridocyclitis.

Clinical Signs

(a) **Pulmonary form**: Granulomatous pneumonia is the feature of this form in man and animals. High temperature, accelerated shallow breathing, grunting and groaning, nasal discharge and moist type of cough are the signs of pulmonary form. A chronic disease with respiratory complications and not responding to normal therapy should be suspected for aspergillosis. Pneumonia is the cardinal sign.

(b) **Myocardial form**: It is a fatal condition in human beings debilitated by cytotoxic or umiga-suppressive drugs and is rarely seen in animals.

(c) **Allergic form**: Inhalation of spores of *A. umigates* causes high temperature, asthma, malaise and prostration.

(d) **Otomycotic form**: *A. umigates* grow in cerumen and debris of ear canal in human and produces otorrhoea with foul odored exudation. Dogs may also suffer from this form.

(e) **Cellulolytic form**: Found to produce cellulitis of face and corneal region.

(f) **Cerebral form**: Rarely meningitis, meningo-encephalitis and paralysis set up in central nervous system infection.

(g) **Abortive form**: It is more common in adult cow, mare and ewe. From the lungs the fungi traverse the haematogenous route and from there it reaches the gravid uterus in 3rd month of pregnancy. Expulsion of aborted dead fetus, retained placenta and sometimes the aborted fetus born with cutaneous Aspergillosis.

(h) **Toxic form**: Mycotoxicosis is a very acute, fatal disease of birds, animals, human produce patent toxin known as aflatoxin $B_{1,}B_{2,}G_{1,}G_{2,}M_{1,}M_{2.}$ *A. flavus* produces toxins known as "flavotoxins". Toxins are produced in aspergillus affected corns and cereals. Consumption of these toxins through feed, fodder and forage cause toxicosis in birds, animals, human beings, cattle, sheep, pigs and mortality. Vascular haemorrhages, hepatic necrosis, proliferation of bile duct and umigate. Fungal toxicosis causes the reduction in growth rate and lower feed efficiency.

Cattle

Clinical signs develop in 15 days, slight cough to umigat breathing, bloody and foul smelling umigate.

Horse

Infection restricted to nasal sinuses and umigate pouches.

Sheep

Catarrhal pneumonia, death usually occurs long time after infection, conidiophores present in sputum and in discrete, calcified nodules (1-7mm dia) in lungs.

Pigs

The aspergillosis is rare in pigs, in affected pigs, persistent cough with lobar pneumonia.

Wiild Animals

Pneumonia and respiration problems.

Brooder Pneumonia

Mortality in infected flocks may be biphasic. Acute respiratory disease causes 5-50 per cent mortality in first 1-3 wks of age of birds. Chronic pulmonary insufficiency, ascites, blindness, neurological fungal metastasis causes up to 5 per cent mortality.

At Hatchery

In first 3-5 days neonates are dyspnoeic, ploypnoeic and open mouth breathing/ gasping due to progressive air way obstruction.

Adult Birds

Birds remain sub clinically infected for sometimes. Slow progressive respiratory embarrassment. Increase body weight, demands on reduced functional pulmonary mass. Asphyxiated due to blockage of syrinx or the trachea.

Necropsy Findings

Thick crusted cutaneous lesions formed on the head, ears and neck. In asymptomatic pulmonary aspergillosis a small grey, raised lesions develop in lungs. Acute mycotic pneumonia will show blood tinged fluid in pleural cavity and fibrinous pneumonia. The abortive form will produce necrotizing placentitis with yellow grey colored cotyledons. Necrotic cotyledons with leathery appearance of placenta showed are suspected for mycotic abortion in cattle.

Cattle

Sub-pleural nodules and interlobular emphysema. Inflammation in small intestine. Generalised interstitial haemorrhage is a typical feature and in lungs centres of heaptization without nodule formation.

Horses

Nodule formation in lungs, involvement of meninges and interstitial haemorrhage with caseous nodules in the kidneys.

Sheep

Bluish-grey nodules are surrounded by narrow haemorrhagic zone in lambs (2-3 mm dia). Bronchitis, granulomatous lesion in lungs of a day old lamb which indicates the develop of disease in utero.

Pigs

Nodule formation in lungs, spleen and kidney enlarged and congested, nodule formation in mesenteric lymphndoes.

Wild Animals

Miliary nodule formation in lungs and through out viscera. Tumor like growths containing hyphae in conchal, ethmoid bones and in lungs arise.

Brooder Pneumonia

Lesions in meninges, leading to large superficial white plaques over the caudal cerebral cortex and in umiga and iris leading to fungal ophthalmitis and iridocyclitis.

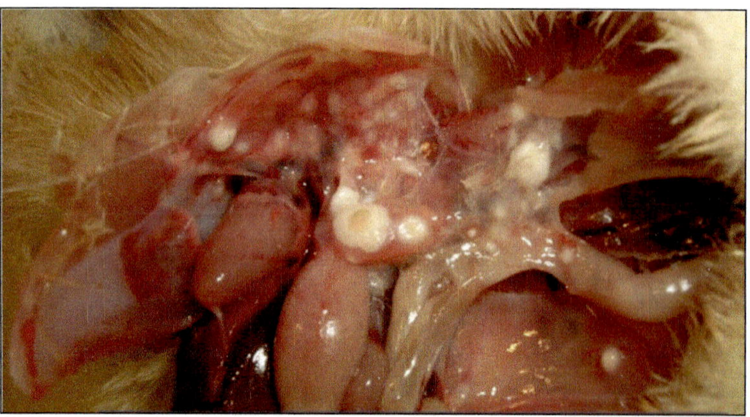

Figure 3.1. Aspergillosis in the air sacs of a chick.

Diagnosis

Based on clinical signs, and necropsy findings. Isolation of organism by culture: Direct culture of eexudates can be done. Glucose peptone chloramphenicol slants incubating at room temperature. Microscopic examination will reveal presence of Aspergillus mycelia. Suspected specimen can also be cultured in Sabouraud's dextrose agar containing antibiotics but not cyclohexamide. Rapidly growing flat white fuzzy colonies will be observed. Antigen of *A. umigates* is commercially available and is used in human skin test and several serological tests have been made against invasive and wide spreaded aspergillosis. Bronchi, bronchioles and alveoli of lungs may reveal the presence of mycelia, fibrin, leukocytes, Langhan's giant cells, exudative cellular inflammation with penetrative mycelia may be present. In the necrotic areas neutrophils may aggregate around clumps of hypae.

Differential Diagnosis

Brucellosis, campylobacteriosis, leptospirosis, tuberculosis, sporotrichosis, candidiasis, coccidioidomycosis, histoplasmosis.

Brooder Pneumonia

Based on clinical signs and necropsy findings. Identification of organism: Examination of branched septate Aspergillus hyphae. Add one or two drops of 10 per cent KOH in smears taken from lesions and heat it gently and examine under microscope. Routine observation of hyphae stained with H and E. Periodic Acid Schiff special fungal stain, Grocott's Methenamine Silver (GMS) stain or Calcofluor white. Demonstration of Conidiospore morphology and speciation made from (granuloma or plaques) culture grown in Sabourauds Dextrose Agar with Antibiotics.

Differential Diagnosis

Other fungal diseases, *Coliform* infection, *Staphylococcal* infection, *Salmonella* infection, chronic bacterial pneumonia.

Treatment

No effective treatment is available against aspergillosis of birds, animals and human. Control depends on reducing exposure to fungus. Eggs should be collected and stored so as to reduce sweating and exposure to spore laden dust. Hatchery equipment and air ducts should be cleaned, disinfected and monitored by cultures. Brooding house, wet or previously wet litter or soil, mouldy or dusty feeds avoided. Feed, water lines, soil should be disinfected. Amphotericin B Injectable lotions 3 per cent daily for long treatment. Clinafarm (Griseofulvin, Fulcin, Fulvicin, Griseo 100)- 7.5 per cent Powder feed additive bolus, liquid powder-Foal- 15 mg D kg D day 2–4 weeks and for Pony- 10 mg D kg D day 1–2 weeks.

Prevention

No successful immunization method has so far been developed against this mycotic problem.

Control

The spores of Aspergilli remain as potential threat to animals. All attempts should be made to prevent proliferation of umigates in animals' sheds on surroundings. Methods of sterilization, sanitation and good management practices may be adopted to control this fungal infection. Richard *et al.*, 1984 used a vaccine prepared from spores, germinated spores, mycelium and cultured filtrates of *A. fumigatus* and injected in birds via aerosol method for immunization was found not sufficient enough for protection.

3.2. Candidiasis

Synonyms

Moniliasis, Thrush, Candidiasis, crop mycosis and Oidiomycosis.

Candidiasis is a localized mucocutaneous disease caused by species of the yeast-like fungus *Candida*, most commonly *C. albicans*. It is distributed worldwide in a variety of animals. *C. albicans* is a normal inhabitant of the nasopharynx, GI tract, and external genitalia of many species of animals and is opportunistic in causing disease. Factors associated with candidal infections are disruption of mucosal integrity; indwelling, intravenous, or urinary catheters; administration of antibiotics; and immunosuppressive drugs or diseases. The organism most frequently infects birds, in which it involves the oral mucosa, esophagus, and crop. Superficial infections limited to the mucous membranes of the intestinal tract have been described in pigs and foals. Systemic candidiasis has also been described in cattle, calves, sheep, and foals secondary to prolonged antibiotic or corticosteroid therapy. In cats, candidiasis is rare but has been associated with oral and upper respiratory disease, pyothorax, ocular lesions, intestinal disease, and urocystitis. Infections are rare in dogs and horses. However, *Candida* spp have been considered a cause of arthritis in horses and mastitis and abortion in cattle. Fungemia and *Candida* peritonitis have been noted in dogs with perforating intestinal lesions after surgery, and mucosal and cutaneous candidiasis has been noted in immunosuppressed dogs and in dogs with diabetes mellitus. It is a fungal disease caused by yeast, *Candida albicans*, and has been manifested by the development of mucocutaneous mycoses in skin, hair and nail. More commonly superficial infection such as oral thrush, vaginitis and life threatening candidemia in animals and human as well. Oesophageal or Crop Candidiasis occurs very frequently but clinical signs are rarely exhibited by the affected birds. Candida organisms mainly affect birds below 3 weeks of age but cause low to nil mortality.

Etiology

The genus candida comprises 150 various species. Candida albicans is the most pathogenic species followed by *C. tropicalis, C. labrata, C. krusei, C. parapsilosis, C. dubliniensis* in human. *Candida* is small, oval, thin walled dimorphic, budding type yeast like cells (blastospheres), measuring 2-6 mm, 3-5 mμm dia, most frequently causes crop mycosis, found on epithelial surfaces and deeper tissues as a branching septate hyphae or pseudohyphae. Less frequently caused by *Oidium pullorum* and *Candida krusei*. Candida species are ubiquitous in the environment.

Epidemiology

Predisposing Factors

Continued use of antibiotics, corticosteroids, vitamin A and B deficiency and high level of glucose in diet. External use of detergents or douches or internal disturbances by hormone can disturb the normal vaginal flora such as *Lactobacilli.* Pregnancy and use of oral contraceptives are considered as risk factors in human. Diabetes mellitus, HIV, AIDS, mononucleosis, cancer therapy and stress. Wearing of wet swim wears also increases the incidence of yeast infections.

Transmission

Infected feces loaded with organisms spread the disease. Man acquires the infection by eating contaminated meat and food. Human acquires the infection through in-utero and venereal contact.

Host Affected

Chickens, turkeys, cattle, buffaloes, horses, goats, sheep, pigs, dogs, cats, including human are susceptible to infection.

Pathogenesis

Animals

The candida species produces the enzyme known as leucine amino peptidase which causes damage to the tissues and thereby induce the development of disease. The presence of high levels of antibiotics, maltose and dextrose cause cutaneous and systemic mycoses in pigs and candida endometritis in mares, panleukopenia in cats due to repeated use of antibiotics. The organism also invades the vital organs and set up mmunea, pneumonia, nephritis, endocarditis, mastitis, repeat breeding and abortion. The organism can be isolated from semen, aborted materials, uterine mucus of repeat breeders and mastitis milk and from the environment.

Poultry

The organisms lives in mouth, oesophagus and crop as a normal resident and also acquired by ingestion. Inhibition of normal microflora and immunosuppression allow the yeast to invade and proliferate on the superficial epithelial layers which results in development of epithelial hyperplasia, pseudo or diptheritic membrane formation. Crop appears to have a sticky and adhesive multifocal, confluent mats of white cheesy materials which may be found less in oesophagus and pharynx. Severely affected birds may have ulcers otherwise very mild inflammatory response will be seen in mucosal candidiasis. Inflammatory response to mucosal candidiasis is mild unless ulceration is prolonged.

Clinical Signs

(a) **Mucocutaneous form:** The tongue, gums, buccal mucosa of the infected animals are filled up with whitish creamy pseudomembranous mmunea which contains yeast cells are known as thrush.

(b) **Cutaneous form**: Thrush in rumen, sub-clinical and acute mastitis, anorexia, lameness, and decrease milk yield may be developed in adult cattle. In calves, gastroenteritis, profuse watery mmunea, anorexia, dehydration and death noticed. Mycotic mastitis and abortion in cows and buffaloes are produced. In pigs, lesions from mouth, esophagus, skin and stomach may spread from vagina of pregnant and non pregnant sows.

Human

Both in children and adults lesions in interdigital space, intra-mammary folds, groins and axillae could be seen. The skin and nails of the whole body of the human are affected. In children and adult lesions found in interdigital space, intramammary folds, groins and axillae. Itching is a very important signs.

Systemic Form

Cattle and calves suffer from inflammation of the stomach and intestine and leads to profuse watery mmunea.

Poultry

Candidiasis is the most common infection, nevertheless, clinical signs seen in severely infected birds. Birds having infection in superficial region of oral cavity, oesophageal and crop become dehydrated and fail to gain body weight. *Candida* spp. invade into nervous system, renal, intestinal area but rarely shows symptoms.

Necropsy Findings

Pseudomembranes and diptheritic membranes in the crop, oesophagus and mouth are highly suggestive of candidiasis but can be produced after ingestion of caustic substances, trichothecare mycotoxicosis and in severe cases oral trichomoniasis. Visualization of hyphae and pseudohyphae microscopically in hair and/or scrapings. Histological section will confirm diagnosis.

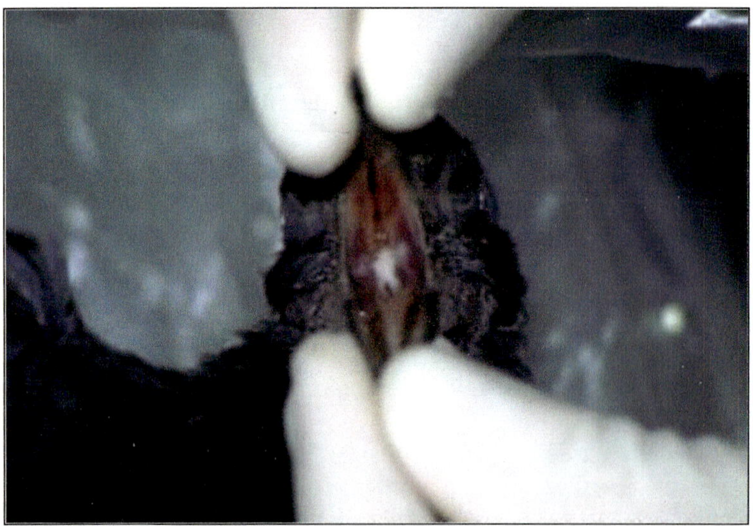

Figure 3.2. Candidiasis oral plague in pigeon.

Diagnosis

Based on clinical signs and necropsy findings. Animal Inoculation: In mice and rabbit One ml antigen in 15ml saline solution is suspended and injected intravenously or intra peritoneally causes death in a rabbit within 4-5 days of injection because of the abscess formation in kidney. The kidney smear show budding cells. Antigen and antibody detection by mmune-diffussion, counter mmune-electrophoresis, tube and latex agglutination test can be done to detect candidia antibody. Speciation requires culture in Sabouraudes dextrose agar but many normal birds may be positive.

Sample Collection

Hair, pus discharges, swab from tissue lesions, blood and serum.

Differential Diagnosis

Histoplasmosis, other mycotic infection.

Treatment

Most candidial infections respond to the treatment with antibiotics. The commonly used antifungal drugs are topical Clotrimazole, Nystatin, Fluconazole and Ketoconazole. Diflucan (Fluconazole): A single dose of 150mg tablet/oral give 90 per cent control in a vaginal yeast infection. (It is also essential to take care of persons allergic for azole group of medicines). It is only useful for vaginal yeast infection. In hospitalized patients, Amphotericin B, Caspofungin or voriconazole can be used. Local treatment with vaginal suppositories or medicated douches. Gentian violet used for breastfeeding thrush, but when used large quantities it can cause mouth and throat ulcerations in nursing babies, and has been linked to mouth cancer in humans and to cancer in the digestive tract of other animals.

3.3. Histoplasmosis

Synonyms

Epizootic Lymphangitis, Pseudo-glanders, Equine blastomycosis, and Equine histoplasmosis.

Histoplasmosis is a chronic, noncontagious, disseminated, granulomatous disease of people and other animals caused by the dimorphic fungus *Histoplasma capsulatum*. The organism is commonly found in soil that contains bird and bat manure. It produces ibropl growth in the soil and in culture at room temperature and grows in a yeast form in tissues and in cultures at 37°C. Histoplasmosis is found worldwide. Endemic areas in the USA include the Mississippi and Ohio River valleys. Infection has been described in many animal species, but disease is uncommon to rare in all but dogs and cats. Infection is commonly via aerosol contamination of the respiratory tract, and the lungs and thoracic lymph nodes are the sites of primary infection, although the GI tract may be a primary site of infection, especially in dogs. The organisms enter the bloodstream from a primary focus and become disseminated throughout the body; they may localize in bone marrow or the eyes, where they produce chorioretinitis or endophthalmitis. It is a chronic, fungal disease affecting different species of animals and persists for 3-12 months. It is a zoonotic disease.

Etiology

It is caused by a dimorphic fungus, *Histoplasma capsulatum*. Gram-positive, yeast like cells with a characteristic double walled capsule are easily found in discharges. Organisms are located both intracellularly and extracellularly in giant cells and macrophages.

Epidemiology

Prevalence of Infection

The course of the disease is prolonged with mortality rate of 10-15 per cent. Disease occurs as outbreak during winter when large numbers of horse are gathered together for military or other purposes. It is a rare systemic mycosis of farm animals such as horses, cattle and pigs occurs with a high prevalence in specific geographic localities. Its occurrence has been noticed in parts of Iran, Asia, India, Northern Africa, and the Mediterranean littoral.

Source of Infection

The fungus is able to survive for the period as long as 4 months in soil and water. Bedding, grooming, utensils, horse blankets or harness acts as medium for spread of infection. Both animate and inanimate objects and environment gain access into abrasions in lower limbs.

Transmission

Infection generally occurs by inhalation of contaminated dust. Direct contact with bedding, grooming, utensils, horse blankets or harness acts as conduit for spreading infection. Fungal spores carried in both animate and inanimate objects and environment gain access into abrasions in lower limbs. The isolation of organism from alimentary tract of biting flies indicates that the biting flies also contribute the spread of infection.

Host Affected

Affects solipede animals such as horse, donkeys and mules. The disease rarely affects cattle and camels.

Pathogenesis

Histoplasmosis is the most common cause of mediastinitis and these remains as a relatively rare disease. Severe infections can cause hepatospleenomegally and lymphadenopathy. Lesions have a tendency to calcify as they heal. Ocular histoplasmosis causes damage to the retina of the eyes. Scar tissue is left on the retina which can experience leakage, resulting in a loss of vision not unlike macular degeneration. This lung infection develops gradually over several weeks, causing a cough and increased difficulty breathing. Symptoms include weight loss, a mild fever, and a general feeling of illness.

Clinical Signs

Initially, lesions are ulcerative, suppurative, pyogranulomatous dermatitis and in many cases lymphangitis developed.

Ocular Form

Keratitis, conjunctivitis, sinusitis and pneumonia occur in other form of the disease. Lesions usually develop on the limbs, particularly about the hocks, and may be present on the back sides of neck, vulva and scrotum. Occasionally lesions appear on the nasal mucosa, inside the nostrils without involving nasal septum. An indolent ulcer develops at the portal of entry making its appearance several weeks to 3 months after infection occurs. A spreading dermatitis, lymphangitis is evident as corded lymphatic with intermittent nodules develops. Nodules rupture and discharge thick creamy pus. Local lymphnodes also enlarged and can rupture. Thickening of the skin in the areas and general swelling of the whole limb is common but with painless lesions.

Pulmonary Signs

Fever, pneumonia, chronic cough, nasal discharge, lethargy, dyspnoea, tachypnoea and pleural effusion are seen.

Extrapulmonary Signs

Ocular discharge, ophthalmitis, wasting, abscess formation, icterus, ibropla, lymphnadenitis, hepatic insufficiency with jaundice and anasarca, placentitis, abortion, widespread lesions in neonates especially in foals.

Zoonosis

Infection is transmissible to human beings. Upon entry in to wounds, the fungus invades subcutaneous tissues and develop a local granuloma/ulcers and from there spread along the lymphatic vessels. Ocular form of disease ensues due to injection of organism into eyes by biting flies.

Necropsy Findings

Pulmonary consolidation and granulomatous pneumonia, enlargement of splanchnic lymphnodes. Gross enlargement of liver containing necrotic foci observed. Lesions are usually confined to the skin, subcutaneous tissues lymphatic vessels and lymphnodes. Granulomatous lesions may be found in lungs, liver and spleen. Histological lesions are quite characteristic and consist of pyogranulomatous inflammation with ibroplasias.

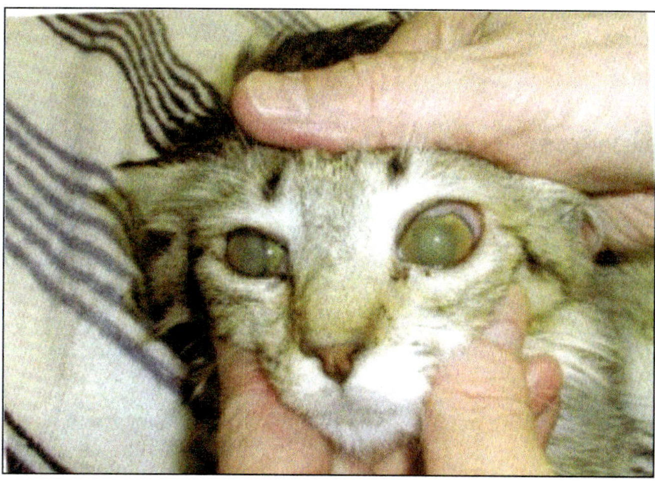

Figure 3.3. Histoplasmosis in cat.

Diagnosis

Based on clinical signs and necropsy findings. For screening the herd, histoplasmin skin test appears satisfactory. *Mullein test is negative but a sterile filtrate of a culture of H. capsulatum var farciminosum, has been used in a cutaneous sensitivity test. Radiography:* Miliary nodules. *Immunology:* CFT, Latex agglutination test. FAT. Antibody to *H. capsulatum var farciminosum* are detectable in serum before or at the time of development of lesions. BUN level should be judged because BUN level should not be exceed 75 mg per cent.

Sample Collection

Sample should be collected in a solution containing 500 units/ml penicillin.

Differential Diagnosis

Glanders. Ulcerative Lymphangitis. Sporotrichosis.

Treatment

Parentral Iodides are as effective in some cases as amphotericin-B. Sodium Iodide is administered as a 10 per cent solution at 1ml/5kg intra-venously once weekly for 4 weeks. Amphotericin B is the drug of choice 0.125 to 0.25ng/lb b.w. slowly intra-venously every 48 hours 3 treatment or 0.1 per cent solution in 5 per cent dextrose slow intra-venously as the drug is nephrotoxic. Supportive treatment with sodium bicarbonate, B vitamins and analgesic is done.

3.4. Aflatoxicosis

Aflatoxins are produced by toxigenic strains of *Aspergillus flavus* and *A. parasiticus* on peanuts, soybeans, corn (maize), and other cereals either in the field or during storage when moisture content and temperatures are sufficiently high for mold growth. Usually, this means consistent day and night temperatures >70°F. The toxic response and disease in mammals and poultry varies in relation to species, sex, age, nutritional status, and the duration of intake and level of aflatoxins in the ration. Earlier recognized disease outbreaks called "moldy corn toxicosis," "poultry hemorrhagic syndrome," and "*Aspergillus* toxicosis" may have been caused by aflatoxins. Aflatoxicosis occurs in many parts of the world and affects growing poultry (especially ducklings and turkey poults), young pigs, pregnant sows, calves, and dogs. Adult cattle, sheep, and goats are relatively resistant to the acute form of the disease but are susceptible if toxic diets are fed over long periods. Experimentally, all species of animals tested have shown some degree of susceptibility. Dietary levels of aflatoxin (in ppb) generally tolerated are dikhu 50 in young poultry, dikhu100 in adult poultry, dikhu 50 in weaner pigs, dikhu200 in finishing pigs, <50 in dogs, <100 in calves, and <300 in cattle. Approximately two times the tolerable levels stated is likely to cause clinical disease, including some mortality. Dietary levels as low as 10–20 ppb result in measurable metabolites of aflatoxin (aflatoxin M_1 and M_2) being excreted in milk; feedstuffs that contain aflatoxins should not be fed to dairy cows. Acceptable regulatory values in milk may range from 0.05 ppb to 0.5 ppb in different countries; individual state or federal regulatory agencies should be consulted when contamination occurs. Aflatoxins are metabolized in the liver to an epoxide that binds to macromolecules, especially nucleic acids and nucleoproteins. Their toxic effects include mutagenesis due to alkylation of nuclear DNA, carcinogenesis, teratogenesis, reduced protein synthesis, and immunosuppression. Reduced protein synthesis results in reduced production of essential metabolic enzymes and structural proteins for growth. The liver is the principal affected organ. High dosages of aflatoxins result in hepatocellular necrosis; prolonged low dosages result in reduced growth rate, immunosuppression, and liver enlargement.

Mycotoxicoses are the poisonous condition resulting from consumption of these toxic chemicals released by fungus that grows in food grains prior to harvest, during storage or after inclusion in finished feed stuff. Fungus produces large number of chemical substances as by products. Many of these fungus products are toxic but some of them have medicinal effects. Mycotoxins produced by fungus are stable in nature and their toxic effects are not eliminated following milling or storage. Thousands of chemically varying mycotoxins have been identified but the toxin producing capacity and the amounl produced may vary depends on the factors such as strain of fungus, temperature of the atmosphere where in the fungus growing, moisture, types of fungus, degree of stress on the host plant, *etc.* Aflatoxicosis, ochratoxicosis and trichothecene mycotoxicosis are the most common mycotoxicoses affects commercial poultry. Aflatoxin is released in corn (maize), peanuts, cottonseed, millet, sorghum and other food grains while the plant grow in them.

Etiology

Aspergillus flavus-produce majority of the toxins. *A. parasiticus produce* mainly alflatoxin. *Aspergillus* species are ubiquitous in the natural environment. Possess both toxigenic and non-toxigenic strains. Produce Aflatoxin in warm (30-35°C) and high humidity (90-99 per cent). Aflatoxicosis is caused by aflatoxins, produced by *Aspergillus flavus* and *Aspergillus parasiticus*. Aflatoxins are commonly found in corn, milo, cottonseed and peanuts. Aflatoxin concentrations in grains produced contain enough aflatoxin to cause acute aflatoxicosis. There are five important aflatoxins, called aflatoxin B_1, B_2, G_1, G_2, and M_1. Aflatoxin M_1 is a metabolite of aflatoxin. B_1 found in milk and urine. It is not found in feed. Aflatoxin $B_1$is found most frequently and in the highest concentrations in naturally contaminated feed.

Epidemiology

Prevalence of Infection

Problems occur worldwide, but especially climates with high temperature and humidity and where grain is harvested with high water content.

Predisposing Factors

High grain humidity and damage due to insects, as well as poor storage conditions are major predisposing causes. The following factors increase the release of Aflatoxin. Plant stress by insects damage, poor nutrition, harvest delay, postharvest storage in cold. B_1, B_2, G_1, G_2 but B_1 are the toxins naturally produced

Aflatoxins. B_1 toxin present in highest concentration and is the most toxic not degraded by food processing and storage. Young birds are more susceptible to Aflatoxin than adults. Ducks are 10 times more susceptible than chickens. Turkeys are moderately affected than chicken and ducks.

Economic Impact

Economic impact is considerable in some countries.

Pathogenesis

Mycotoxins are ingested and then absorbed through the skin, mucous and airways. Once ingested, it compromises the immune system and damage body functions. Metabolites bind to DNA and RNA genetic materials thereby reduce the synthesis of protein and cause decrease cell mediated immunity and humoral immunity. Changes in these metabolites develops enlargement of liver, kidney and spleen. Atrophy of bursa, thymus and testes. Exposure to high concentration leads to accumulation of fat as clear vacuoles in the cytoplasm of hepatocytes produce enlarged friable yellow liver. The continued exposure causes intra hepatic biliary epithelial hyperplasia and extra modullary haemotopoiesis. Toxin also induce anemia. Petechial haemorrhages or bruises increased due to decreased clotting factors and increased capillary fragility. Aflatoxin is excreted rapidly in bile and urine but not accumulated or stored in the body tissues. Hypersensitivity – an allergic reaction to moulds and spores. Aflatoxin is a liver poison (hepatotoxin) in all species. Ruminants tolerate the aflatoxin better than monogastrics or poultry. It causes liver damage at higher doses and liver cancer at lower doses. Aflatoxin exposure can depress the immune system. It may cause abortions in some instances; however the circumstances necessary for abortions to occur are not well defined. By ingestion of B_1 Aflatoxin undergoes biotransformation to numerous highly reactive metabolities with diverse negative effects on metabolism.

Clinical Signs

Acute exposure of all species it causes depression, anorexia, reduced gain or milk production, subnormal body temperature. Chronic exposure in poultry leads to decreased growth rate reduced feed efficiency, steatorrhoea (fat in feces) and bruising. Chronic exposure in swine develops anorexia, unthriftiness, slow growth, icterus, mild anemia, ascites, increased susceptibility to infection. Chronic exposure in cattle causes slow rumen motility for 24 to 48 hours.

Necropsy Findings

Acute Exposure

Hemorrhages and ascites.

Chronic Exposure

Pale, soft, clay-colored liver, mild anemia, icterus and ascites.

Histopathological

Hepatocyte degeneration and necrosis; centrilobular hemorrhagic hepatic necrosis, fatty changes and regeneration of hepatocytes; bile duct epithelial proliferation progressing to interlobular ncongruous and extensive proliferation; Karyomegaly, atypical nuclei, hepatocytic vacuolization and bile retention.

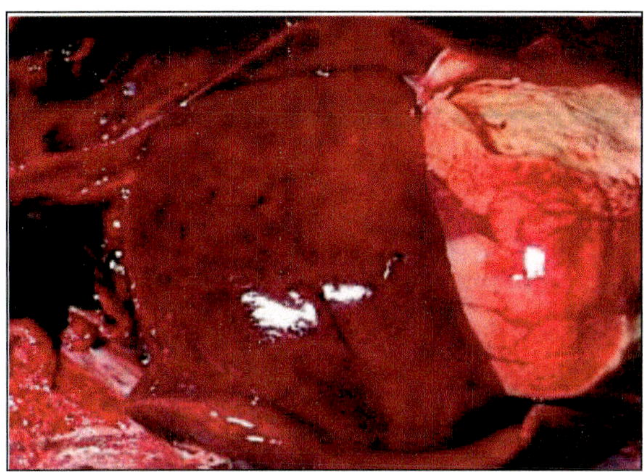

Figure 3.4. Hemorrhagic liver from a bird with an acute aflatoxicosis.

Diagnosis

Based on clinical signs and blood biochemical parameters such as anemia, elevated liver enzymes, serum bile acids, albumin: globulin ratio; prothrombin activity. Tissue or fluid analysis: Aflatoxin M1 present in milk or urine. Parent compound may be present in kidney or liver. Grain or feed analysis: Aflatoxins are present in corn, peanuts or cotton seed. Decreased performance may occur at concentrations as low as 200 ppb in young, sensitive species. At 200 ppb immunity may be impaired. At 200 to 400 ppb hepatic lesions become evident. At 400 ppb clinical illness becomes obvious. Violative residues in milk can occur at concentrations at or near 50 ppb aflatoxin M1.

Differential Diagnosis

Other mycotoxicoses. Other fungal infections.

Treatment

Stop exposure to fungus. Stop feeding contaminated ration and replace with noncontaminated ration. Supportive treatment. Provide supportive treatment as clinical situation dictates.

3.5. Oomycosis

Synonyms

Pythiosis, Lagenidiosis.

Oomycosis is caused by pathogens in the class Oomycetes. These organisms are not true fungi but are aquatic pathogens in the kingdom Stramenopila. They are more closely related to algae than fungi but cause disease that closely resembles zygomycosis. Organisms of significance in veterinary medicine include various species of *Saprolegnia* and *Achyla* (*e.g.*, *S. diclina*), which are the common agents of cutaneous disease in fishes; *Pythium insidiosum*, the cause of a cutaneous and subcutaneous mycosis in horses (bursatti, swamp cancer, leeches), a cutaneous, subcutaneous, and GI disease in dogs, and a cutaneous and paranasal disease of cats; and *Lagenidium* spp, the cause of cutaneous and systemic lesions and large-vessel aneurysms in dogs. Pythiosis is a common disease of domestic animals in some tropical and subtropical areas of the world. In dogs, pythiosis is most often encountered in Southeast Asia, eastern coastal Australia, South America, and in the USA, especially along the Gulf coast. In the USA, the disease most often is seen in fall and winter months.

Clinical Findings and Lesions

In horses, lesions are large, roughly circular, granulomatous, ulcerated, fistulated nodules, or subcutaneous swellings with yellow-gray necrotic masses or cores. The lesions are most common on the legs (especially the lower limbs), abdomen, chest, and genitalia. Distribution of lesions is attributable to the aquatic nature of the organism. The lesions are pruritic, discharge a mucosanguineous ncongru, and often are self-traumatized. The granulomas contain firm, yellowish, coralliform masses of necrotic tissue known as "kunkers," which may be removed intact. Kunkers are foci of coagulative necrosis in vessels that have become sequestered from the surrounding tissue; they contain broad, branching aseptate hyphae and are 1–10 µm in diameter. Bone involvement may be a feature of chronic pythiosis. Enteric pythiosis in horses is characterized by fibrosing and stenotic GI lesions containing intralesional foci of caseous material and fungal hyphae.

Specimens removed at surgery or necropsy consist of fibrous tissue with irregularly spaced, firm, focal areas of necrosis that vary in size and color. Microscopically, alterations vary from foci of acute exudative inflammation with numerous eosinophils to a granulomatous reaction with sequestered areas of necrosis and a framework of hyphae that are thick-walled, branching, and slightly irregular in width.

GI and cutaneous forms of pythiosis are seen and are characterized by severe granulomatous and eosinophilic inflammation. *P. insidiosum* infection is seen most often in the GI tract of young adult dogs, especially Labrador Retrievers. The stomach, proximal small intestine, and ileocolic junction are affected most commonly, but any part of the intestine, esophagus, and colon can be diseased. Clinical signs include vomiting, weight loss, and anorexia. The weight loss can be severe, but affected dogs usually do not appear systemically ill until late in the disease. The lesions are typically characterized by severe transmural thickening of the gastric or intestinal wall, with mesenteric lymphadenopathy in which the lymph nodes are embedded in a large, firm granulomatous mass involving the surrounding mesentery. Bowel ischemia, infarction, or acute hemoabdomen may develop due to extension of disease into mesenteric vessels. Enteric pyogranulomas typically consist of necrotic foci infiltrated and surrounded by neutrophils, eosinophils, epithelioid macrophages, plasma cells, and multinucleated giant cells. Etiologic agents may not be apparent on sections stained with H and E. Sections stained with Gomori methenamine silver show branching, rarely septate hyphae. Cutaneous pythiosis is typified by nonhealing wounds, invasive masses, and ulcerated nodules with draining tracts. The extremities, tail head, ventral neck, or perineum are affected most commonly. Pythiosis in cats is rare and typified by either cutaneous or nasopharyngeal lesions.

Lagenidiosis is an oomycotic infection of dogs characterized by progressive, multifocal cutaneous and subcutaneous lesions, most often affecting the extremities, mammary region, perineum, or trunk. Regional lymphadenopathy is common. At least two species of *Lagenidium* have been shown to affect dogs. One of the *Lagenidium* spp causes more aggressive cutaneous infection with systemic involvement, whereas a less aggressive *Lagenidium* spp tends to cause more slowly progressive cutaneous disease. Cutaneous lesions are characterized as firm dermal or subcutaneous nodules, or as ulcerated, thickened, edematous areas of deep cellulitis with regions of necrosis and numerous draining tracts. In contrast to the clinical course of cutaneous pythiosis, in dogs with aggressive *Lagenidium* spp, involvement at distant sites is often seen. Thoracic and abdominal lymph nodes, lungs, and especially great vessels may be affected. Animals with great vessel or sublumbar lymph node involvement typically have cutaneous or subcutaneous lesions on the hindlimbs and often develop hindlimb edema. Great vessel aneurysms may acutely rupture, resulting in hemoabdomen and sudden death.

Diagnosis

In horses, lesions of pythiosis are similar to those of zygomycosis and may be confused with cutaneous habronemiasis, excessive granulation tissue, and certain equine neoplasms. In pythiosis, the necrotic cores are distinct from the surrounding tissue, and a seropurulent discharge from the sinus tracts is prominent. The lesions contain irregular, branching (at right angles), rarely septate hyphae, 4–8 µm in diameter.

In dogs, diagnosis can be made by isolation of *P. insidiosum* from infected tissues. Culture identification or PCR has been used. Immunoblot serology for detection of anti-*P. insidiosum* antibodies is available and appears to be both sensitive and specific. Immunoblot serology for detection of anti-*Lagenidium* antibodies in canine serum can provide a presumptive diagnosis of lagenidiosis but must be interpreted in conjunction with results of serologic testing for *P. insidiosum* infection because of the potential for cross-reactivity in serum from dogs with pythiosis. The histologic features of lagenidiosis are similar to those of pythiosis and zygomycosis. However, *Lagenidium* hyphae are usually much larger and visible on H and E-stained tissues. Definitive diagnosis of lagenidiosis and pythiosis is best made by culture and PCR identification.

Treatment

The prognosis for pythiosis or lagenidiosis is poor if surgical excision cannot be done. Complete surgical excision is the treatment of choice, but the disease is often too extensive at the time of diagnosis to allow complete resection. In animals with lesions limited to a single distal extremity, amputation is recommended.

Medical therapy for pythiosis should include itraconazole (10 mg/kg/day) and terbinafine (5–10 mg/kg/day). Steroids may decrease inflammation and improve clinical signs in the short term. Treatment with amphotericin B lipid complex can also be attempted. Approximately 20 per cent of dogs with pythiosis respond to longterm antifungal therapy. Lagenidiosis appears to be poorly responsive to medical therapy. In horses, the prognosis is guarded, and timely recognition and treatment are essential for successful management. Factors that influence prognosis include size and site of lesion and duration of infection. Small lesions of short duration that have not invaded critical structures usually respond best to treatment. Surgical excision, immunotherapy, or a combination of both may be effective. Immunotherapy consists of a series of intradermal or SC injections of killed, sonicated, whole-cell hyphal antigens or precipitated soluble antigens of the causative fungus. Subcutaneous abscesses at the sites of injection, osteitis, or deep-seated laminitis may be a complication of such therapy. Surgical removal plus systemic or local administration of amphotericin B may be a satisfactory treatment if the disease is localized.

3.6. Blastomycosis

Blastomycosis, caused by the dimorphic fungus *Blastomyces dermatitidis*, is characterized by pyogranulomatous lesions in various tissues. It is most common in people, dogs, and cats but has also been described in such widely divergent species as horses, ferrets, deer, wolves, African lions, bottlenosed dolphins, and sea lions. It appears not to be a disease of cattle, sheep, or pigs. Blastomycosis is generally limited to North America, and most cases have occurred in the Mississippi, Missouri, Tennessee, and Ohio River basins and along the Great Lakes and the St. Lawrence Seaway. There is an endemic area in the Pacific Northwest. Even within these river basins, the organism is found in geographically restricted areas. Beaver dams and other habitats where soil is moist, acidic, and rich in decaying vegetation may serve as the ecologic niche for the organism, but it is often difficult to find in the environment. The organism has also been recovered from pigeon and bat feces. Rain, dew, or fog may play a critical role in liberating the infective conidia, which then are aerosolized and inhaled. When respiratory defenses are overwhelmed or immunosuppressed, disseminated disease occurs via hematogenous spread from the lungs. Cutaneous lesions may result from a primary entry through the skin or, more commonly, by dissemination from a pulmonary focus. Needle-stick injuries to veterinary personnel after aspiration of cutaneous lesions from infected animals have resulted in primary cutaneous infection. Ocular lesions tend to develop first in the posterior segment, resulting in granulomatous chorioretinitis and retinal detachment. Anterior segment involvement often follows, resulting in anterior uveitis and panophthalmitis.

Clinical Findings: The signs vary with organ involvement and are not specific. Weight loss may be accompanied by coughing, anorexia, lymphadenopathy, dyspnea, ocular disease, lameness, skin lesions, and fever. Dry, harsh lung sounds from lung lesions are common in dogs with blastomycosis. Signs of pulmonary involvement are seen in as many as 85 per cent of affected dogs. Severe pulmonary involvement results in hypoxemia, which indicates a poor prognosis. Lymph node involvement is seen in approximately half of affected dogs, which is about the same proportion of dogs that have cutaneous involvement. Skin lesions may include proliferative granulomas and subcutaneous abscesses that ulcerate and drain a serosanguineous discharge. The skin lesions are often very small and multifocal in dogs, but large abscesses are occasionally seen, especially in cats. The planum nasale, face, and nail beds are most often involved. Signs of ocular blastomycosis are seen in 30 per cent –50 per cent of affected dogs and include blindness, uveitis, glaucoma, and retinal detachment. Lameness associated with fungal osteomyelitis or severe paronychia occurs in approximately one quarter of affected dogs. CNS signs are uncommon, occurring in <5 per cent of dogs, but they may be more common in cats. The pattern of systemic involvement is similar in cats, but cats are affected far less commonly than dogs. Hematuria and dysuria may be seen with urogenital blastomycosis.

Lesions

Gross lesions consist of few to numerous, variable-sized, irregular, firm, gray to yellow areas of pulmonary consolidation and nodules in the lungs and thoracic lymph nodes. Dissemination may result in nodular lesions in various organs but especially the skin, eyes, and bone. Cutaneous lesions are single or multiple papules, or chronic, draining, nodular pyogranulomas.

Diagnosis

Blastomycosis should be considered in dogs with draining cutaneous nodules and signs of respiratory disease. In cats, respiratory tract involvement is seen most frequently, followed by involvement of the CNS, regional lymph nodes, skin, eyes, and GI and urinary tracts. Radiographic findings in the lungs include noncalcified nodules or consolidation, with enlargement of the bronchial and mediastinal lymph nodes. The predominant patterns on thoracic radiographs are those of diffuse nodular interstitial and peribronchial densities. Commonly, the bronchial lymph nodes are greatly enlarged and appear in radiographs as dense masses. Diagnosis can be made from biopsy of tissue or aspirated specimens taken from cutaneous lesions or other involved organs by the presence of thick-walled yeast that often have daughter cells budding from a broad base. These round to ovoid, pale pink (H and E) blastospores measure 8–25 µm and have a refractile, double-contoured wall. They may be empty or contain basophilic nuclear material and have single, broad-based buds. An antibody response, detected by agar gel immunodiffusion, usually occurs, but this response is neither sensitive nor specific when attempting to make a definitive diagnosis. An enzyme immunoassay for antibodies to rBAD-1 repeat has shown improved sensitivity. A recently developed antigen enzyme immunoassay has been used in both serum and urine to detect cell-wall galactomannan that is immunologically indistinguishable in histoplasmosis and blastomycosis. Although the titer is not useful in differentiating between the two infections, it helps to diagnose the presence of one of these two systemic mycoses.

Treatment

Itraconazole (5 mg/kg/day) is the treatment of choice for dogs and cats with blastomycosis. A minimum of 2 mo of treatment is necessary, and the drug should be continued until active disease is not apparent. Clinical cure can be expected in ~70 per cent of dogs, with recurrence months or years after treatment noted in ~20 per cent of treated dogs. Most dogs will respond to retreatment with itraconazole. Other azoles such as fluconazole and ketoconazole are not as effective as itraconazole, but a study evaluating cost-effectiveness of fluconazole showed it to be a less expensive alternative, despite longer treatment times. In fulminating cases of blastomycosis, especially those with evidence of hypoxemia, combination therapy with amphotericin B and itraconazole is recommended. Short courses of anti-inflammatory dosages of glucocorticoids have been advocated during the first few days of treatment by some, but steroid use is controversial and may actually worsen the prognosis. The prognosis is best for dogs with only mild lung disease, is more guarded for dogs with moderate to severe lung disease, and is poorest for dogs with CNS involvement.

3.7. Coccidioidomycosis

Synonyms

Valley Fever.

Coccidioidomycosis (Valley Fever) is a dustborne, noncontagious infection caused by the dimorphic fungus *Coccidioides immitis*. Infections are limited to arid and semiarid regions of the southwestern USA and to similar areas of Mexico and Central and South America. Although many species of animals, including people, are susceptible, only dogs are affected significantly. Placental infection leading to abortion and osteomyelitis has been described in horses. Ruminants and pigs may have subclinical infections with lesions restricted to foci in the lungs and to thoracic lymph nodes. Inhalation of fungal spores is the only established mode of infection, and spores may be carried on dust particles. Epidemics may occur when rainy periods are followed by drought, resulting in dust storms. Most bovine infections are contracted in dusty feedlots.

Clinical Findings and Lesions

The disease varies from inapparent (cattle, sheep, pigs, dogs, cats) to progressive, disseminated, and fatal (dogs, nonhuman primates, cats, and people). Coccidioidomycosis is primarily a respiratory disease that ranges from self-limiting to chronic. Dissemination occurs in ~20 per cent of canine infections, with many tissues, especially eyes, joints, and bone, affected. Clinical signs can vary greatly, depending on organ involvement and severity of infection. Dogs with disseminated disease may have chronic cough, anorexia, cachexia, lameness, enlarged joints, fever, and intermittent diarrhea. Dissemination to the skin with draining ulceration may occur, but primary infection through the skin is rare. Cats infected with *C. immitis* most often present with dermatologic signs (draining skin lesions, subcutaneous granulomatous masses, abscesses), fever, inappetence, and weight loss. Less common clinical signs in cats include respiratory (dypsnea), musculoskeletal (lameness), neurologic, and ophthalmologic abnormalities. Approximately 50 per cent of infected cats appear to have disseminated disease.

Gross lesions may be limited to the lungs, mediastinum, and thoracic lymph nodes, or may be disseminated to various organs. Lesions are discrete, variable-sized nodules with a firm, gray-white cut surface, and resemble those of tuberculosis. The nodules are pyogranulomas composed of epithelioid and giant cells, and the center of some foci may contain purulent ncongru and fungal organisms. Some lesions may have mineralized foci.

Diagnosis

In endemic areas, coccidioidomycosis should be considered in dogs with chronic bronchopulmonary disease and when pulmonary nodules and enlarged lymph nodes are found on thoracic radiographs. The lesions are pyogranulomas that contain *C. immitis* free in the ncongru and in epithelioid and multinucleate giant cells. The organisms vary in size and appear as relatively large (20–80 µm, up to 200 µm) spherules with a double-contoured wall. The mature spherules (sporangia) contain endospores (sporangiospores) 2–5 µm in diameter. Diagnosis is established by demonstrating the spherules in tissues. Serum can also be tested by agar gel immunodiffusion (AGID) assays for detection of precipitin and complement-fixing antibodies. Currently, most commercial laboratories run AGID assays for IgG and IgM antibodies; results of these assays are specific but relatively insensitive. An enzyme immunoassay for *Coccidioides* galactomannan antigen useful in human infections has proved insensitive in dogs. A presumptive diagnosis can be made when serology is positive in an animal with consistent clinical signs. Attempts to culture the fungus should be restricted to those laboratories equipped to handle such dangerously infective cultures.

Treatment

Disease is often self-limiting, but if chronic respiratory signs or multisystemic disease are present, longterm antifungal therapy is needed; with disseminated infection, treatment of at least 6–12 mo is typical. **Fluconazole** (2.5–10 mg/kg/day) is the most commonly used drug to treat disseminated or chronic respiratory infections. **Ketoconazole** (10–30 mg/kg/day) and **itraconazole** (10 mg/kg/day) are also commonly used to treat dogs with coccidioidomycosis but are more expensive and have a higher incidence of adverse effects. Amphotericin B may be the most effective antifungal drug, but it is highly nephrotoxic. It may be indicated in animals that either do not improve or are unable to tolerate the azole antifungals.

3.8. Cryptococcosis

Cryptococcosis is a systemic fungal disease that may affect the respiratory tract (especially the nasal cavity), CNS, eyes, and skin (particularly of the face and neck of cats). The causal fungi, *Cryptococcus neoformans* and *C gattii*, exist in the environment and in tissues in a yeast form. Infection occurs worldwide. The fungi are found in soil and fowl manure, especially in pigeon droppings. Transmission is by inhalation of spores or contamination of wounds. In avian droppings, it may occur in a noncapsulated form as small as 1 µm, which can be inhaled into the deeper portions of the lungs. Cryptococcosis is most common in cats but also is seen in dogs, cattle, horses, sheep, goats, birds, and wild animals. In people, many cases are associated with a defective cell-mediated immune response.

Clinical Findings and Lesions

Bovine cryptococcosis has been associated only with cases of mastitis, and many cows in a herd may be infected. Affected cows have anorexia, decreased milk flow, swelling and firmness of affected quarters, and enlarged supramammary lymph nodes. The milk becomes viscid, mucoid, and gray-white, or it may be watery with flakes. The disease in horses almost invariably is a respiratory ailment with obstructive growths in the nasal cavities.

Cryptococcosis, Cat

In cats, upper respiratory signs secondary to nasal cavity infection are most common and include sneezing; mucopurulent, serous, or hemorrhagic unilateral or bilateral chronic nasal discharge; polyp-like mass(es) in the nostril; and/or a firm, subcutaneous swelling over the bridge of the nose. Cutaneous lesions are also common and are characterized by papules and nodules that are fluctuant to firm. Larger lesions tend to ulcerate, leaving a raw surface with a serous ncongru. Neurologic signs associated with cryptococcosis of the CNS may include depression, changes in temperament, seizures, circling, paresis, and blindness. Ocular abnormalities may also develop, including dilated unresponsive pupils and blindness due to exudative retinal detachment, granulomatous chorioretinitis, panophthalmitis, and optic neuritis.

In contrast to cats, dogs often have disseminated disease with CNS or ocular involvement. Clinical signs are often related to meningoencephalitis, optic neuritis, and granulomatous chorioretinitis. Lesions in the nasal cavity of many dogs have been reported, but they are usually not the primary finding or reason for presentation. Approximately 50 per cent of dogs have lesions in the respiratory tract, usually the lungs, and most have granulomas present in multiple systems. Structures often involved in order of decreasing frequency are kidneys, lymph nodes, spleen, liver, thyroid, adrenals, pancreas, bone, GI tract, muscle, myocardium, prostate, heart valves, and tonsils.

Lesions associated with cryptococcosis vary from a gelatinous mass, consisting of numerous organisms with minimal inflammation, to granuloma formation. The lesion is usually composed of aggregates of encapsulated organisms within a connective tissue reticulum. The cellular response is primarily macrophages and giant cells with a few plasma cells and lymphocytes. Epithelioid giant cells and areas of caseous necrosis are less common than with the other systemic mycoses.

Diagnosis

The most rapid method of diagnosis is cytologic evaluation of nasal ncongru, skin ncongru, CSF, or samples obtained by paracentesis of the aqueous or vitreous chambers of the eye or by impression smears of nasal or cutaneous masses. Gram stain is most useful; the organism retains the crystal violet, whereas the capsule stains lightly red with safranin. India ink is also used to visualize the organism, which appears unstained and silhouetted against a black background. It is not as definitive as Gram stain unless budding is seen, because lymphocytes, fat droplets, and aggregated India ink particles may be confused with the organism. Wright stain has been used most often in diagnosing canine and feline cases, but this stain can cause the organism to shrink and the capsule to become distorted. New methylene blue and periodic acid-Schiff (PAS) stains are better than Wright stain for this reason. Because cytologic evaluation is rapid, impression smears or potassium hydroxide preparations should always be made of suspected cryptococcal lesions.

If no organisms are seen, a biopsy of the lesion can be taken; part of the sample can be used for culture and the rest processed for routine histology. The organism can be stained with H and E, but the capsule does not stain. The organism is more easily visualized with PAS and Gomori methenamine silver stains, but the capsule does not stain with these, either. The best stain for *Cryptococcus* is Mayer mucicarmine because of its ability to stain the capsule. Immunofluorescent staining can also be used. The large capsule and thin cell wall of *Cryptococcus* differentiate it from *Blastomyces*. *Cryptococcus*, by its budding and lack of endospores, can be distinguished from *Coccidioides immitis*.

Detection of cryptococcal capsular antigen in serum, urine, or CSF is a useful, rapid method of diagnosis in those suspected cases in which the organism is not identified. A latex agglutination test is commercially available in kit form. The antigen titer can also be used to help determine response to therapy.

The organism can be cultured from ncongru, CSF, urine, joint fluid, and tissue samples if a large enough sample volume is available. Sabouraud agar with antibiotics is used if bacterial contamination is likely.

Treatment

Fluconazole (2.5–10 mg/kg/day) or itraconazole (10 mg/kg/day) are considered the treatments of choice. Amphotericin B can be given SC (0.5–0.8 mg/kg diluted in 0.45 per cent saline containing 2.5 per cent dextrose; 400 mL for cats, 500 mL for dogs <20 kg, 1,000 mL for dogs >20 kg), 2–3 times per wk. Amphotericin B lipid complex (1–2 mg/kg for cats or 2–3 mg/kg for dogs) can also be given 3 times/wk for 12–15 treatments. Flucytosine can be used alone; however, drug resistance may develop, so combination therapy with amphotericin is recommended.

3.9. Epizootic Lymphangitis

Epizootic lymphangitis is a chronic granulomatous disease of the skin, lymph vessels, and lymph nodes of the limbs and neck of Equidae caused by the dimorphic fungus *Histoplasma farciminosum*. The disease is seen in Asian and Mediterranean areas but is unknown in the USA. The fungus forms mycelia in nature and yeast forms in tissues and has a saprophytic phase in soil. Infection probably is acquired by wound infection or transmission by bloodsucking insects.

Clinical Findings and Lesions

The disease is characterized by freely movable cutaneous nodules, which originate from infected superficial lymph vessels and nodes and tend to ulcerate and undergo alternating periods of discharge and closure. Affected lymph nodes are enlarged and hard. The skin covering the nodules may become thick, indurated, and fused to the underlying tissues. Lesions also may be present in the lungs, conjunctiva, cornea, nasal mucosa, and other organs. The nodules are pyogranulomas with a thick, fibrous capsule and contain thick, creamy ncongru and the causative organisms.

Diagnosis

The clinical features are highly suggestive. Diagnosis can be confirmed by microscopic examination of eexudates and biopsy specimens. The yeast forms of the organisms distend the cytoplasm of macrophages and appear in H and E sections as globose or oval bodies (3–4 µm) with a central basophilic body surrounded by an unstained zone. The organism closely resembles *H capsulatum*. Serologic testing is available with serum agglutination titers of 1:80 or higher reported to be positive. Positive titers may be reflective of past exposure, with specificity for current infection being low.

Treatment

No completely satisfactory treatment is known. Surgical excision of lesions combined with antifungal drugs (amphotericin B) could be used.

3.10. Hyalohyphomycosis

Hyalohyphomycosis is infection caused by nonpigmented fungi (other than the genera *Aspergillus* or *Penicillium* or the class Zygomycetes) that in tissue form hyphal elements with hyaline or clear walls. Examples of genera causing hyalohyphomycosis in people and other animals include *Acremonium*, *Fusarium*, *Geotrichum*, *Paecilomyces*, *Pseudallescheria*, *Sagenomella*, *Phialosimplex*, *Geosmithia*, *Geomyces*, and *Scedosporium*. Hyalohyphomycosis is far less common than phaeohyphomycosis.

Clinical Findings

Lesions range from local cutaneous, subcutaneous, corneal or nasal mucosal disease to disseminated disease involving the lungs and multiple other organ systems. Disseminated and corneal forms have been reported most commonly. Animals presenting with cutaneous lesions should be evaluated for systemic disease. Animals being treated with immunosuppressive drugs for immune-mediated disease may develop cutaneous hyalohyphomycosis and not have lesions at other sites, whereas immunocompetent animals that develop hyalohyphomycosis most often do have disseminated disease, or at least disease that is not confined to the skin.

Diagnosis

The several causative fungi cannot be identified by their histologic features in tissues; culture isolation and/or PCR are required.

Treatment

Surgical removal with or without azole antifungal therapy is the treatment of choice for local disease. Disseminated disease typically carries a grave prognosis.

Treatment with newer azole antifungals and/or amphotericin B lipid complex may be attempted and is most likely to be effective if immunosuppressive drugs can be tapered.

3.11. Mycetomas

Mycetomas are granulomatous nodules of the subcutaneous tissues that contain tissue grains or granules. Within the grains are dense colonies of the organism. When such lesions are caused by fungi, they are known as eumycotic mycetomas. The causal agents of eumycotic mycetomas include a variety of saprophytic geophilic fungi. Eumycotic mycetomas caused by pigmented fungi such as *Curvularia* spp and *Madurella* spp are called black- or dark-grain mycetomas. White-grained mycetomas are caused by unpigmented fungi such as *Acremonium* spp and *Scedosporium apiospermum* (the asexual state of *Pseudallescheria boydii*).

Clinical Findings and Lesions

Most eumycotic mycetomas are confined to the subcutaneous tissue, but white-grain mycetomas may be extensions of abdominal cavity disease. Peritonitis or abdominal masses are typically seen in white-grain mycetomas. Black-grain mycetomas are usually characterized by relatively poorly circumscribed cutaneous nodules on the extremities or face. The lesions may ulcerate or form fistulas. When the feet or limbs are involved, the infection may extend to the underlying bone.

The fungal mycelia proliferate in the lesions and organize into aggregates known as granules or grains. In these granules, the mycelium is compact and frequently bizarre and distorted in form. Chlamydospores are frequent, especially at the periphery, and the mycelium may or may not be embedded in an amorphous, cement-like substance. Histologically, the granules are frequently surrounded by eosinophilic deposits. Granules may be of various colors and sizes, depending on the species of fungus involved.

Diagnosis

A presumptive diagnosis can be made if there are grains within the ncongru of draining tracts. For cytology, the grains should be examined for the presence of fungal elements. If no tissue grains are found in the ncongru, a biopsy of the lesion should be taken for histopathologic examination. Cultures should be performed to confirm cytologic findings and to identify the causative agent. Either tissue grains or biopsy specimens should be cultured.

Treatment

The prognosis for abdominal mycetomas is guarded, because tissue involvement is usually extensive. Cutaneous mycetomas, while not life-threatening, are often difficult to resolve. Radical surgical excision, including limb amputation, may be effective for some cases of cutaneous mycetomas. Effectiveness of antifungal chemotherapy has been reported in only a few cases. In one report, fluconazole, 50 mg/day for 6 wk, was used to successfully treat a dog with intra-abdominal maduromycosis. In another report, longterm treatment with itraconazole, 5–10 mg/kg/day, failed to resolve a disseminated *Acremonium* infection in a dog.

3.12. Penicilliosis

Infections with *Penicillium* spp are rare in domestic animals. In dogs, infections of the nasal cavity, lungs, lymph nodes, and bones have been reported. Nasal disease is most common and behaves similar to nasal aspergillosis. In cats, the fungus has been isolated from the nasal cavity, orbital cellulitis and sinusitis, and lungs. It has also been reported to cause systemic disease in captive toucanets (*P. griseofulvum*) and bamboo rats (*P. marneffei*) in Southeast Asia. *Penicillium* spp are widely distributed in nature and are found in soils, grains, and various foods and feeds.

Clinical Findings and Lesions

Dogs with nasal penicilliosis have chronic sneezing and an acute to chronic nasal discharge that varies from intermittent hemorrhagic to intermittent or continuous mucoid or mucopurulent. Radiographic findings include areas of turbinate destruction with increased radiolucency. Grossly, the nasal mucosa has foci of necrosis and ulceration; microscopically, fungal hyphae may form a thick mat over an intact mucosa adjacent to these foci. Systemic disease often affects long bones, resulting in lameness.

Diagnosis

Diagnosis is based on fungal culture, character of the lesions, presence of fungal hyphae, and a positive agar-gel double-diffusion test. Cultural isolation of a *Penicillium* sp must be accompanied by demonstration of tissue invasion by the fungus for confirmation. In tissues, *P marneffei* closely resemble the yeast phase of *Histoplasma capsulatum*.

Treatment

Very little has been reported concerning treatment of penicilliosis. Surgical turbinectomy with curettage has been combined with flushing of the nasal cavity with 1 per cent tincture of iodine or povidone-iodine (10:1) and oral thiabendazole. Fluconazole, 2.5–5 mg/kg/day for 2 months, has been used to successfully treat some dogs with nasal penicilliosis.

3.13. Phaeohyphomycosis

Phaeohyphomycosis refers to chronic cutaneous, subcutaneous, mucosal, cerebral, or systemic infection caused by one of several genera and species of pigmented fungi of the family Dematiaceae. Several fungal genera have been reported to affect people and other animals, including *Alternaria, Bipolaris, Cladophialophora (Xylohypha, Cladosporium), Curvularia, Exophiala, Fonsecaea, Moniliella, Phialophora, Ramichloridium,* and *Scolecobasidium*. Fungi in this category are saprophytic, widely distributed organisms found in soil, water, and decaying vegetable matter. Infection may result from fungal implantation into tissue at the site of an injury.

Clinical Findings and Lesions

Phaeohyphomycosis has been described in cows, cats, horses, and dogs. The most common clinical presentations include ulcerated cutaneous nodules of the digits, pinnae, nasal planum, and nasal/paranasal tissues in cats. The nodules may ulcerate and have draining fistulous tracts. These pyogranulomas contain pigmented, septate hyphae with irregular enlargements and thin-walled, budding, yeast-like forms. Granulomatous meningoencephalitis caused by pigmented fungi has been reported in dogs and cats. Dogs treated with multiple immunosuppressive agents, especially cyclosporine, appear to be predisposed to developing multifocal cutaneous lesions. Systemic dissemination is most likely in animals treated with immunosuppressive drugs.

Diagnosis

Phaeohyphomycosis can be diagnosed by microscopic examination of ncongru and biopsy specimens, which reveals pigmented, dark-walled, irregularly septate filamentous hyphae (2–6 µm in diameter) or yeast-like cells. Infected tissues may be grossly pigmented, giving an appearance of melanoma. The several causative fungi cannot be identified by their histologic features in tissues; cultural isolation and/or PCR are required. The differential diagnosis should include neoplasia, other granulomas, and epidermoid cysts.

Treatment

Phaeohyphomycosis is generally poorly responsive to treatment. Wide excision of cutaneous or subcutaneous lesions is recommended, followed by 6–12 mo of treatment with itraconazole (10 mg/kg/day).

Nonresectable disease should be treated with itraconazole. Voriconazole or posaconazole may be more effective, but voriconazole is not recommended in cats. In dogs being treated with immunosuppressive therapy, the prognosis may be better if the immunosuppressive drugs (especially cyclosporine) can be discontinued.

3.14. Rhinosporidiosis

Rhinosporidiosis is a chronic, nonfatal, pyogranulomatous infection, primarily of the nasal mucosa and occasionally of the skin of horses, cattle, dogs, cats, and aquatic birds, caused by the fungus *Rhinosporidium seeberi*. Uncommon in North America, it is seen most often in India, Africa, and South America. The organism has not been cultured, and its natural habitat is unknown. Trauma may predispose to infection, which is not considered transmissible.

Clinical Findings and Lesions

Infection of the nasal mucosa is characterized by polypoid growths that may be soft, pink, friable, lobulated with roughened surfaces, and large enough to occlude the nasal passages. The cutaneous lesions may be single or multiple, sessile or pedunculated. The nasal polyps and cutaneous lesions have a granulomatous, fibromyxoid inflammatory component and contain the fungal organism.

Diagnosis

Rhinosporidiosis may be confused with other granulomatous lesions of the nasal mucosa and skin, including aspergillosis, entomophthoromycosis, "nasal granuloma," and cryptococcosis. Microscopic demonstration of spherules (sporangia) of *R seeberi* in biopsy specimens confirms the diagnosis. The spherules may be numerous, vary in size (up to 300 µm), have thick walls that stain periodic acid-Schiff positive, and contain endospores 4–19 µm in diameter. Developing stages of varying size without spores are distributed throughout the lesion.

Treatment

Surgical excision of the lesions is considered standard, but recurrence is common. Amphotericin B and itraconazole have been described for medical treatment but are generally not as effective as surgery.

3.15. Sporotrichosis

Sporotrichosis is a sporadic, chronic, granulomatous disease of people and various domestic and laboratory animals caused by *Sporothrix schenckii*. The organism is dimorphic and forms mycelia on vegetation and in Sabouraud dextrose agar at 25°–30°C (77°–86°F) but is yeast-like in tissue and media at 37°C (98.6°F). It is ubiquitous in soil, vegetation, and timber; is distributed worldwide; and in the USA is most commonly found in coastal regions and river valleys. Infection usually results from direct inoculation of the organism into skin wounds via contact with plants or soil or penetrating foreign bodies. Disseminated disease caused by inhalation of spores is rare.

Sporotrichosis has been reported in dogs, cats, horses, cows, camels, dolphins, goats, mules, birds, pigs, rats, armadillos, and people. Zoonotic infections can occur. The cat may be the species with the greatest zoonotic potential, and transmission from cats to people has been reported without evidence of trauma. In contrast, transmission from other infected species appears to require inoculation of previously traumatized skin. The large number of organisms shed from the wound and in the feces of infected cats is believed to be responsible for the increased zoonotic potential of feline sporotrichosis. Epidemics of sporotrichosis have been reported in Brazil. Data from these studies support the importance of cats in the zoonotic transmission of the organism. Caretakers of infected cats were four times more likely to become infected than others living in the same household.

Clinical Findings and Lesions

Sporotrichosis may be grouped into three forms: lymphocutaneous, cutaneous, and disseminated. The lymphocutaneous form is the most common. Small, firm dermal to subcutaneous nodules, 1–3 cm in diameter, develop at the site of inoculation. As infection ascends along the lymphatic vessels, cording and new nodules develop. Lesions ulcerate and discharge a serohemorrhagic ncongru. In cats, lesions are most often seen on the head, especially on the bridge of the nose and pinnae. Although systemic illness is not seen initially, chronic illness may result in fever, listlessness, and depression. Respiratory signs may be apparent. The cutaneous form tends to remain localized to the site of inoculation, although lesions may be multicentric. Disseminated sporotrichosis is rare but potentially fatal and may develop with neglect of cutaneous and lymphocutaneous forms or if the animal is inappropriately treated with corticosteroids. Infection develops via hematogenous or tissue spread from the initial site of inoculation to the bone, lungs, liver, spleen, testes, GI tract, or CNS.

Diagnosis

Diagnosis can be made by culture (samples obtained from unopened lesions) or microscopic examination of the ncongru or biopsy specimens. In tissues and ncongru, the organism is present as few to numerous, cigar-shaped, single cells within macrophages. The fungal cells are pleomorphic and small (2–10 × 1–3 µm); buds may be present and give the appearance of a ping-pong paddle. A fluorescent antibody technique has been used to identify the yeast-like cells in tissues. In species other than cats, *Sporothrix* organisms are often sparse in ncongru and infected tissue, so that diagnosis usually requires culture. In cultures, a true mycelium is produced, with fine, branching, septate hyphae bearing pear-shaped conidia on slender conidiophores.

Treatment

Itraconazole (10 mg/kg/day) is considered the treatment of choice for sporotrichosis. Treatment should be continued 3–4 wk beyond apparent clinical cure. Terbinafine has also been used successfully. Alternatively, a supersaturated solution of potassium iodide, administered PO, has been used with some success; therapy is continued 30 days beyond apparent clinical cure. During treatment, the animal should be monitored for signs of iodide toxicity: anorexia, vomiting, depression, muscle twitching, hypothermia, cardiomyopathy, cardiovascular collapse, and death. Cats are especially sensitive to iodides and the development of iodism.

Zoonotic Risk

Sporotrichosis is an important zoonosis, with animal-to-human transmission well documented. Strict hygiene must be observed when handling animals (especially cats) with suspected or diagnosed sporotrichosis. People in contact with infected animals should be informed of the contagious nature of the disease when therapeutic options are discussed.

3.16. Zygomycosis

Zygomycosis is used to describe infection with fungi in the class Zygomycetes and two genera in the order Entomophthorales, *Basidiobolus* and *Conidiobolus*. True zygomycete infections are rare, but conidiobolomycosis and basidiobolomycosis are more common and cause pyogranulomatous lesions grossly and histologically similar to those caused by pythiosis and lagenidiosis. This is primarily an infection of the nasopharyngeal mucosa and subcutaneous tissue of horses and rarely other animals (llamas, sheep) by *C. coronatus*, *C. ncongruous*, *C. lamprauges*, or *B. ranarum*. These ubiquitous fungi are present in soil and decaying vegetation and, in the case of basidioboli, the GI tracts of amphibians, reptiles, and macropods. *C. coronatus* affects almost exclusively the mucosa of the nose and mouth. *Basidiobolus* infects the lateral aspects of the head, neck, and body. *C. coronatus* is also an important insect pathogen.

Clinical Findings

Ulcerative pyogranulomas of the mucous membrane of the nasopharyngeal tissue, mouth, or nodular growths of the nasal mucosa and the lips may be seen with conidiobolomycosis, resulting in mechanical obstruction of the nasal cavity, dyspnea, and nasal discharge. Local dissemination into the retropharyngeal, retrobulbar, or other tissues of the face may be noted. Lesions in basidiobolomycosis are usually single, circular, ulcerative, pruritic nodules of the skin of the upper body. Fistulous tracts discharge a serosanguineous fluid from the lesions, which frequently are traumatized. Extension to regional lymph nodes results in swelling of the nodes and development of yellow necrotic foci. Lesions may contain a creamy, yellow central core of necrotic tissue. Disseminated basidiobolomycosis is rare but has been described in dogs and a mandrill.

Lesions

In excised tissues or necropsy specimens, a thickened fibrotic dermis has scattered, red or creamy white areas. The lesions, which contain hyphal forms, a heavy infiltrate of eosinophils, and sequestered areas of necrosis, have histologic features of infectious granulomas.

Diagnosis

Clinically, zygomycosis may be confused with cutaneous habronemiasis and oomycosis but can be differentiated by microscopic examination of tissues. In H and E sections, the fungus appears as holes and elongated channels, and many hyphae have a wide eosinophilic cuff; in sections stained for fungi, the organism consists of large, branching, sometimes septate, 2.5–25 μm hyphae. Cultural examination is required to identify the causative fungus.

Treatment

Longterm itraconazole administration is recommended for treatment of nasopharyngeal infection. Although lesions often regress, recurrence is common after treatment is discontinued. Cutaneous zygomycete infections should be treated with wide surgical resection followed by longterm itraconazole.

Chapter 4

Rickettisial Disease

Rickettsiae are an unusual type of bacteria that cause several diseases, including Rocky Mountain spotted fever. Rickettsiae differ from most other bacteria in that they can live and multiply only inside the cells of another organism (host) and cannot survive on their own in the environment.

Each of the rickettsiae has its own hosts and vectors (organisms that carry parasites to other organisms). Although some rickettsiae are found primarily in people, the usual host for most species is an animal. The population of animals that can serve as hosts is called the reservoir of infection. Animals in the reservoir may or may not be ill from the infection. People usually become infected through the bites of ticks, mites, fleas, and lice (vectors) that previously fed on an infected animal.

4.1. Anaplasmosis

Anaplasmosis, formerly known as gall sickness, traditionally refers to a disease of ruminants caused by obligate intraerythrocytic bacteria of the order Rickettsiales, family Anaplasmataceae, genus *Anaplasma*. Cattle, sheep, goats, buffalo, and some wild ruminants can be infected with the erythrocytic *Anaplasma*. Anaplasmosis occurs in tropical and subtropical regions worldwide (~40°N to 32°S), including South and Central America, the USA, southern Europe, Africa, Asia, and Australia. The *Anaplasma* genus also includes *A. phagocytophilum* (compiled from species previously known as *Ehrlichia phagocytophila, E. equi,* and human granulocytic ehrlichiosis agent,), *A. bovis* (formerly *E. bovis*), and *A. platys* (formerly *E. platys*), all of which invade blood cells other than erythrocytes of their respective mammalian hosts. Bovine anaplasmosis is of economic significance in the cattle industry.

Order: Rickettsiales; Genus: Anaplasma

It is an infectious haemoparasitic disease caused by *Anaplasma* spp. in cattle, sheep and goat and entralceed by fever, anaemia, jaundice and emaciation. It is usually subclinical in sheep and goats.

Distribution

Worldwide in tropics and subtropics; also in temperate areas of USA.

Sl.No.	Parasite	Host	Pathogenecity
1	*A. marginale*	Cattle, wild ruminants, sheep and goat (inapparent)	Pathogenic
2	*A. entral*	Cattle, wild ruminants, sheep and goat (inapparent)	Mild anaplasmosis

Intermediate host/vectors: One host tick *Boophilus* spp- transtadial transmission and little evidence on transovarian transmission. Tabanids- Mechanical transmission. 20 tick species are involved.

Location: Red blood cells.

Morphology

Anaplasma marginale: A small round, dark red inclusion bodies within RBCs on Giemsa staining. One organism in the RBC characteristically in the outer margin.

Anaplasma entral: Similar but are commonly found in the centre of RBCs.

Life Cycle

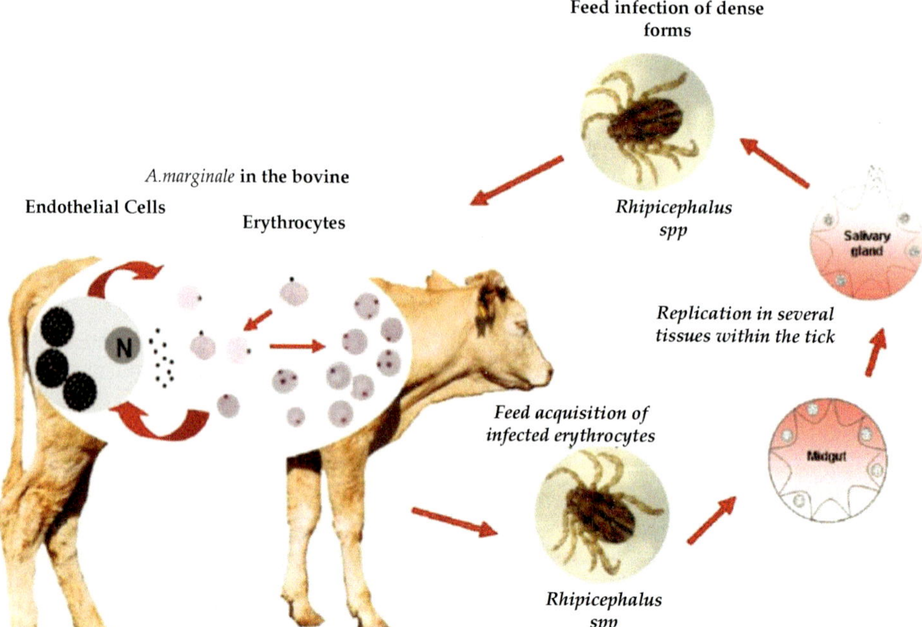

Figure 4.1. Life cycle of *Anaplasma marginale*.

Epidemiology

Age: Over 3 years of age group are commonly affected; Young animals are relatively resistant; Mortality-80 per cent. *Breed:* British breeds and Zebu cattle are equally susceptible but are not commonly affected due to their relative resistance to the ticks.

Transmission: By developmental transtadial transmission by Ixodidae ticks-*Boophilus* spp. Mechanical transmission by tabanid flies. Mechanical transmission by infected hypodermic needles, castration, dehorning, spaying, blood transfusion, vaccination, embryo transfer and blood sampling. Congenital transmission: Less frequent.

Carrier status: Infected cattle are carriers for many years or for life. Sheep, goats, wild ruminants may act as carriers. Cattle in endemic areas are less susceptible due to previous exposure.

Immunity: Acquired immunity in cattle due to previous infection.

Risk factors: Low plane of nutrition- clinical disease is less severe; thin hungry cattle – less susceptible than fat and well fed cattle. Cattle introduced in feed lots –highly susceptible.

Pathogenesis: Incubation period: 15 to 36 days; mortality-80 per cent in imported cattle. In endemic areas, seasonal death rate – 10 per cent.

Acute cases: 10 – 90 per cent RBCs are parasitized resulting in anaemia and death. Phagocytosis of parasitized RBCs with the release of inflammatory reactants and development of fever. Appearance of anti-erythrocytic antibodies in late acute stage exacerbates the anaemia. Fall in haematocrit level, RBC level and appearance of immature RBCs.

Clinical Signs

Very mild in cattle of less than 1 year.

(a) Per acute: Fatal in cattle of less than 3 years of cattle and death within a day of onset of clinical signs. Sudden onset of high fever, anaemia, icterus, severe dyspnoea, hyper excitability and death within 24 hours; Abortion in pregnant cows. Urine –normal colored; Milk yield-reduced.

(b) Sub acute: In young animals and recovery is slow in more chronic cases. Sheep and Goats: Usually sub clinical, but may be severe in goats with the clinical signs similar to goats.

Diagnosis

Clinical Signs: Detection of organisms in peripheral blood smear, Presence of insect vectors, History of entralce of outbreak, Nucleic acid probes.

Serological tests: Capillary tube agglutination test, CFT, IFA, Rapid card agglutination test, Dot- ELISA (highly sensitive and specific) and Antigen capture ELISA.

Differential Diagnosis

Babesiosis- More acute and haemoglobinuria.

Treatment

Tetracyclines: OTC and CTC @ 6-10 mg/kg, single dose or daily for 10 –16 days; effective in elimination of carriers. Long acting TC-20 mg/kg, I/V, every week, 2-4 injections.

Imidocarb: 3 mg/kg, effective for classic cases, no sterility of carriers.

Amicarbalide: 20 mg/kg, S/c, no sterility of carriers.

Control

Control is not practicable because of Wide spread insects, Long period of infectivity of carrier animals; inability to detect infection and carrier status in wild animals. Control of ticks by acaricides. Control of vector flies. Prevention of artificial transmission by instruments/surgical operations by disinfection. Elimination of carriers by screening the animals entering into areas by capillary agglutination tests/CFT. Elimination of carriers by a series of 4 injections at 3 days intervals of long acting TC.

Immunization: Killed *A. marginale* in an adjuvant vehicle as a vaccine (Anaplaz) in U.S.A. Dose- 2 vaccinations at 6 weeks apart. Immunity- at least for 5 months.

Demerit- Not completely protective and development of carriers and isoerythrolysis in neonates.

Live virulent vaccine: Limited to relatively resistant age group below 1 year of age. Demerit- development of carrier status.

Live attenuated vaccine: Use of attenuated virulent strain, irradiated organisms and a virulent strain adapted for growth in sheep/deer and the vaccine is frozen in liquid nitrogen.

Modified live vaccines: Effective and limited to mature cattle; induces resistance to clinical diseases.

Infection and Treatment

Administration of susceptible stock with small quantities of small blood containing mildly pathogenic *A. centrale* or a relatively avirulent *A. marginale* with or without subsequent administration of drug (OTC) is practiced in several countries.

4.2. Ehirlichiosis

In the past, a number of obligate intracellular organisms that infect eukaryotic cells were classified in the genus *Ehrlichia* on morphologic and ecologic grounds. With newer genetic analyses, these agents have been reclassified into the genera of *Ehrlichia*, *Anaplasma*, and *Neorickettsia*, all of which are in the family Anaplasmataceae. However, usage of the term "ehrlichiosis" to broadly describe these infections may still persist.

Ehrlichiosis is the rickettsial disease caused by the genus of *Ehrlichia* found in blood WBCs as intracytoplasmic inclusions and is charecterized by a short febrile illness associated with leuopenia and transmitted by ticks.

Morphology

Small pleomorphic, coccoid to ellipsoidal intracytoplasmic forms in circulatory WBCs of various mammals. Organisms occur singly or in compact colonies as a morula which is characteristic of the organism.

Epidemiology

Transmission: Non- contagious and is transmitted by bite of ticks. Experimentally by parenteral inoculation of organisms in horses.

Age: Very young lambs; Adult sheep and cattle newly entered in endemic areas.

Complications: Disease predisposes sheep- lambs to Louping ill, tick pyaemia (Enzootic staphylococcosis) and pasteurellosis.

Carrier status: Puppies for long time and stress precipitate the disease; Recovered animals.

Pathogenesis: Organisms invade in monocytes, macrophages and epithelial cells and they multiply and the entire cytoplasm is filled with organisms causing destruction of leucocytes and thrombocytes. This results in leukopenia, thrombocytopenia, anaemia, bone marrow depression. Horse - Invasion of intestinal epithelial cells by organisms causing colitis and typhilitis.

***Ehrlichia* in Livestock**

Sl.No.	*Species*	*Host*	*Location*	*Vector*	*Disease*
1	*E. bovis* (India)	Cattle	Mononuclear cells	*Hyalomma spp, Rhipicephalus sp.*	Bovine Ehrlichiosis (Nofel/ Nobi)
2	*E. canis*	Dog	Monocytes	*R. appendiculatus, R. sanguneus*	Tropical canine Pancytopenia, Canine Rickettsiosis, Nairobi bleeding disease, Lohore disease, Lahopi caninme fever
3	*E. ovina*	Sheep	Mononuclear cells	*R. bursa*	Mild disease
4	*E. equi*	Horse	Neutrophils and Eosinophils	Not known	Rarely fatal
5	*E. risticii*	Horse	Monocytes and Macrophages	Dermacentor sp?	Potomoc Horse Fever, Equine Ehrlichial Colitis

Clinical Signs

Cattle: Asymptomatic, Incubation period: 1-6 weeks.

Acute cases: Fever, tremor, incoordination, convulsion, anorexia, pale visible mucous membrane, lymph node enlargement, salivation and lacrimation, diarrhoea, frequent micturition, ocular and nasal disharge, nervous signs, death during convulsive phase of illness; abortion or temporary sterility in males may result.

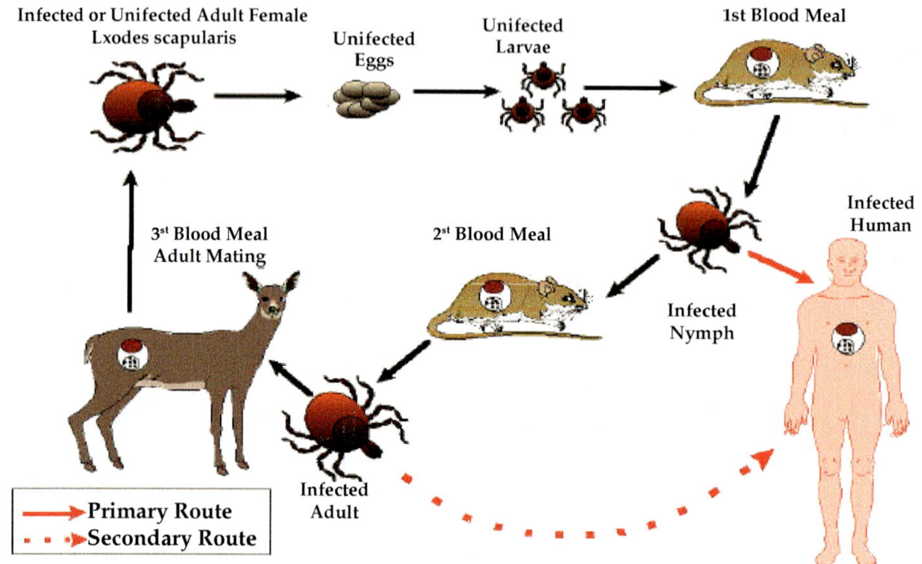

Figure 4.2. Life cycle of *Ehrlichia.*

Horses: Inapparent disease, in severe cases, high fever, anorexia, congested mucous membrane, severe diarrhoea of projectile in nature, colic, signs of dehydration, shock and signs of laminitis.

Subacute- Mild colic and subcutaneous oedema.

Sheep: Long incubation period, High fever persisting for long time, depression, anorexia, profound anaemia, ataxia, paraphlegia, sternal recumbency followed by death. Abortion may occur in sheep newly introduced in endemic areas.

Dogs: Undulating fever, lymph node enlargement, anorexia, depression, pale mucous membrane, haemorrhage and clotting abnormalities result in haematemesis, epistaxis, haematuria and haemorrhagic diarrhoea; Polyarthritis, polydypsia, polyuria and uraemia occur. Eye- haemorrhagic ophthalmitis is common. Death is due to secondary infection resulting from lekopenia, mucosal/serosal haemorrhages due to platelet deficiency (ecchymoses); also due to anaemia.

Lesions: Subcutaneous edema, enlarged spleen and lymph node, haemorrhage in liver and kidney, alimentary tract and many organs including joints and eyes.

4.3. Rocky Mountain Spotted Fever (*Rickettsia rickettsii* infection)

Etiology

Rocky Mountain spotted fever (RMSF) is a disease of people and dogs caused by *Rickettsia rickettsii*. *R. rickettsii* and closely related members of the spotted fever group of rickettsiae are considered endemic throughout much of North, South, and Central America. These pathogens are transmitted primarily through the bites of infected ticks. The ability of genetically similar rickettsial organisms, such as *R. parkeri*, to cause clinically similar disease in dogs is unknown. Because of their susceptibility to *R. rickettsii* and relatively higher rates of tick exposure, dogs may serve as excellent sentinels of risk for *R. rickettsii* infection in people. Clusters of disease are frequently reported in defined geographic areas, and temporally associated infections may be seen in both dogs and their owners.

Epidemiology

In the USA, *Dermacentor variabilis* (the American dog tick) and *D. andersoni* (the Rocky Mountain wood tick) are considered the primary vectors for *R. rickettsii*. In South America, several *Amblyomma* spp of ticks have been implicated in transmission. The organism has also been isolated from *Rhipicephalus sanguineus* ticks (the brown dog tick), which appear to be the primary vector in some focal areas of Arizona, particularly on American Indian tribal lands, and may also play an as-yet unappreciated role in outbreaks elsewhere in the USA. *R. sanguineus* ticks are also associated with transmission of *R. rickettsii* in Central America and with large city-based outbreaks in Mexico. The pathogen is acquired by larval and nymph stages of ticks while feeding on infected vertebrate hosts and is also passed from female ticks to progeny through transovarial transmission. An estimated <1 per cent of *Dermacentor* spp. ticks carry *R. rickettsii*, even in areas considered highly endemic. In highly enzootic regions of Arizona where *R. rickettsii* is transmitted by the brown dog tick, as many as 5 per cent of ticks may be infected.

Seroprevalence in dogs from endemic areas ranges from 4.3 per cent –77 per cent, but these values do not accurately reflect infection rates because of the detection of cross-reacting antibodies to other genetically similar rickettsiae. RMSF transmission through blood transfusion has been documented in a single human case and should be considered when selecting canine blood donors. Direct transmission from dogs to people has not been reported, although human infection may occur after contact of abraded skin or conjunctiva with tick hemolymph or excreta during removal of engorged ticks from pets.

Clinical Findings

Dogs are highly susceptible to clinical infection with *R rickettsii*; in contrast, it is rarely diagnosed in cats. Early signs in dogs may include fever ([up to 105°F 40.5°C]), anorexia, lymphadenopathy, polyarthritis, coughing or dyspnea, abdominal pain, vomiting and diarrhea, and edema of the face or extremities. Petechial hemorrhages of the conjunctiva and oral mucosa may be seen in severe cases. Focal retinal hemorrhage may be seen during the early course of disease. Neurologic manifestations such as altered mental states, vestibular dysfunction, and paraspinal hyperesthesia may occur.

Thrombocytopenia is common. Leukopenia develops during the early stages of infection and, in untreated cases, is followed by progressive leukocytosis. Serum biochemical abnormalities may include hypoproteinemia, hypoalbuminemia, azotemia, hyponatremia, hypocalcemia, and increased liver enzyme activities. Case fatality rates of ~1 per cent –10 per cent are expected.

Lesions

Vascular endothelial damage is due to direct cytopathic effects of the rickettsiae. Severity of the necrotizing vasculitis can be directly correlated to the infective dose. Vascular endothelial damage and thrombocytopenia contribute to development of petechiae and ecchymoses. Necrosis of the extremities (acryl gangrene) or disseminated intravascular coagulation can develop in severely affected dogs.

Diagnosis

Currently, there are no in-house diagnostic tests available for diagnosis of acute RMSF in dogs. Indirect fluorescent antibody titer (IFA) is preferred for serologic testing. However, because of the high incidence of cross-reacting antibodies to a variety of nonpathogenic spotted fever group rickettsiae, as well as long term persistence of antibodies after acute RMSF infection, demonstration of a 4-fold rise in titer should be documented in conjunction with a compatible clinical syndrome. Differential diagnoses include other causes of fever of unknown origin. The therapeutic response is usually dramatic, as it is in other canine rickettsial diseases. Animals with neurologic dysfunction may have residual deficits. Immunity appears to be lifelong after natural infection; therefore, recurrent episodes should not be attributed to RMSF.

Treatment

Antibiotic treatment should be administered based on clinical suspicion without waiting for results of serologic tests, because delayed administration of antibiotics may result in higher rates of severe or fatal outcome. Doxycycline is the treatment of choice, regardless of age of the dog, and should be administered at a dosage of 5–10 mg/kg/day, PO or IV, for 10–21 days. Tetracycline at 22 mg/kg, PO, tid for 2 wk is also effective. Chloramphenicol has been used to treat RMSF in the past, but its use is associated with higher rates of fatal outcome in human patients, and it is not recommended. Other broad-spectrum antibiotics are ineffective against *R. rickettsii* infection, and there is some evidence in human cases that use of fluoroquinolones may actually worsen infection. Early seronegative tests should not be considered a reason to stop therapy, because antibodies may take dikhuaaa1 wk to develop in acute cases. Supportive care for dehydration and hemorrhagic diathesis may be necessary. Because of alterations in vascular integrity, conservative rates of fluid administration are advised. Precautions should be taken for the safe removal and control of ticks. In settings in which *R rickettsii* transmission from *R sanquineus* is suspected, medications and products with proven efficacy against this tick species are important to use. Because *R sanguineus* infestations can be problematic in kennels and around homes, and longterm tick control is needed for outbreak control, use of effective long-acting tick collars on all susceptible dogs might be considered; collars containing propoxur, amitraz, or flumethrin have proven activity against *R. sanguineus*.

Zoonotic Risk

R. rickettsii is considered a zoonotic pathogen. The potential for household clustering and large urban outbreaks, particularly in areas with transmission by brown dog ticks, makes RMSF a disease of significant public health concern. Although clinical disease occurs in both animals and people, the involvement of a required intermediate tick vector for transmission means dogs and other infected animals do not pose a direct transmission risk in normal circumstances. Infection in dogs indicates a heightened risk of human infections related to tick exposure in a given area, and serologic studies of dogs in emerging areas may help predict human risk of infection. Particularly in areas where transmission occurs *via R. sanguineus*, close cooperation between veterinary, medical, and public health officials is important to achieve control.

4.4. Murine Typhus (*Rickettsia typhi* infection, *R. felis* infection)

Rickettsia typhi, the causative agent of murine typhus, and *R. felis* are zoonotic pathogens maintained primarily in rodent reservoirs (rats, mice) that may also be associated with enzootic cycles involving opossums and domestic cats. Infection is transmitted to people and other animals through contact with infected fleas.

Epidemiology

Infection in people is primarily thought to occur through exposure of abraded skin with infectious flea feces; aerosolization of infectious materials may occur in limited settings. Dogs and cats are presumably exposed in a similar fashion. Although known to occur worldwide, currently fewer than several hundred human cases of murine typhus are reported in the USA each year. Enzootic infection is the most commonly reported from southern Texas, California, and Hawaii, although the disease is believed to be underreported.

Clinical Findings

Clinical illness associated with canine and feline infection with *R. typhi* and *R. felis* is not well documented, but evidence of exposure based on presence of antirickettsial antibodies has been noted, particularly in association with outbreaks of human disease. Although a role as a possible reservoir for infection has been suggested, particularly for cats, the importance of domestic animals in maintenance of enzootic cycles has not been well elucidated. Nonetheless, dogs and cats may, at a minimum, serve as a source of fleas that may pose a transmission risk to people. Regular flea control is recommended to reduce risk of flea-associated transmission to people.

Diagnosis

An indirect fluorescent antibody (IFA) titer assessed in paired sera is preferred for serologic testing and is most commonly used in conjunction with environmental assessments around a human outbreak. There is some degree of antibody cross-reactivity with antibodies from other rickettsial infections, including *R. rickettsii*, so assessments should ideally be made with paired sera. PCR of whole blood may also be used, but its utility in assessing canine and feline infection is unknown because the animals may not exhibit clinical signs during periods of rickettsemia, making it difficult to determine the optimal time for assessment.

Treatment

In the absence of clinical signs, specific treatment is not recommended. If clinical illness associated with *R. typhi* or *R. felis* infection is suspected in a dog or cat, doxycycline may be administered at a dosage of 5–10 mg/kg/day, PO or IV, for 10–21 days. Animals should be provided with routine preventive treatments to control fleas. Control programs involving animal removal from an area of enzootic activity should be accompanied by pesticide treatment of the environment to prevent fleas feeding on people after the removal of preferred blood-meal hosts.

Zoonotic Risk

R. typhi is considered a zoonotic pathogen. Serologic evidence of exposure or past infection in dogs or cats indicates a heightened risk of human infections in a given area, and flea control for pets is an essential component of disease control.

4.5. Salmon Poisoning Disease and Elokomin Fluke Fever (*Neorickettsia* spp. infection)

Salmon poisoning disease (SPD) is an acute, infectious disease of canids, in which the infective agent is transmitted through the various stages of a fluke in a snail-fish-dog life cycle. The name of the disease is misleading, because no toxin is involved. Elokomin fluke fever (EFF) is an acute infectious disease of canids, ferrets, bears, and raccoons that resembles SPD but has a wider host range. In people, *Neorickettsia sennetsu* causes a disease known as Sennetsu ehrlichiosis, and in horses *N ristici*i causes a disease known as Potomac horse fever; these have not been reported as a cause of illness in dogs except for one report of *N. risticii* in Illinois.

Etiology

SPD is caused by *N. helminthoeca* and is sometimes complicated by a second agent, *N. elokominica*, which causes EFF. The vector for these *Neorickettsia* agents is a small fluke, *Nanophyetus salmincola*. Dogs and other animals become infected by ingesting trout, salmon, or Pacific giant salamanders that contain the encysted metacercaria stage of the rickettsia-infected fluke. In the dog's intestine, the metacercarial flukes excyst, embed in the duodenal mucosa, become gravid adults, and transmit the rickettsiae to monocytes-macrophages. The fluke infection itself produces little or no clinical disease. A recent report of SPD in two captive Malayan sun bears underscores the need to consider this etiology in non-native exotic species with compatible exposure and clinical histories.

Epidemiology

The life cycle of *Neorickettsia helminthoeca* is maintained by the release of infected fluke ova in the feces of the mammalian host. Infected miracidia develop from these ova and infect the snails *Juga plicifera* and *Juga silicula* to form infected rediae. Rediae develop into infected cercariae that are released from the snail, penetrate the salmon or trout, and develop into encysted metacercariae infected with *Neorickettsia*. The cycle is completed when mammals eat the fish, and infected metacercariae become infected gravid adults and pass *Neorickettsia* to fluke eggs. Although *Neorickettsia* infection of dogs is not required for the life cycle of *Neorickettsia*, mammalian infection is required to maintain the trematode life cycle. Transmission by cage-to-cage contact, rectal thermometers, or aerosols is rare.

There are no age, sex, or breed predilections; however, the disease prevalence is higher when the availability of trematode-infected fish is greater. Infected fish are found in the Pacific Ocean from San Francisco to the coast of Alaska, but SPD is more prevalent from northern California to Puget Sound. It is also seen inland along the rivers of fish migration. SPD also has been reported in southern California and Brazil. The snail is the primary factor for geographic limitation, but dogs fed undercooked or raw fish from the supermarket may have developed SPD.

Clinical Findings

In SPD, signs appear suddenly, usually 5–7 days after eating infected fish, but may be delayed as long as 33 days, and persist for 7–10 days before culminating in death in up to 90 per cent of untreated animals. Body temperature peaks at 104°–107.6°F (40°–42°C) 1–2 days later, then gradually declines for 4–8 days and returns to normal. Frequently, animals are hypothermic before death. Fever is accompanied by depression and complete anorexia in virtually all cases. Persistent vomiting usually occurs by day 4 or 5. Vomiting occurs in most cases, and diarrhea, which develops by day 5–7, often contains blood and may be severe. Dehydration and extreme weight loss occur. When severe, the GI signs are clinically indistinguishable from those of canine parvoviral infection. Generalized lymphadenopathy develops in ~60 per cent of cases. Nasal or conjunctival exudate may be present and mimic signs of distemper. Neutrophilia is common, but a marked, absolute leukopenia with a degenerative left shift may occur. Thrombocytopenia is reported in 94 per cent of the cases. Serum chemistry values are normal.

Clinically, EFF is a milder infection than SPD. Severe GI signs are less commonly seen in EFF infections, and lymphadenopathy may be a more pronounced finding. Case fatality rates with EFF are lower, at ~10 per cent of untreated cases.

Lesions

Infection appears to chiefly affect the lymphoid tissues and intestines. There is enlargement of the GI lymph follicles, lymph nodes, tonsils, thymus, and to some extent, the spleen, with microscopic necrosis, hemorrhage, and hyperplasia. Remarkable abdominal or mesenteric lymphadenomegaly may be seen. Variable but often severe nonhemorrhagic enteritis is seen throughout the intestine with SPD but is less commonly seen with EFF. Microscopic foci of necrosis also appear apart from the follicles. Nonsuppurative meningitis or meningoencephalitis has been identified in some dogs.

Diagnosis

Fluke ova are found on fecal examination in ~92 per cent of cases, which supports the diagnosis. The ova are oval, yellowish brown, rough-surfaced, and ~87–97 × 35–55 μm, with an indistinct operculum and a small, blunt point on the opposite end. During the first day or two, few ova may be passed. Intracellular organisms have been demonstrated by Romanowsky staining on lymph node aspirates in ~70 per cent of cases. PCR testing to detect DNA-specific *N. helminthoeca* (or *Neorickettsia* genus) is recommended for accurate diagnosis. Serologic testing using the *N. helminthoeca* organism has been developed. Other causes of fever of unknown origin, generalized lymphadenopathy, vomiting, and diarrhea are differential diagnoses. When diarrhea and exudative conjunctivitis occur, distemper should be considered.

Prevention and Treatment

Currently, the only means of prevention is to restrict the ingestion of uncooked salmon, trout, steelhead, and similar freshwater fish. In animals that recover, a profound humoral immune response persists, but there is no cross-resistance between *N. helminthoeca* and *N. elokominica*. Sulfonamides are not effective and may exacerbate the clinical disease. Recommended treatment is parenteral oxytetracycline (7 mg/kg, IV, tid for 5 days) or doxycycline (10 mg/kg, bid for 7 days). Oral tetracycline or doxycycline is contraindicated because of impinging GI signs. Animals usually succumb because of dehydration, electrolyte and acid-base imbalances, and anemia. Therefore, general supportive therapy to maintain hydration and acid-base balance, while meeting nutritional requirements and controlling diarrhea, is often essential. Judicious use of whole blood transfusions may be helpful.

Chapter 5

Parasitic Diseases

The clinical signs associated with GI parasitisms are shared by many diseases and conditions; however, a presumptive diagnosis based on signs, grazing history, and season is often justified. Infection usually can be confirmed by demonstrating nematode eggs or tapeworm segments on fecal examination. However, in clinical evaluation of fecal examinations, two points should be remembered: 1) a fecal worm egg count (number of worm eggs per gram (EPG) of feces is not always an accurate indication of the number of adult worms present, and 2) specific identification of certain nematode eggs (*e.g.*, "strongyles") is impractical except in specialized laboratories. EPG counts can be negative or deceptively low in the presence of large numbers of immature worms; even when many adult parasites are present, the count can be low if egg production has been suppressed by host immune reaction or recent anthelmintic treatment. Variations in the egg-producing capability of different worms (significantly lower for *Trichostrongylus*, *Ostertagia*, and *Nematodirus* than for *Haemonchus*) may also distort the true picture. The ova of *Nematodirus*, *Bunostomum*, *Strongyloides*, and *Trichuris* are distinctive, but reliable differentiation of the more common species of ruminant strongyle ova is difficult. Fecal culture of strongyle eggs can produce distinctive third-stage larvae if differentiation is important premortem.

The advent of safe and effective broad-spectrum anthelmintics has largely reduced the need to differentiate the genera and species of these parasites. In areas where *Ostertagia* spp predominate, the analysis of sera for increased plasma pepsinogen levels is a useful diagnostic aid. Generally, increased levels of pepsinogen activity (tyrosine levels >3 IU) are associated with clinical abomasal parasitism. Problems of interpretation may arise in immune animals under challenge, in which there are no clinical signs but the pepsinogen levels may be increased because of a hypersensitivity-type reaction in the abomasal mucosa. Where *Haemonchus* spp predominate, the traditional estimation of PCV as an indicator of anemia has been largely replaced by use of the FAMACHA test. In some countries, serologic diagnosis (ELISA) of important species, such as *Ostertagia* in cattle, is also used and based on antibody titers in bulk tank milk samples in dairy herds. Such information is used as an indicator of pasture challenge at a herd level, as an indirect indicator of productivity, and is linked with the effectiveness of parasite control strategies.

In many management situations, high levels of infection can be expected, particularly after favorable temperature and rainfall conditions. "Diagnostic drenching" may be recommended when eggs are few or absent, yet history and signs suggest infections, although care should be taken not to treat animals indiscriminately to minimize the risk of anthelmintic resistance developing. Routine postmortem examinations can provide valuable parasitologic data about the status of the rest of the herd or flock. On necropsy, *Haemonchus, Bunostomum, Oesophagostomum, Trichuris,* and *Chabertia* adults (or advanced immature worms) can be seen easily. *Ostertagia, Trichostrongylus, Cooperia,* and *Nematodirus* are difficult to see except by their movement in fluid digesta, and clinically important infections are easily overlooked. In such cases, the total contents and all washings should be combined to a known volume, and a worm count established to evaluate the severity of the infection. The number of worms found in aliquots of the gut contents and scrapings of the mucosa will enable the total worm count to be calculated. However, the smaller nematodes may be difficult to see against a background of digesta, so they can be stained (5 min) with a strong iodine solution. Once the digesta and any tissue have been decolorized with 5 per cent sodium thiosulfate, the iodine-stained worms can be seen easily. The significance of the numbers of worms present varies according to worm and host species. For example, only 100 *Haemonchus* are of clinical significance in lambs, whereas 5,000–10,000 *Ostertagia* are typically required before clinical signs are seen. If the animals have been diarrheic for a few days, worms may have been expelled and so the location, type, and severity of gross lesions may also be of considerable diagnostic value.

Mixed parasite infections should be considered when evaluating clinical, laboratory, and necropsy findings, because grazing animals rarely have monospecific infections in the field.

The diagnosis of ostertagiosis in cattle during the period of larval inhibition (aka arrested development, hypobiosis, diapause) presents technical problems, particularly for the feedlot industry in the USA. Fecal egg counts and plasma pepsinogen analysis do not provide useful information because inhibition occurs within a few days of larval ingestion, before either the egg-laying adult stage has been reached or plasma pepsinogen levels increase. Predisposing factors for inhibition of larvae include age and geographic source of cattle, time of year or season of arrival, previous grazing history and management, weather conditions prevailing during the last grazing period, and prevalence of *Ostertagia ostertagi* in the source region.

Information on such factors is not usually available for feedlot cattle. If cattle have arrived after spring grazing in the south of the USA or fall grazing in the north, they could have heavy burdens of inhibited larvae. Lighter calves from areas where prevalence of parasites is high may also have such a problem. It is becoming more widely accepted that a significant cause of clinical disease or feed efficiency problems in feedlot cattle is parasitism, possibly ostertagiosis. When cattle are brought in from a suspect area and at a suspect time of year, it may be advisable to treat the new arrivals promptly with an anthelmintic effective against inhibited larvae.

5.1. Amphistomiasis

Stomach flukes are parasite of ruminants which particularly affect cattle and sheep. The flukes are often found in small numbers but only seriously affect livestock under certain conditions, in heavy infections, and in certain growth stages. The disease is characterized by severe enteritis. Young cattle are the usual subjects of the disease. Heavy infection with immature flukes in the upper intestine can cause serious ill-health and death. Amphistomiasis or paramphistomiasis (alternatively spelled amphistomosis or paramphistomosis) is a parasitic disease of livestock animals, more commonly of cattle and sheep, and humans caused by immature helminthic flatworms belonging to the order Echinostomida. The term amphistomiasis is used for broader connotation implying the disease inflicted by members of Echinostomida including the family Paramphistomidae/Gastrodiscidae (to be precise, the species *Gastrodiscoides hominis*); whereas paramphistomiasis is restricted to that of the members of the family Paramphistomatidae only. *G. discoides* and *Watsonius watsoni* are responsible for the disease in humans, while most paramphistomes are responsible in livestock animals, and some wild mammals. In livestock industry the disease causes heavy economic backlashes due to poor production of milk, meat and wool.

Morphology

Small, conical in shape and pink in colour.

Epidemiology

Factors influencing ourbreak of amphistomiasis: Management, environmental factors, intermediate host, definitive host, and the egg contain the miracidium when passed in the faeces.

Management: Animals are reared in extensive systems of management, grazing near pond area/other natural resources, especially - drier months, snail population - concentrated more fresh palatable grasses are more favour for encystation of metacercariae, attracts animals.

Environmental factors: Season – drier months, high rain fall, temperature – embryonation (miracidium) and maturation of cercariae (27°C), light - strong light influences release of cercariae from snail intermediate host, availability of suitable snail, young snails are highly susceptible than adult, multiplication of snails take places in warm, watery environment.

Definitive host: Young animals are highly susceptible than adult, preinfection – give resistant, the egg contain the miracidium when passed in the faeces, the egg do not hatch.

Name of the Snail	*Name of Trematode*
Indoplanorbis exustus	*Gigantocotyle explanatum, Cotylophoron cotylophorum* and *Gastrodiscus secundus*
Gyraulus convexiculus	*Gastrothylax crumenifer*
Lymnaea luteola	*Fischoederius elongatus* and *Fischoederius cobboldi*

Intermediate host for Amphistomes: *Planorbis, Bulinus Pseudosuccinea, Fossaria Indoplanorbis, Lymnaea, Pygmanisas, Glyptanisus* and *Cleopatra.*

Life Cycle

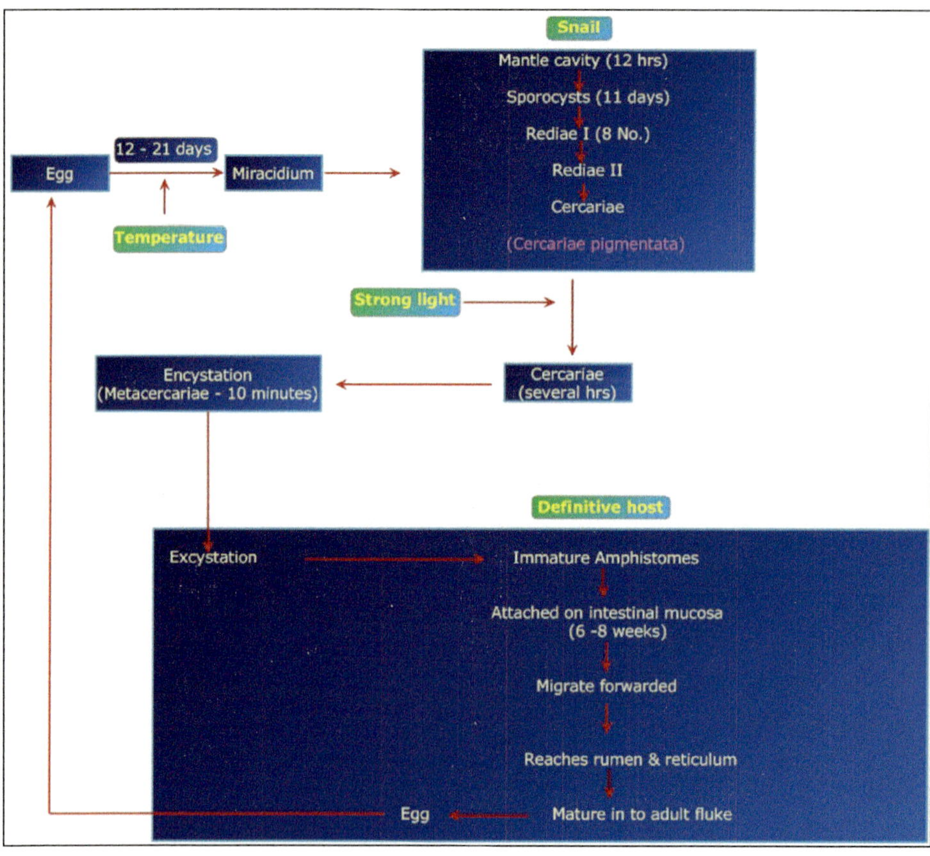

Figure 5.1. Life cycle of Amphistomiasis.

Pathogenesis

Adult flukes: Fore stomach–large numbers of worms–not much pathogenic changes, bile duct and gall bladder–superficial haemorrhage.

Liver–Fibrosis: Immature flukes (pitto), duodenum, upper ileum-plug feeder: plug intestinal mucosa–haemorrhages and necrosis (haemorrhagic duodenitis), embedded in mucosa/muscularis.

Clinical signs: fetid diarrhoea, marked weakness, thirsty and drink more water.

Different Species of Amphistomes

Amphistomes are called as Stomach flukes or conical flukes.

Name of Trematodes	*Host*	*Location*
Paramphistomum gotoi	Cattle	Fore stomach
Paramphisomum cervi	Cattle	Fore stomach
Cotylophoron cotylophorum	Sheep, Goat and Cattle	Rumen and Reticulum
Calicophoron calicphorum	Sheep and Cattle	Rumen and Reticulum
Ceylonocotyle streptocoelium	Cattle, Sheep and Antelope	Rumen and Reticulum
Ceylonocotyle scoliocoelium	Cattle, Sheep and Antelope	Rumen and Reticulum
Gigantocotyle explanatum	Buffalo and Cattle	Bile duct, Gall bladder and Duodenum
Gastrothylax crumenifer	Sheep, Cattle and Buffalo	Rumen and Reticulum
Fischoederius elongatus	Cattle and other Bovidae	Rumen
Fischoederius cobboldi	Zebu cattle	Rumen
Carmyerius spatiosus	Cattle and Antelope	Rumen
Carmyerius gregarius	Cattle and Buffalo	Rumen
Gastrodiscus aegyptiacus	Equine and Pig	Large and Small intestine
Gastrodiscus secundus	Horse and Elephant	Colon
Gastrodiscoides hominis	Man and Pig	Colon
Pseudodiscus collinsi	Horse	Colon

Diagnosis

It is based on history and clinical signs, faecal examination, gross – presence of immature worms in fluid faeces, microscopic - presence of typical egg.

Treatment

Bithionol sulphoxide – 40 mg/kg (activity against Immature – 100 per cent), Resorantol – 65 mg/kg (Immature – 65 per cent and Mature – 100 per cent), Niclosamide - 90 mg/kg (Immature – 99.9 per cent and Mature – 8 per cent), Niclofolan - 6 mg/Kg (Immature – 96 per cent and Mature – 43 per cent), Oxyclozanide – 18.7 mg/kg for two days (Immature and Mature - 100 per cent), Hexachlorophene – 20 mg/kg - single dose, Resorantol and Oxyclozanide are the drug of choice for both immature and mature Amphistomes.

Control

Avoid grazing near pond area, prevent access of natural water resources – fencing of water resources, provide wholesome water supply at convenient places, drainage of water pools and swampy area, snail control, prophylactic deworming.

5.2. Anchylostomatidae

The Ancylostomatidae are a family of worms that includes the hookworms. The family Ancylostomatidae (Hook worms) includes the genus *Ancylostoma, Bunostomum, Agriostomum, Gaigeria.*

Epidemiology of *Ancylostoma*

Infection rate: Adult female lay - 16,000 egg/day (egg laying inversely proportional to worm load).

Bionomic: Similar to Strongyles, Slightly sandy and moist soil suitable for survivability, Direct sunlight lethal to larvae.

Housing: Soiled bedding with damp, porous or cracked floor – leads to massive infection, arrested larval development inside the host (in L_3 form), exposed to sudden chilling. Depends upon immunological status.

Host: Young puppies are highly susceptible (due to translacteal infection). One year old age groups are highly susceptible, Smaller breeds are highly susceptible than heavier breeds. Nutritional status - well nourished animal with stand the infection and poor iron reserves in the body leads to severe infection (Milk is the poor source of iron). Stress and corticosteroid therapy precipitate the infection from dormant larvae in muscle. Infection of definitive host, Paratenic host, Rodents (L3) —> passive ingestion —> Definitive host.

Life Cycle

A. braziliense – failure to induce prenatal infection - Intrauterine infection is absent. *A. duodenale*, skin penetration is important mode of infection, arrested larval development occurs during unfavorable condition.

Pathogenesis

Anemia: Due to blood sucking activity of worm, stages of worm - L4 mainly followed by L5 and adult, 8 days of post infection (DPI)– starts to suck blood, 10 –15 DPI peak blood loss and 20 DPI egg out put and heavy blood loss. Death occurs within 10 –24 DPI in untreated cases. Types of anemia – initially normocytic and normochromic followed by microcytic and hypochromic anemia due to loss of iron reserves.

Clinical Signs

(a) **Acute cases:** Hydremia, oedema, general weakness, emaciation, stunted growth. Diarrhoea – 4 DPI and fresh blood mixed with watery mucus on 8 DPI. Skin lesion. Associated with percutaneous infection ranges from moist eczema to ulceration. Cutaneous larval migration or creeping eruption. Damage in feet occurs due to severe infection. Lesion aggravated by licking and self biting (after rain when allowed on wet grass or sand in endemic areas).

    Haemorrhagic pneumonitis: Due to translacteal migration.

(b) **Chronic cases:** Reduced appetite, poor growth, poor hair coat. *A. braziliense* – blood loss insignificant (0.001 ml), hypoproteinaemia and protein losing gastroenteropathy.

Immunity: Natural age resistance occurs on 8th month of age in female and 11th months of age in male. Acquired immunity - Crisis – similar to self cure phenomena occurred in *H. contortus*. Graded doses of gamma irradiated L3 larvae when given

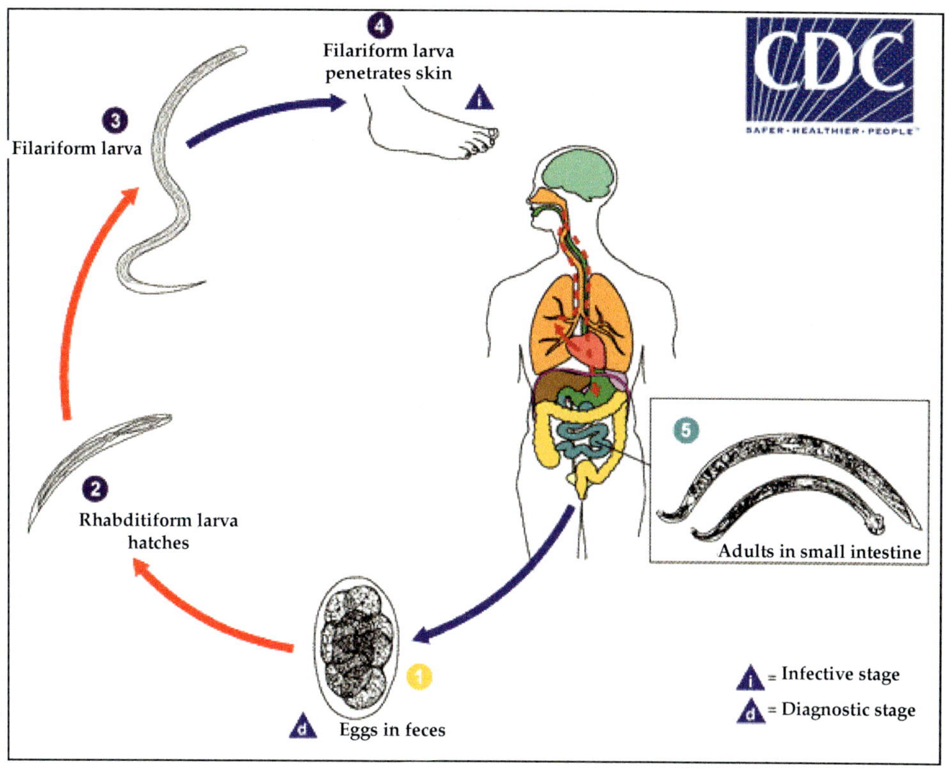

Figure 5.2

Eggs are passed in the stool–1, and under favorable conditions (moisture, warmth, shade), larvae hatch in 1 to 2 days. The released rhabditiform larvae grow in the feces and/or the soil–2, and after 5 to 10 days (and two molts) they become filariform (third-stage) larvae that are infective–3. These infective larvae can survive 3 to 4 weeks in favorable environmental conditions. On contact with the human host, the larvae penetrate the skin and are carried through the blood vessels to the heart and then to the lungs. They penetrate into the pulmonary alveoli, ascend the bronchial tree to the pharynx, and are swallowed–4. The larvae reach the small intestine, where they reside and mature into adults. Adult worms live in the lumen of the small intestine, where they attach to the intestinal wall with resultant blood loss by the host–5. Most adult worms are eliminated in 1 to 2 years, but the longevity may reach several years.

S/C or orally, egg count increases upto 2 months after challenge there after marked reduction of egg count and large number of adult worm expelled through faeces. Dose: 1,000 larvae. Age of administration – 72 hours after birth (Presence of maternal antibodies (colostral) will not interfere). Duration of immunity – 7 months in absence of reexposure. **Species:** *A. caninum, A. braziliense, A. ceylanicum, A. duodenale.*

Ancyclstomum caninum

Host: Dog and other carnivores; **Location**: Small intestine.

Distribution: Cosmopolitan in tropical and subtropical countries.

Morphology: Male: 1 cm and female – 1.5 cm. Fairly rigid and grey or reddish in colour (Depending on the presence of blood in the alimentary canal).

Egg: Similar to *Oesophagostomum*.

Ancyclstomum braziliense

Host: Dog, cat and wild carnivores; **Location**: Small intestine

Bunostomum **(Hook Worms of Ruminants)**

Bunostomum trigonocephalum

Host: Sheep, goat and cattle (rarely); **Location**: ileum and jejunum

Life cycle: Similar to *Ancylostoma*, prepatent period: 30 – 56 days

Epidemiology: Similar to *Ancylostoma*.

Occurrence is more common in warmer climate than cold climate, mixed infection Strongyles and *Bunostomum*.

Clinical Signs

Anaemia, oedema on intermandibular region – "Bottle jaw". Diarrhoea – not infrequent, faeces dark in colour due to altered blood pigments. Prostration and finally death.

Diagnosis

Based on clinical signs, faecal examination.

Treatment

Fenbendazole - 5 mg/kg. Albendazole –7. 5 mg/kg. Parbendazole – 15 5 mg/ kg. Cambendazole - 20 5 mg/kg. Thiabendazole -75 mg/kg.

Control

Avoid wet floor shelter – larvae highly susceptible to dryness. Similar to *Ancylostoma*.

Bunostomum phlebotomum

Host: Young calves, Sheep are rarely affected; **Location**: Duodenum.

Clinical Signs

Anaemia, diarrhoea, submandibular oedema. In stabled cattle itching and stamping of legs.

Diagnosis

Based on clinical signs, Faecal examination: EPG > 1,000 - severe infection.

Treatment

For anaemia: Blood transfusion, haematinics and iron therapy, protein rich foods.

Anthelmintics: Dichlorvos - 12 –15 mg/kg (choline esterase inhibitor), Tetramisole – 7.5 mg/kg S/C, 20 mg/kg oral, Mebendazole - 40 mg/kg (total or divided doses), Fenbendazole - 20 mg/kg (immature and mature), Nitroscanate - 50 mg/kg oral.

Prophylaxis: Kennel floor should keep as clean and dry. Floor should treat with salt such as sodium borate @ 2 kg/10 liter -destroys the larvae. Floor should make up of impervious cement concrete. Faeces removed and disposed off properly. Deworming regimen similar to Toxocara. In pregnant bitches - 3 weeks before whelping to 2 days after whelping daily with fenbendazole @ 7.5 mg/kg. Nourishing litters, first dose - 1 – 2 weeks of age, second dose - 3- 4 weeks of age, weaned puppies - once in three months.

5.3. Ascariasis

Roundworms are a type of parasitic worm. Infections caused by roundworms are relatively common. Ascariasis is the most common roundworm infection. About 10 per cent of the developing world is infected with intestinal worms, according to the World Health Organization (WHO). However, infections with parasitic worms are not as common in the United States, according to the Centers for Disease Control and Prevention (CDC). Ascariasis is most common in places without modern sanitation. It's transmitted through unsafe food and water. The infection usually causes no symptoms, but heavier infestations can lead to problems in the lungs or intestines.

Epidemiology

Hosts: Pigs

Age: Young pigs (<4 months) are highly susceptible.

Cattle: Infection occurs due to rising of cattle on piggery shed and grazing of cattle on pasture land fertilized with infected pig manure.

Sheep: Especially young lambs grazed on pasture land fertilized with infected pig manure.

Human beings: Only few reports.

Paratenic host: Earth worm and dung beetle.

Parasite

Infection rate: Adult worm lay 2,00,000 - 20,00,000 eggs per day. Eggs contains infective larvae resist adverse conditions like freezing, disinfectant like 2 per cent formalin - so viable upto 5 years or even more. Susceptible to dry hot environmental temperature (>40°C).

Environment: Embryonation - optimal temp - 22 - 26°C, high relative humidity and oxygen tension. Cropping and ploughing - no effect on infective egg.

Suitable Season: Temperate countries: warmer months - 22-26°C. Tropical countries: warmer months - 30-33°C. Egg in the environment can be transported through wind, uncooked vegetables, fruits, *etc.*

Ascaris, Gastrointestinal Nematodiasis

Ascaris: *A. suum, Parascaris: P. equorum, Toxocara: T. canis; T. cati and T. vitulorum, Toxascaris: T. leonine.*

General Morphology

Adult: Generally larger worms.

Females: Oviparous, produce large No. of eggs.

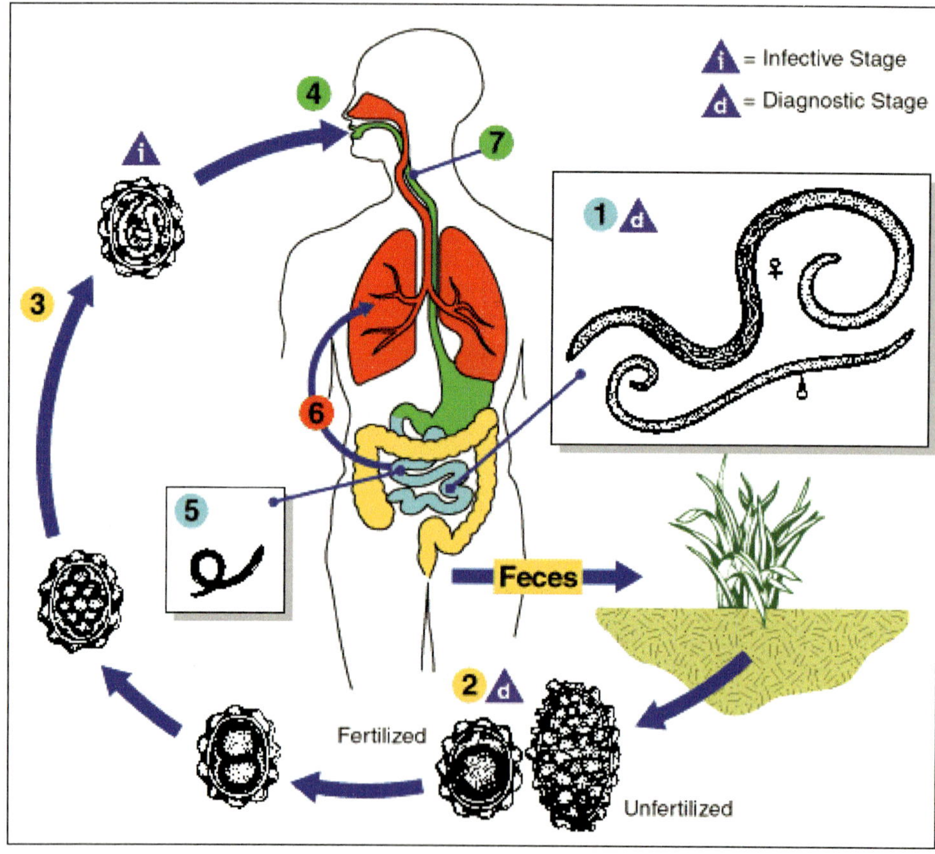

Figure 5.3

Adult worms–1 live in the lumen of the small intestine. A female may produce up to 240,000 eggs per day, which are passed with the feces–2. Fertile eggs embryonate and become infective after 18 days to several weeks–3, depending on the environmental conditions (optimum: moist, warm, shaded soil). After infective eggs are swallowed–4, the larvae hatch–5, invade the intestinal mucosa, and are carried via the portal, then systemic circulation to the lungs–6. The larvae mature further in the lungs (10-14 days), penetrate the alveolar walls, ascend the bronchial tree to the throat, and are swallowed–7. Upon reaching the small intestine, they develop into adult worms–1. Between 2 and 3 months are required from ingestion of the infective eggs to oviposition by the adult female. Adult worms can live 1 to 2 years.

Egg: Unsegmented when laid, the eggs are oval or subglobular and the shell is in most cases thick. Inner -thin and lipid layer, middle layer -tough and chitin layer, outer layer -thick and protein layer, hatching of egg.

Ascaris suum

Host: Pig.

Morphology: 40 cm long. Immature some times called as *A. ovis* occasionally found in sheep, dog and cattle.

Egg: Albumin layer (outer) bears prominent projections "Knob" which is brownish yellow in colour.

Life cycle: Direct.

Prepatent period: 2 months. No prenatal infection.

Pathogenesis

Pigs

Migration of larvae - migratory haemorrhagic tracts

Lungs: Transient Pneumonia - Ascarids Pneumonia

Liver: Milk spots (observed in all age groups) - migration with molting - whitish cloudy spots up to 1 cm in diameter. Which represents fibrous repair of inflammatory reactions to the passage of larvae in liver of previously sensitized pigs?

Adults: Presence of numerous worms in the intestine may be twisted - become solid mass which cause obstruction - perforation – peritonitis. Some worms wander enter into stomach and voided through vomitus. If enter liver through bile duct - causing biliary stasis - obstructive jaundice.

Cattle: Acute interstitial pneumonia.

Sheep: Pneumonia as well as milk spots.

Clinical Signs

In pigs

Signs of pneumonia - cough - retarded growth. Migration of *A. suum* larvae in the pig may enhances latent infections of Enzootic pneumonia (Viral) and swine influenza.

Adult worm - heavy infection - diarrhoea - reduced weight gain. Breakdown of immunity in hog cholera vaccination with live virus are often attributed to this cause. *Concurrent infection*: *A. suum* with Salmonellosis.

Diagnosis

Based on clinical signs - some time larvae in sputum.

Characteristic egg - EPG: >1000 indicative of significant infection

Treatment

Ascarids pneumonia - levamisole - 7.5 mg/kg and Ivermectin, Intestinal stage: Benzimidazole and Imidazole compounds are drug of choice, *Levamisole HCl*: s/c -

7.5 mg/kg; drenching - 8 mg/kg and through feed - 0.72 g/kg of feed, *Tetramisole Hcl*: - immature and mature, oral - 15 mg/kg and through feed 5 kg/500 kg of feed. *Parbendazole* - 30 mg/kg. *Cambendazole* - 20 mg/kg. *Fenbendazole* - 5 mg/kg - ovicidal effect. *Dichlorvos* - sows - 10 mg/kg and weaned pigs - 40 mg/kg. *Morantel citrate:* weaner - 5 mg/kg and older - 12.5 mg/kg. *Piperazine:* 100 - 400 mg/kg.

Control

Contaminated pens*:* use solutions of hot caustic soda or live steam. *Pasture management:* rotational cultivation.

McLean County System: It is most important preventive measures are those concentrated with protection of the young pigs immediately after birth or later against Ascarids infection. Basic principles of McLean County System, clean sow, clean farrowing pen, clean pasture, few hours before furrowing, the pregnant sows are thoroughly washed and scrubbed in order to remove any egg adhering to the body and is then placed in furrowing pen, the furrowing pen should made up of concrete floor. The floors and walls should be thoroughly scrubbed with boiling water and caustic soda by hard broom, with in 10 days after furrowing the sow and it litters are removed to an Ascarids - free field, planted with a suitable crop, after weaning the sow is removed and the young pigs are grow up which are able to resist the major effect of infection.

Factors impeding control measures: The worms are prolific egg layers, the infective eggs are very resistant and long lived, Young animals are most susceptible.

5.4. Babesiosis

Babesiosis is caused by intraerythrocytic protozoan parasites of the genus *Babesia*. Transmitted by ticks, babesiosis affects a wide range of domestic and wild animals and occasionally people. Although the major economic impact of babesiosis is on the cattle industry, infections in other domestic animals, including horses, sheep, goats, pigs, and dogs, assume varying degrees of importance throughout the world.

Two important species in cattle—*B. bigemina* and *B. bovis*—are widespread in tropical and subtropical areas and are the focus of this discussion. However, because there are many common features of the diseases caused by different *Babesia*, much of this information can be applied to other species.

Family: Babesidae

First vector borne disease caused by *Babesia* spp in cattle, sheep, pigs, horses and dogs and is characterized by fever, intravascular haemolysis causing a syndrome of anaemia, haemoglobinuria, and haemoglobinaemia and are transmitted by ticks.

Morphology

In RBC- seen singly as ovoid, round, elongate or amoeboid trophozoites; as pyriform merozoites (pairs)/cruziform (tetrads) merozoites; characteristically they are pear shaped; large forms lie with their narrow ends at an acute angle and small forms at obtuse angle.

Life Cycle of *Babesia* Sp.

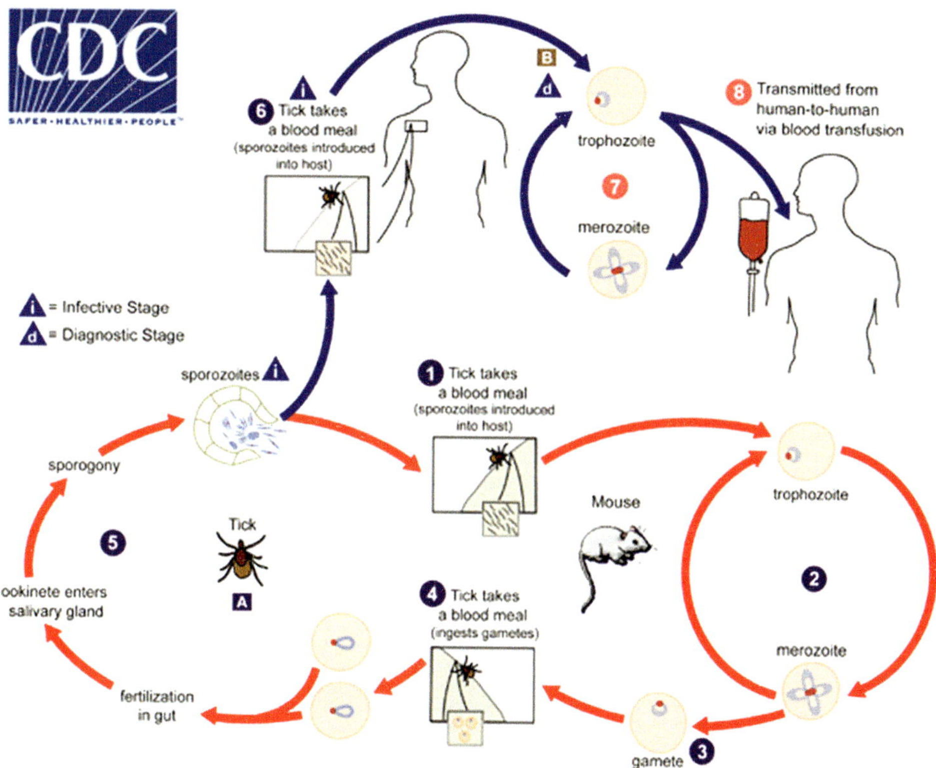

Figure 5.4

The *Babesia microti* life cycle involves two hosts, which include a rodent, primarily the white-footed mouse, *Peromyscus leucopus,* and a tick in the genus *Ixodes*. During a blood meal, a *Babesia*-infected tick introduces sporozoites into the mouse host–1. Sporozoites enter erythrocytes and undergo asexual reproduction (budding)–2. In the blood, some parasites differentiate into male and female gametes, although these cannot be distinguished by light microscopy–3. The definitive host is the tick. Once ingested by an appropriate tick–4, gametes unite and undergo a sporogonic cycle resulting in sporozoites–5. Transovarial transmission (also known as vertical, or hereditary, transmission) has been documented for "large" *Babesia* species but not for the "small" *Babesia*, such as *B. microti*–A. Humans enter the cycle when bitten by infected ticks. During a blood meal, a *Babesia*-infected tick introduces sporozoites into the human host–6. Sporozoites enter erythrocytes–B and undergo asexual replication (budding)–7. Multiplication of the blood-stage parasites is responsible for the clinical manifestations of the disease. Humans usually are dead-end hosts. However, human-to-human transmission is well recognized to occur via contaminated blood transfusions–8.

Pathogenesis

Highly pathogenic and death rate is higher in adults. Intra vascular haemolysis is the principal pathogenic effect due to the multiplication of *B. bigemina* and *B. bovis* in peripheral and visceral blood vessels respectively thus resulting in profound anemia, (hypochromic normocytic), jaundice and haemoglobinuria. Death is due to destruction of RBCs by auto-antibody mechanism, failure to recoup blood loss, cerebral anoxia and accumulation of toxic by-products.

***B. bovis*:** Production of vaso active substances, kinin and kallikrein results in vasodilatation accompanied by increased vascular permeability leading to circular stasis and shock. Disseminated intravascular coagulation (DIC) due to break down products resulting in fatal pulmonary thrombosis in calves. Ischaemic changes in skeletal and cardiac muscles in survivors.

Haematology: TEC - less than 2 million/cmm and neutrophilia.

Biochemical changes: Reduced calcium, phosphorous, total serum protein; Increase in blood glucose, total serum bilirubin and SGOT in liver damage.

Necropsy Findings

Urinary bladder containing reddish, pink or coffee colored urine; Enlargement and congestion of lymph nodes.

Clinical Findings

Incubation period: 2-3 weeks; Subclinical infection infection in young cattle. Fever, anorexia, brick red conjunctiva which becomes anaemic, depression, weakness, cessation of rumination, salivation, dryness of muzzle, lachrymation, dropped milk yield. Profound diarrhoea followed by constipation. Advanced stages: Severe anaemia, haemoglobinuria, jaundice, dark red to brown urine with a very stable froth and death after 24 hours.In survivors - course is 3 weeks. Abortion in pregnant animals. Cerebral form (*B.bigemina*): In coordination, posterior paralysis, mania, convulsions, coma, fever, death within 12-36 hours after clinical signs.

Chronic cases: Extend for several weeks with intermittent temperature.

B. divergens: Similar to above. Also spasm of anal sphincter muscles causing the passage of Pipe-stem liver.

Diagnosis

Detection of piroplasms in peripheral blood smears which is not always possible. Both thick and thin blood smears may be used for demonstration of organisms in RBCs. Presence of heavy infestation with ticks. FAT- Acridine orange fixed with blood smear appeared red with yellow nucleus; DNA probes.

Necropsy: Splenomegaly, jaundice, haemoglobinuria, myocardial ecchymoses –highly suggestive. Immunodiagnosis in subclinical infections. IHA- 80 per cent effective in field infections. IFA, CFT, IHA and Capillary agglutination tests (specific and no cross reaction).

Others: Latex agglutination tests, Card agglutination test, ELISA, Microplate enzyme immuno assay. IFA differentiates antibodies due to vaccination and natural infection.

Babesia **sp. in Livestock**

Sl.No.	Babesia spp .	Vectors	Transmission	Disease
		Cattle, Buffalo and Zebu		
1	*B. bigemina* (India)	*Boophilus annulatus* *B. microplus* *R. appendiculatus* *R. bursa* *Haemophysalis punctata*	Transovarian and Transtadial, also Intra uterine	Cattle Tick Fever Red Water Disease Bovine Piroplasmosis Texas Fever Triteza
2	*B. bovis* (India)	*B. microplus* *B. calcaratus* *R. bursa* *Ixodes ricinus* *I. persulcatus*	Transovarian and Transtadial, also Intra uterine	Bovine Babesiosis Piroplasmosis Red Water Disease
3	*B. major*	*Ixodes ricinus*	Transovarian and Transtadial	Less severe than *B. bigemina*
4	*B. divergens*	*B. calcaratus* *Haemophysalis punctata*	Transovarian	Less severe than *B. bovis*
		Sheep and Goats		
1	*B. motasi*	*Dermacenter silvarian* *Haemophysalis punctata* *R. bursa*	Transovarian and Transtadial	Pathogenic
2	*B. ovis*	*R. bursa*	Transovarian and Transtadial Transplacental	Less severe than *B. motasi*
		Sheep		
1	*B. foliata* (India)	Not known	Not known	Not known
		Goat		
1	*B. taylori* (India)	Not known	Not known	Benign type disease
		Dogs		
1	*B. canis*	*R. sanguineus*	Transtadial	Biliary Fever Malignant jaundice Canine Piroplasmosis Canine babesiosis
2	*B. gibsoni* (India)	*R. sanguineus* *Haemophysalis bispinosa*	Transtadial and Transovarian	Slightly Pathogenic
		Cats		
1	*B. felis* (India)	Not known	Not known	Less pathogenic than dog
2	*B. cati* (India)	Not known	Not known	Less pathogenic than dog

Sl.No.	Babesia spp .	Vectors	Transmission	Disease
		Equines		
1	*B. equi* (India)	*Dermacenter spp* *R. sanguineus* *R. bursa* *Hyalomma anatolicum*	Transovarian and Transtadial, also Intra uterine	More pathogenic
2	*B. cabbali*	*Dermacenter spp* *R. sanguineus* *R. bursa* *Hyalomma anatolicum*	Transovarian and Transtadial, also Intra uterine	Less pathogenic
		Pigs		
1	*B.trautamanni*	*Boophilus spp* *R. sanguineus* *Dermacenter spp*	Transovarian	Mild/Fatal
2	*B. peroncittoi*	Not known	Not known	Mild/Fatal

Babesiosis in Cattle

Disease: Cattle tick fever, Red water disease or Piroplasmosis or Texas fever.

Morphology: A large piroplasm, round, pyriform, oval or irregular form or characteristically pear shaped and lie in pairs forming an acute angle in RBCs.

Life cycle: The spherical forms in the ovary of *B. microplus* occur with parasitophorous vacuole formed by host cells where they are transformed into folded kinetes. The sporozoites in tick salivay gland are pyriform.

Epidemiology

Virulence of parasite: *B. divergens* and *B. canis* – relatively pathogenic; *B.major* and *B.ovis* – mildly pathogenic producing transient anaemia.

Age of the host: Inverse age resistance; Greatest infection rate in animals in the age 6-12 months age group and infection is uncommon in animals over 5 years of age. *B. bigemina*: Under 1 year age are susceptible and *B. bovis* - Over 2 years of age are susceptible.

Breed: *B. bigemina*- All races of cattle are equally susceptible; *B. bovis*- Zebu and Africander cattle are more resistant than British and European breeds and Santa Getrudis- intermediate position.

Transmission: Transovarian transmission-one host tick and Transtadial transmission- two or three host tick. Transmission by several generations of ticks is possible. Intrauterine transmission- B. bigemina and *B.ovis*. Physical-By contaminated needles and surgical instruments, *e.g.*, *B. bigemina* and *B. equi*. also *B. bovis*.

Carrier status: Infected adult animals like sheep act as carriers for over 2 years; if the are constantly infected, they act as carriers for life.

Reservoir status: White tailed deer and African buffaloes.

Premunity: Cattle are immuned to reinfection due to exposure to continuing low grade infection. for example, premunity occurs for more than 1 year. Immunity is species specific. In endemic areas, calves acquire colostral immunity.

Risk factors: Endemic areas-Outbreak is associated with stress due to parturition, tick borne fever/starvation. Break down of immunity occurs if there is superimposed infection with *A. marginale*/FMDV in cattle and canine distemper in dog.

Season: Greatest incidence occurs soon after the peak of tick population which varies with temperature, humidity and rainfall.

Enzootic instability: It occurs when there is sudden increase in the tick population due to favourable climatic conditions; the incidence of the clinical cases may increase sharply.

Babesiosis in Dogs

Disease: Biliary fever/Malignant jaundice.

Pathogenesis: *B. canis*

Incubation period: 10-20 days; fever, anaemia, icterus, inappetence, marked thirst, weakness, prostration and frequent death.

Peracute cases: Haemoglobinuria, bilirubinuria.

Acute cases: Acute respiratory failure, extensor spasms and death within 4-5 days.

Atypical signs: Catarrhal bronchitis, pneumonia, subcutaneous edema, ascites, purpura, red urine or blood clots in faeces.

CNS signs: Locomotor disturbances, paresis and epileptic fits.

Lesions: Petechial hemorrhages in various organs and mucous membrane; icterus; edema in pleural and peritoneal cavities.

B. gibsoni: Chronic type of disease with relapses of fever, progressive anaemia, haemoglobinuria, jaundice - less common, staggering gait and death.

Treatment: Berenil.

Babesiosis in Horses

Life cycle: Similar to *B. bigemina.*

B. equi

Incubation Period: 10-21 days. Severe in young and new born foal, Course-8-10 days. Chronic cases survive for months and carries persists for 4 years. Mixed infections with *B. cabbali* can occur. Fever, reluctance to move, edema of fetlock, head and ventral abdomen, frequent colic, jaundice, anaemia.

***B. caballi*:** Nervousness, Walking in circle, Incoordination and paralysis of hind quarters, Haemoglobinuria - rare.

Treatment: Imidocarb-@ 4mg/Kg on 4 occasions at 72 hrs intervals.

Babesiosis: Epierythrozoonoses –anemia, Theileriosis-haemoglobinuria, Leptospirosis- severe in young ones. Anaplasmosis, Trypanosomosis, Bacillary haemoglobinuria, Rabies. Copper toxicity.

Treatment Aromatic diamidines: Imidocarb dipropionate (Imizol), @ 1 mg/kg, S/C; 2 mg/kg, Most effective against B. bigemina; therapeutic and prophylactic; completely eliminates the parasites with some residual activity.

Merit: Noninfected cattle develops one month resistance; To protect cattle during pregnancy where vaccination is contraindicated. Quinuronium derivatives (Acaprin, Babesan, piroplasmin. Piruvan). Effective against *B. bigemina* and other larger spp; 1 ml/50 kg but with a maximum dose of 6 ml, S/C.

Other Aromatic diamidines: Diamprone -@ 10 mg. kg, deep I/M. Phenamidine-@ 12 mg/kg, S/C in 40 per cent aqueous solution. Pentamidine-Chemo immunizing agent against *B. bigemina* in cattle.

Others: Tryphan blue solution (1-2 per cent) - 100 ml, I/V. Acriflavin (5 per cent)- 20 ml. Amicarbalide - effective in cattle and horses; @ 5-10 mg/kg, but I/M at 24 hrs interval. Primaquine - 0.5 mg/kg; I/M.

Control

Control of ticks- acaricides, repellants; dipping of animals at regular intervals. Segregation and treatment of animals harbouring infection. Chemoprophylaxis-Imidocarb for 2 months which allows animals infected gradually. Killed vaccine-with incomplete Freund's adjuvant and irradiated *Babesia* spp. Chemoimmunization-vaccination with virulent organisms and simultaneous subsequent challenge with Babesia spp. Live attenuated vaccine- less virulent and attenuated babesia are suspended in a cell free plasma are used after passing through spleenectamized calves. Vaccine contains 10^3 *B. bovis* organisms/dose are the minimum infective dose. Live attenuated tissue culture vaccines are also effective. Vaccination with non-living antigens, antigenic proteins produced in blood stream or culture medium as a part of the growth process of *Babesia* spp. Subunit vaccine from monoclonal technology. Blood transfusion- Oldest; immunization by inoculation of infected blood followed by babesidal drugs but transmission of bovine leucosis and other diseases. Diminazene aceturate-@ 3-8 mg/kg, but deep I/M; safe and effective to treat all spp.

5.5. Coccidiosis

Coccidiosis is usually an acute invasion and destruction of intestinal mucosa by protozoa of the genera *Eimeria* or *Isospora*. Clinical signs include diarrhea, fever, inappetence, weight loss, emaciation, and in extreme cases, death. However, many infections are subclinical. Coccidiosis is an economically important disease of cattle, sheep, goats, pigs, poultry, and also rabbits, in which the liver as well as the intestine can be affected. In dogs, cats, and horses, coccidiosis is less often diagnosed but can result in clinical illness. Other genera, of both hosts and protozoa, can be involved.

Eimeridae

Organisms commonly called coccidia are typically intracellular parasites of epithelial cells of intestine of vertebrates with few exceptions. All forms have a single host in which they undergo asexual (Schizogony or merogony) and sexual (Gametogony) cycle of reproduction. Sporulation of fertilized zygote usually takes place outside the host.

Genera of Importance

Coccidiosis is caused by *Eimeria* spp and *Isospora* spp.

Morphology

Oocysts: Most common shapes are spherical, ovoid/ellipsoidal, It have refractile shell and some species with a small pore at one end called micropyle covered with a prominent polarcap. An outer wall enclosing 4 sporocysts each containing 2 sporozoites in the sporulated oocyst which is the infective stage.

Tissue stage: Mature schizonts identified by their location histologially, size and number of merozoites they contain which are arranged in a crescent shaped organism like a sliced onion. In mature microgametocyte, the microgamates are arranged around the periphery in the cell. Macrogametocyte has a large central nucleus and with small granules arranged around the periphery of the cell.

Life Cycle

See Figure 5.5

Prepatent period: In poultry- 5 days.

Three phases: Sporulation, Infection and schizogony, Gametogony and Oocyst formation.

Coccidiosis in Cattle, Pathogenesis and Clinical Signs

Twelve *Eimeria* spp. have been identified in the feces of cattle worldwide, but only three (*E. zuernii, E. bovis,* and *E. auburnensis*) are most often associated with clinical disease. The other *Eimeria* spp. have been shown experimentally to be mildly or moderately pathogenic but are not considered important pathogens. Coccidiosis is commonly a disease of young cattle (1–2 months to 1 yr) and usually is sporadic during the wet seasons of the year. "Summer coccidiosis" and "winter coccidiosis" in range cattle probably result from severe weather stress and crowding around a limited water source, which concentrates the hosts and parasites within a restricted area. Although particularly severe epidemics have been reported in feedlot cattle during extremely cold weather, cattle confined to feedlots are susceptible to coccidiosis throughout the year. Outbreaks usually occur within the first month of confinement. Cows may contribute to environmental contamination of *E. bovis* oocysts through a periparturient increase in fecal oocyst counts. Time to onset of diarrhea after infection is 16–23 days for *E. bovis* and *E. zuernii* and 3–4 days for *E alabamensis;* clinical disease due to coccidiosis does not typically occur in the first 3 weeks of life. Coccidiosis is therefore not considered part of the neonatal diarrhea complex in calves. The most typical syndrome of coccidiosis is chronic

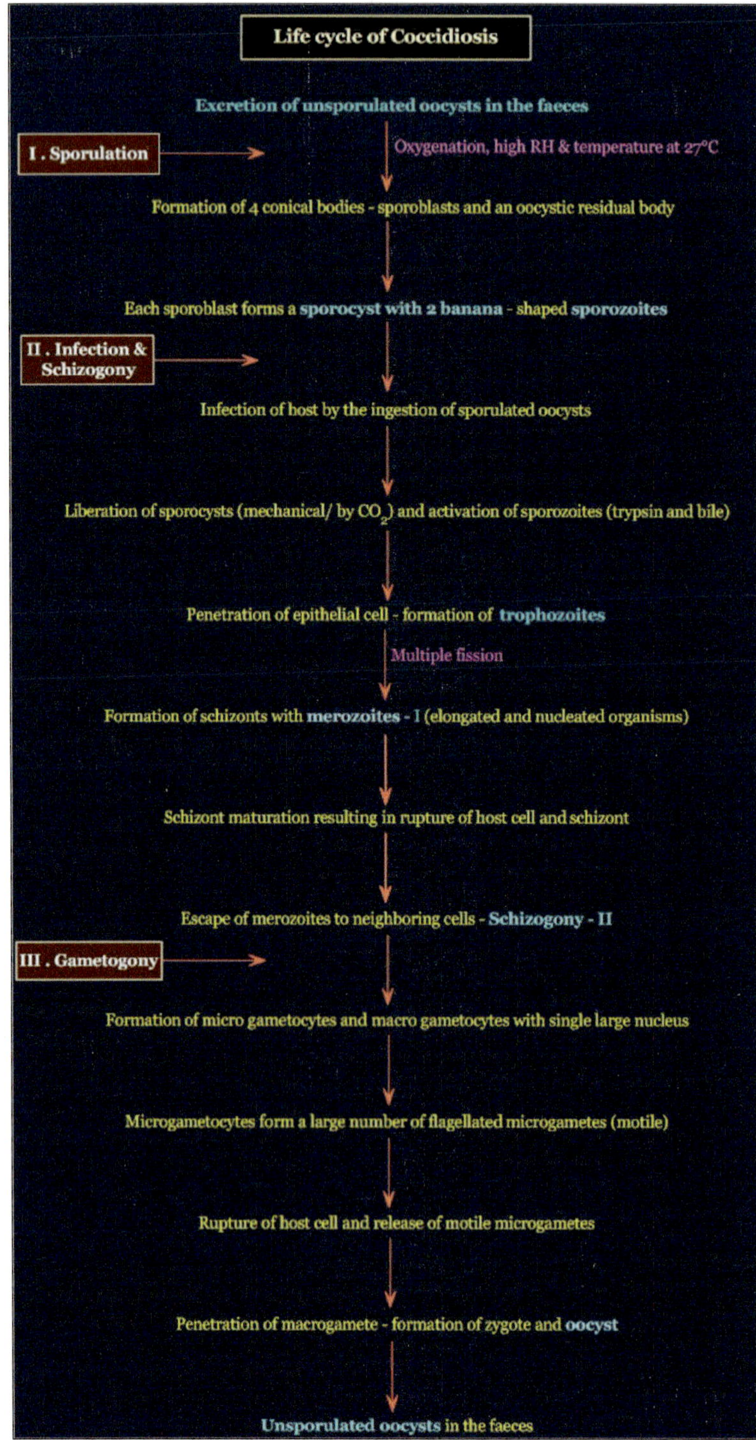

Figure 5.5. Life cycle of Coccidiosis.

or subclinical disease in groups of growing animals. Calves may appear unthrifty and have fecal-stained perineal areas. In light infections, cattle appear healthy and oocysts are present in normally formed feces, but feed efficiency is reduced. The most characteristic sign of clinical coccidiosis is watery feces, with little or no blood, and animals show only slight discomfort for a few days. Severe infections are rare. Severely affected cattle develop thin, bloody diarrhea that may continue for >1 wk, or thin feces with streaks or clots of blood, shreds of epithelium, and mucus. They may develop a fever; become anorectic, depressed, and dehydrated; and lose weight. Tenesmus is common because the most severe enteritis is confined to the large intestine, although pathogenic coccidia of cattle can damage the mucosa of the lower small intestine, cecum, and colon. During the acute period, some calves die; others die later from secondary complications (*e.g.*, pneumonia). Calves that survive severe illness can lose significant weight that is not quickly regained or can remain permanently stunted. Calves with concurrent enteric infections (*e.g.*, *Giardia*) may be more severely affected than calves with coccidia infections alone. In addition, management factors, such as weather, housing, feeding practices, and how animals are grouped, are important in determining the expression of clinical coccidiosis in cattle.

Nervous signs (*e.g.*, muscular tremors, hyperesthesia, clonic-tonic convulsions with ventroflexion of the head and neck, nystagmus) and a high mortality rate (80 per cent –90 per cent) are seen in some calves with acute clinical coccidiosis. Outbreaks of this "nervous form" are seen most commonly during, or after, severely cold weather in midwinter in Canada and the northern USA; there are no reports of the "nervous form" outside this geographic location. Affected calves may die <24 hr after the onset of dysentery and nervous signs, or they may live for several days, commonly in a laterally recumbent position with a mild degree of opisthotonos. Nervous signs have not been reported in experimental clinical coccidiosis in calves, which suggests that the nervous signs may be unrelated to the dysentery or, indeed, even to coccidiosis.

Diagnosis of coccidiosis is by finding oocysts on fecal flotation or direct smear or by the McMaster technique. Quantitative oocyst counts on individual rectal samples from at least five calves in a pen are helpful to confirm coccidiosis as a cause of clinical disease. Differential diagnoses include salmonellosis, bovine viral diarrhea, malnutrition, toxins, or other intestinal parasites.

Coccidiosis is a self-limiting disease, and spontaneous recovery without specific treatment is common when the multiplication stage of the coccidia has passed.

Drugs that can be used for therapy of clinically affected animals include sulfaquinoxaline (6 mg/lb/day for 3–5 days) and amprolium (10 mg/kg/day for 5 days). Sulfaquinoxaline is particularly useful for weaned calves that develop bloody diarrhea after arrival at a feedlot. For prevention, amprolium (5 mg/kg/day for 21 days), decoquinate (22.7 mg/45 kg/day for 28 days) and lasalocid (1 mg/kg/day to a maximum of 360 mg/head/day), or monensin (100–360 mg/head/day) can be used. The major benefits of coccidiostats are through improved feed efficiency and rate of gain.

In an outbreak, clinically affected animals should be isolated and given supportive oral and parenteral fluid therapy as necessary. The population density of the affected pens should be reduced. All feed and water supplies should be high enough off the ground to avoid fecal contamination. Mass medication of the feed and water supplies may be indicated in an attempt to prevent new cases and to minimize the effects of an epidemic. Cattle with coccidiosis and nervous signs should be brought indoors, kept well-bedded and warm, and given fluid therapy orally and parenterally. However, the case fatality rate of calves with coccidiosis and nervous signs is high despite intensive supportive therapy. Parenteral sulfonamide therapy may be indicated to control development of secondary bacterial enteritis or pneumonia, which may be seen in calves with coccidiosis during very cold weather. Corticosteroids are contraindicated, because they increase shedding of oocysts and have induced clinical disease in subclinically infected calves.

Coccidiosis has been difficult to control reliably. Overcrowding of animals should be avoided while they develop immunity to the coccidial species in the environment. Calving grounds should be well drained and kept as dry as possible. All measures that minimize fecal contamination of hair coats and fleece should be practiced regularly. Feed and water troughs should be high enough to avoid heavy fecal contamination. Control of coccidiosis in feeder calves brought into a crowded feedlot depends on management of population density, presence of appropriate feed bunks, or use of chemotherapeutics, to control the numbers of oocysts ingested by the animals while effective immunity develops.

Coccidiostats are used to control naturally occurring coccidiosis. The ideal coccidiostat suppresses the full development of the life cycle of the coccidia, allows immunity to develop, and does not interfere with production performance. Sulfonamides in the feed at 25–35 mg/kg for dikhuaaa15 days are effective to control coccidiosis in calves. Monensin is an effective coccidiostat and growth promotant in calves. Postweaning coccidiosis in beef calves has been controlled using monensin administered via intraluminal continuous-release devices. Lasalocid is related to monensin and is also an effective coccidiostat for ruminants. Mixing lasalocid in the milk replacer of calves beginning at 2–4 days of age is an effective way to control coccidiosis. Lasalocid is also effective as a coccidiostat when fed free-choice in salt at a level of 0.75 per cent of the total salt mixture. A level of 1 mg/kg is the most effective and rapid and is recommended when outbreaks of coccidiosis are imminent. Decoquinate in the feed at 0.5–1 mg/kg suppressed oocyst production in experimentally induced coccidiosis of calves. Decoquinate is most effective in preventing coccidial infections when fed continually in dry feed at 0.5 mg/kg. Monensin, lasalocid, and decoquinate at the manufacturer's recommended levels are equally effective. Toltrazuril administered at 15 mg/kg as a single oral dose, 14 days after animals are moved into group housing, effectively prevents diarrhea due to coccidiosis. Diclazuril (5 mg/kg) is being investigated as an oral anticoccidial in calves.

Control of infection should include changes in management factors that contribute to development of clinical disease. Inadequate housing and ventilation should be corrected, feeding practices adopted that avoid fecal contamination of feed, calves grouped by size, and an "all-in/all-out" method of calf movement from pen to pen adopted.

E. bovis: Diarrhoea, dysentery, tenesmus, increased body temperature and death. Lesion -Thickened, edematous, congested mucosae with haemorrhage of caecum, colon and terminal ileum with large amounts of blood.

E. zuernii: Most pathogenic; causes catarrhal enteritis.

Lesions: caecum and colon are filled with semi fluid haemorrhage material or fresh blood with mucus.

Clinical signs: Watery faeces with unpleasant odour, soiling of posterior part of animals.

Severe cases: animals succumb and die after 7 days of clinical signs.

Chronic cases: Bloody/bloodless pasty mucus faeces, anorexia, convulsions, tremor, weakness, emaciation, death due to pneumonia (secondary bacterial infection).

Winter Coccidiosis: By *E. zuernii* in cattle during cold/stormy weather during winter where concentration of sporulated oocysts increase.

Mixed infections: Abdominal pain, foul smelling diarrhoea, with blood or with soiled strings, drooping ears, rough coat, soiled hind quarters, tenesmus and anaemia. Inability to raise on legs, partial paralysis of anal sphincter; recovery is rare at this stage and death occurs in young calves. Secondary pneumonia, emaciation in severe cases.

Neurological coccidiosis: Caused by *Eimeria* sp., Mortality-70 per cent; Clinical signs are encephalopathy, diarrhoea, tenesmus, haematochezia, CNS dysfunction, twitching, hyperesthesia followed by nystagmus, opisthotonus, tremors, bellowing, snapping of eyelids, occasionally blindness, death within 1 month.

Pathogenesis and Clinical Signs

Caecal Coccidiosis

Pathogenesis: *E. tenella* is primarily responsible for caecal coccidiosis but gametogenous stage of *E. necatrix* and occasionally some stage of *E. brunetti* can cause; Morbidity-100 per cent; Mortality- 80 per cent. Principally in chicks of 3-7 weeks of age after 72 hours of infection. Mortality is produced by a dose of $2x10^5$ oocysts produces mortality in 1-2 weeks age chicks. Severity of the disease varies from indistinct infection to acute/highly fatal depending upon the number of oocysts and virulence; Mortality- upto 100 per cent. Second generation schizonts migrate to the lamina propria and submucosa and rupture of schizonts leads to massive haemorrhage, detachment of mucosal surface, diarrhoea and death within 4-6 days.

Clinical Signs

Clinical form: Occurs due to the ingestion of large number of oocysts over a short period and is characterized by the presence of soft faeces with blood, dullness, listlessness, drooping feathers, anaemias, paralysis and death.

Sub clinical form: Poor weight gain and poor conversion rate.

Lesions

Presence of dilated caeca with mixture of clotted and unclotted blood, caseous caecal contents adherent to mucosa, caseous plugs detached from mucosa and shed in the faeces; White spots and petechiae in caeca.

Intestinal Coccidiosis

Pathogenesis: Both acute and chronic coccidia can occur by *E. necatrix* but sub-clinical form is more common. Death can occur within 5-7 days.

Clinical Signs

Similar to caecal coccidiosis.Chronic watery diarrhoea with blood (mucus droppings in *E. maxima* infection); stunted growth, reduced egg production, listlessness, anorexia, soiling of vent and feathers; recovered birds are unthrifty and emaciated for a long time.

Lesions in the midgut: Second generation schizonts accumulation in deep mucosa as minute grayish white spots. Balooning of intestine filled with clots of blood/fresh blood and severe haemorrhage at 5-6 days after infection. Intestine greatly thickened, dull red with fragile lining and friable with gangrene. *E.maxima* - Salmon pink eexudates and haemorrhage.

Rectal Coccidiosis: Occur by *E. brunetti* in small intestine to cloaca. White fluid droppings mixed with blood and mucosa. Coagulative necrosis and slight haemorrhage. Loss of body weight and reduced feed intake and in appetence.

Coccidia of Livestock and Poultry

Sl.No.	*Species*	*Location*	*Pathogenicity*
		Chicken	
1	*E. tenella*	Caeca	Most pathogenic - Caecal Coccidiosis
2	*E. brunetti*	Lower small intestine, Caeca, rectum, Cloaca	Most pathogenic- Rectal Coccidiosis
3	*E. necatrix*	Jejunum, mid-gut and other parts of large intestine	Most pathogenic- Intestinal coccidiosis
4	*E. maxima*	Mid-gut	Medium/highly pathogenic intestinal Coccidiosis
5	*E. acervulina*	Duodenum	Mildly pathogenic
6	*E. mivati*	Duodenum and Rectum	More pathogenic
7	*E. mitis*	Duodenum and jejunum	Mild pathogenic
8	*E. praecox*	Duodenum	Mild/Non- pathogenic
9	*E. hagoni* (uncommon)	Duodenum	Slightly pathogenic
		Turkey	
1	*E. adenoides*	Small intestine and large intestine	Most pathogenic
2	*E. gallopavonis*	Lower small intestine, Caecum, Rectum	Moderately pathogenic/Non-pathogenic

Sl.No.	Species	Location	Pathogenicity
3	*E. meleagridis*	Small intestine, Caecum and Rectum	Mildly pathogenic
4	*E. meleagrimitis*	Small intestine	Markedly pathogenic
5	*E. dispersa*	Small intestine	Mildly pathogenic
		Geese	
1	*E. truncata*	Kidney	Highly pathogenic
2	*E. anseris*	Small intestine	Low pathogenic
3	*E. nocens*	Posterior small intestine	Moderately pathogenic
		Cattle	
1	*E. zuernii*	Small intestine and large intestine	Highly pathogenic
2	*E. bovis*	Ileum, caecum and colon	Common pathogenic - clinical coccidiosis
3	*E. alabamensis*	Small intestine, caecum and upper colon	Non- pathogenic
		Sheep	
1	*E. ovinoidalis*	Caecum and colon	Highly pathogenic
2	*E. crandallis*	Caecum and colon	Mildly pathogenic
		Goat	
1	*E. arloingi*	Caecum and colon	pathogenic
		Rabbit	
1	*E. steidae*	Liver	Pathogenic
2	*E. intestinalis*	Intestine	Pathogenic
3	*E.flavescens*	Intestine	pathogenic
		Horse	
1	*E. leukarti*	Small intestine	Pathogenic in heavy infections
		Pigs	
1	*I. suis*	Jejunum and small intestine	Pathogenic, not frequent
2	*E. debliecki*	Jejunum and small intestine	Pathogenic, not frequent
		Dog	
1	*I. canis*	Small intestine and large intestine	Mildly Pathogenic
		Cat	
1	*I. rivolta*	Small intestine and large intestine	Pathogenic
2	*I. felis*	Small intestine and caecum	Mildly Pathogenic

Coccidiosis in Cattle

Morphology: Oval oocysts. Presence of micropyle and absence of micropyle cap and residual cysts. Sporocysts are elongate and ovoid with banana shaped sporozoites.

Life cycle: P.P.P- 15 to 21 days. Schizonts is seen in the central lacteals of the intestinal villi.

Epidemiology

Agent: Delay in the lifecycle may occur due to the arrestment of schizogony stage and resumption occurs several months later with subsequent shedding of oocysts. Pathogenesis is done by gamont stage of oocysts.

Age of the host: Primarily in young calves of 21 days old to 6 months age; adults are also affected.

Risk factors: Massive intake of oocysts. Overcrowding in unhygienic yards. Pasture where congregation of livestock around the water holes. Lack of sanitation.

Coccidiosis in Dogs, Horses and Pigs

Coccidiosis in Dogs: Many species of coccidia infect the intestinal tract of cats and dogs. All species appear to be host-specific. Cats have species of *Isospora, Besnoitia, Toxoplasma, Hammondia,* and *Sarcocystis*. Dogs have species of *Isospora, Hammondia,* and *Sarcocystis*. Neither dogs nor cats have *Eimeria*.

Hammondia has an obligatory two-host life cycle with cats or dogs as final hosts and rodents or ruminants as intermediate hosts, respectively. *Hammondia* oocysts are indistinguishable from those of *Toxoplasma* and *Besnoitia* but are nonpathogenic in either host. The most common coccidia of cats and dogs are *Isospora*. Some *Isospora* spp. of cats and dogs can facultatively infect other mammals and produce in various organs an encysted form that is infective for the cat or dog. Two species infect cats: *I. felis* and *I. rivolta*; both can be identified easily by oocyst size and shape. Almost every cat eventually becomes infected with *I. felis*. Four species infect dogs: *I. canis, I. ohioensis, I. burrowsi,* and *I. neorivolta*. In dogs, only *I. canis* can be identified by the oocyst structure; the other three *Isospora* overlap in dimensions and can be differentiated only by endogenous developmental characteristics.

Clinical coccidiosis, although not common, has been reported in kittens and puppies. In kittens, it is seen primarily during weaning stress. The most common clinical signs in severe cases are diarrhea (sometimes bloody), weight loss, and dehydration. Usually, coccidiosis is associated with other infectious agents, immunosuppression, or stress.

Treatment may be unnecessary in cats, because they usually spontaneously eliminate the infection. In clinically affected cats, trimethoprim-sulfonamide (30–60 mg/kg/day for 6 days) can be used.

In kennel conditions when the need for prophylaxis might be predicted, amprolium is said to be effective, although it is not approved for use in dogs. In severe cases, in addition to supportive fluid therapy, sulfonamides such as sulfadimethoxine (50 mg/kg the first day and 25 mg/kg/day for 2–3 wk thereafter) can be used. Sanitation is important, especially in catteries and kennels, or where large numbers of animals are housed. Feces should be removed frequently. Fecal contamination of feed and water should be prevented. Runs, cages, and utensils should be disinfected daily. Raw meat should not be fed. Insect control should be established. Young puppies and kittens are more prone.

Risk factors - Overcrowding and poor sanitation. Infection by predator- prey relationship. Usually carry coccidiosis infections but rarely severe disease occur; causes diarrhoeic syndrome. Treatment is rarely practiced.

Coccidiosis in Horses

Causes diarrhoea and death in heavy infections only.

Coccidiosis in Pigs

Eight species of *Eimeria* and one of *Isospora* infect pigs in North America. Piglets 5–15 days old are characteristically infected with only *I. suis*, which produces enteritis and diarrhea. These agents must be differentiated from viruses, bacteria, and helminths that also cause scours in neonatal pigs. *I. suis* is prevalent in neonatal pigs. Infection is characterized by a watery or greasy diarrhea, usually yellowish to white and foul smelling. Piglets may appear weak, dehydrated, and undersized; weight gains are depressed, and sometimes piglets die. A contributing factor to mortality is that piglets become covered with diarrheic feces and stay damp. Oocysts are usually shed in the feces and can be identified by their size, shape, and sporulation characteristics; however, in peracute infections, diagnosis must be based on finding stages of the parasite in impression smears or histologic sections of the small intestine, because pigs can die before oocysts are formed. In severely affected piglets, histologic lesions confined to the jejunum and ileum is characterized by villous atrophy, blunting of villi, focal ulceration, and fibrinonecrotic enteritis with parasite stages in epithelial cells.

Preventive control by feeding anticoccidials to sows from 2 wk before farrowing through lactation or to neonatal pigs from birth to weaning has been reported; however, effectiveness of the latter has not been confirmed. Although the sow is a logical source of infection for piglets, this has not been well documented. Thorough removal of feces and disinfection of farrowing facilities between litters greatly decreases infection. Piglets that recover from infection are highly resistant to reinfection.

Although less commonly associated with clinical coccidiosis, *E debliecki, E neodebliecki, E scabra*, and *E spinosa* have been found in pigs ~1–3 months old with diarrhea. Illness may last 7–10 days, with pigs remaining unthrifty.

Treatment of coccidiosis may include sulfamethazine in drinking water. The control of coccidiosis in newborn piglets infected with *I. suis* has been unreliable. The use of coccidiostats in the feed of the sow for several days or a few weeks before and after farrowing has been recommended and used in the field, but the results are variable. Amprolium and monensin are ineffective for prevention of experimental coccidiosis in piglets. A control program designed to decrease the number of oocysts has been recommended and consists of proper cleaning, disinfection, and steam cleaning of the farrowing housing. Amprolium (25 per cent feed grade) at the rate of 10 kg/tonne of sows' feed started 1 wk before farrowing and continued until the piglets are 3 wk of age has been recommended, but the results are unsatisfactory. A single dose of toltrazuril (20 mg/kg, PO) decreased oocyst excretion, the incidence of diarrhea, and weight gain impairment in piglets with experimentally induced coccidiosis. Diclazuril (5 mg/kg) is being investigated as an oral anticoccidial in piglets.

Clinical condition is not frequent. Enteritis in piglets (1-2 weeks age groups) and diarrhoea. Older animals are carriers.

Epidemiology

Agent

Production of oocysts: Immediately after prepatent period, oocysts are passed in very large number in the faeces, *e.g., E. tenella*. Number of oocysts voided falls rapidly and cannot be found easily unless reinfection. Occasionally small number of oocysts is found in the faeces several months after a single infection. Reproduction potential of a species of coccidium after ingestion by a susceptible host influences the number of oocysts, *e.g.*, high biotic potential of *E. tenella*. Number of viable sporulated oocysts ingested by a host influences the oocyst production. Light infection produces relatively more number of oocysts. Increased resistance of host influences depressed oocysts production. Caecal plugs in caecal coccidiosis retard the passage of oocysts in the faeces.

Causation of disease: It depends on, virulence of coccidium, *e.g., E. tenella and E. necatrix*, Number of oocysts ingested. Oocysts introduced in empty crop causes a more severe infection. Feeding calcium carbonate in excess of 3 per cent in feed.

Host

Age: 1 to 2 weeks- less susceptible and 4 to 6 – most susceptible. More than 6 weeks – resistant. Susceptibility increases with age in *E.tenella.*

Breed: White Leghorn, Rhode Island and Newhampsire are resistant. Barred Plymouth Rock, Gersey White Giant and Light Sussex are susceptible. Breeder and Layer pullets are at greatest risk.

Transmission: It depends on the type of housing and management and by ingestion of oocysts.

Risk factors: In intensive management system, incidence is more common. Reduced incidence in birds kept on wire floors and solid floor houses. Dirt condition, overcrowding of stock results in greater accumulation of oocysts and spread of infection. In broiler production, overcrowding with high temperature.

Carriers: Mechanical carriers- sparkling beetles, migratory birds and birds recovered from infection.

Immunity: Previous exposure results in species - specific resistance. Some species induces a solid immunity, other species need several infections and is self – limiting in nature. Both CMI and humoral immunity are elicited. Immunity is due to 2nd generation schizogony; Trickle infection: Continuous level of ingestion of oocysts induces very strong immunity but cause damage the intestine. Severity of disease increases with concurrent infections; Marek's disease increases the severity of coccidiosis.

Environment

Favourable conditions: Optimum temperature and RH: Temperature: 25- 32°C; RH – 90 per cent. Survival of oocysts in the soil is about a year and during winter.

Unfavorable conditions: Both unsporulated oocysts and sporulated oocysts are extremely sensitive to desiccation (greater than 56°C is lethal) Direct sunlight is lethal to the parasite. Below 10°C, cool and dry conditions, freezing kill the oocysts. Bacterial or fungal growth kills/lethal to parasite. Chemical disinfectant: 10 per cent ammonia or methyl bromide kills the oocysts.

Coccidiosis in Rabbits

Epidemiology

Age: Commonest around weaning and young rabbits are highly susceptible

Risk Factors: Intensive breeding and rearing under poor sanitation.

Pathogenesis

Hepatic Coccidiosis: P.P.P- 18 days; Appear 12 days after infection, rabbits die without sign in heavy infections.

Clinical signs -Diarrhoea, distension of the abdomen, meteorism, inappetence, constipation, icterus and oedema of the body.

Lesions: Enlargement of bile ducts; haemorrhage and enlargement of liver.

P.P.P- 7 days; occurs frequently.

Clinical signs –Diarrhoea, indigestion, bloating, inappetence, reduced weight gain, sudden death without symptoms or convulsion and paralysis.

Lesions: Acute/subacute, rarely chronic, thickened wall with grayish white deposits, contents are pasty, diarrhoeic and with blood streaks.

Diagnosis: Demonstration of oocysts in the faeces and postmortem examination.

Treatment: Sulphonamides like sulphamezathine in drinking water @ 0.2 per cent effective.

Coccidiosis in Sheep and Goats

Infection with *Eimeria* is one of the most economically important diseases of sheep. Historically, some *Eimeria* spp. were thought to be infectious and transmissible between sheep and goats, but the parasites are now considered host-specific. The names of some species of goat coccidia are still erroneously applied to species of similar appearance found in sheep. *E. crandallis* and *E. ovinoidalis* (*ninakohlyakimovae*) are pathogens of lambs (usually 1–6 months old); *E. ovina* appears to be somewhat less pathogenic. Older sheep serve as sources of infection for the young. All other *Eimeria* of sheep are essentially nonpathogenic, even when large numbers of oocysts are present in feces.

Signs include diarrhea (sometimes containing blood or mucus), dehydration, fever, inappetence, weight loss, anemia, wool breaking, and death. The ileum, cecum, and upper colon are usually most affected and may be thickened, edematous, and inflamed; sometimes, there is mucosal hemorrhage. Thick, white, opaque patches containing large numbers of *E. ovina* oocysts may develop in the small intestine. Because oocysts are prevalent in feces of sheep of all ages, coccidiosis cannot be diagnosed based solely on finding oocysts. Peak oocyst counts of >100,000/g of feces have been reported in 8- to 12-wk-old lambs that appeared healthy. However, diarrhea with oocyst counts of a pathogenic species of >20,000/g is characteristic of coccidiosis in sheep. Immune complex glomerulonephritis has also been attributed to coccidiosis. Fly strike and secondary bacterial enteric infections may accompany coccidiosis in lambs.

Lambs 1–6 months old in lambing pens, intensive grazing areas, and feedlots are at greatest risk as a result of shipping, ration change, crowding stress, severe weather, and contamination of the environment with oocysts from ewes or other lambs. Because occurrence of coccidiosis under these management systems often becomes so predictable, coccidiostats should be administered prophylactically for 28 consecutive days beginning a few days after lambs are introduced into the environment. A concentrated ration containing monensin at 15 g/tonne can be fed to ewes from 4 wk before lambing until weaning, and to lambs from 4–20 wk of age. The toxic level of monensin for lambs is 4 mg/kg. Lasalocid (15–70 mg/head/day, depending on body weight) may be effective. A combination of monensin and lasalocid at 22 and 100 mg/kg of diet, respectively, is an effective prophylactic against naturally occurring coccidiosis in early weaned lambs under feedlot conditions.

Treatment of affected sheep once coccidiosis has been diagnosed is not effective, but severity can be reduced if treatment is begun early. A single treatment of toltrazuril (20 mg/kg) can significantly reduce the oocyst output in naturally infected lambs for ~3 wk after administration. Diclazuril (1 mg/kg) is an effective oral anticoccidial in lambs and is administered once at ~6–8 wk of age (most common) or twice (at 3–4 wk of age and again 3 wk later). Sulfaquinoxaline in drinking water at 0.015 per cent concentration for 3–5 days may be used to treat affected lambs. In groups of lambs at pasture, frequent rotation of pastures for parasite control also helps control coccidial infection. However, when lambs are exposed to infection early in life as a result of infection from the ewe and a contaminated lambing ground, a solid immunity usually develops and problems are seen only when the stocking density is extremely high.

Numerous species of *Eimeria* are found in goats in North America and elsewhere. The *Eimeria* spp are host specific and are not transmitted from sheep to goats.

E. arloingi, *E. christenseni*, and *E. ovinoidalis* are highly pathogenic in kids. Clinical signs include diarrhea with or without mucus or blood, dehydration, emaciation, weakness, anorexia, and death. Some goats are actually constipated and die acutely without diarrhea. Usually, stages and lesions are confined to the small intestine, which may appear congested, hemorrhagic, or ulcerated, and have scattered pale, yellow to white macroscopic plaques in the mucosa. Histologically, villous epithelium is sloughed, and inflammatory cells are seen in the lamina propria and submucosa. In addition, there have been several reports of hepatobiliary coccidiosis with liver failure in dairy goats. Diagnosis of intestinal coccidiosis is based on finding oocysts of the pathogenic species in diarrheal feces, usually at tens of thousands to millions per gram of feces. It is not unusual to find oocyst counts as high as 70,000/g of feces in kids without overt disease, but weight gain may be affected.

Angora and dairy goats, raised under different management practices, may have similar patterns of exposure of kids. Just after parturition, nursery pens and surrounding areas may be heavily contaminated with oocysts from does. Resistance to infection is decreased just after shipping, changing rations, introducing new animals, or mixing young with older animals. Coccidiostats can be administered to a herd immediately after diagnosis or as a preventive in predictable situations such as those mentioned above.

Diagnosis and treatment are similar to those for cattle and sheep. Sulfadimidine at 55 g/tonne is also effective for control of coccidiosis in goats. In nonlactating goats, adding monensin to the feed at 18 g/tonne is preventive.

Epidemiology

Agent: P.P.P – 15 days; Pathogenicity is by gametogony and schizogony.

Age of the host: Upto 6 months of age in lambs and kids; usually 4-7 weeks of age.

Transmission: Newborn lambs/kids pick up the infection by suckling their soiled dams through soiled litter, drinking water and infected pastures.

Carrier status: Adults are symptomless and transmit infection to the young ones.

Season: Flare-up during onset of rains and winter.

Risk factors: Unhygienic condition, intensive grazing, oocysts contamination around feeding troughs, confinement in feedlots and weaning.

Pathogenesis: Diarrhoea with foul smelling and with or without streaks of blood. Constipation, severe abdominal pain, tenesmus, anaemia, inappetence, unthriftiness, loss of weight, slight rise of body temperature, ailing kids lie down due to abdominal pain, soiling of hind quarters with faeces attracting blow flies.

Diagnosis: Treatment and Control: Similar to cattle.

Coccidiosis in Turkeys and Geese

Pathogenesis

Turkeys: *E. adenoids* is the primary cause of turkey coccidiosis.

Age: Young birds are highly susceptible especially at 4-5 weeks.

Risk Factors: Intensive breeding (result in heavy loss), over crowding, poor sanitation- dampness of house. Sporulation period- 1 day; P.P- 5 days. Pathogenicity by gametogony and schizogony.

Clinical cases: Intestines with catarrhal inflammation with or without haemorrhage. Swollen and oedematous intestine with petechial haemmorhage on the mucosa of caeca. Intestinal contents are pasty and orange coloured, then become compact, caseous, mucoid with blood; tucked head under wings in affected cases.

Geese: Haemorrhagic enteritis by *E. anseris. E. truncata*- Mortality- 100 per cent, marked emaciation, muscular in coordination, enlargement of kidney with light colour, numerous white nodules, streaks and lines and destruction of kidney tubular cells; acute nephritis may be seen.

Diagnosis: Correct and early diagnosis depends on 2 factors, History of the flock, Finding various types of lesions and their locations by P.M. examination.

Others: Faecal examination for the presence of oocysts is of little significance in severe out breaks and clinical cases, as the mortality

Coccidiosis in Cattle, Diagnosis and Treatment

Characteristic signs - Bloody diarrhoea and tenesmus. Faecal examination for oocysts. Post mortem examination if no oocysts are found.

Differential Diagnosis

Bovine winter dysentery - Epidemic and acute. Johne's disease - chronic diarrhoea, Necrotic enteritis - Sudden death, Hypomagnesemia - Hyperaesthesia, prolapse of 3rd eyelid. Cobalt deficiency – Pica, Salmonellosis - Septicaemia.

Treatment: Amprolium - 20-25mg/kg for 4 to 5 days. Sulphamezathine - 0.125 mg/kg for 13 days. Neurological coccidiosis - Calcium boro gluconate and amprolium @ 50mg/kg.

Treatment:Aim of the treatment is to allow sufficient schizogony develop in unaffected birds to stimulate their resistance. for example: sulphonamides have the great effect on II stage schizont without inhibiting I stage schizogony and increases the resistance. Fully recommended dose should be given and withdrawn gradually by reducing half of the dose, otherwise it is lethal.

Sl.No.	*Drug*	*Dose*	*Coccidia*	*Stage of Coccidia*
Coccidiostats				
1	Amprolium	125 ppm in feed/water for 6 days	*E. tenella, E. necatrix* and also *E. maxima*	I and II Schizonts
2	Amprolium + Ethopabate	125 ppm + 8 ppm in feed/ water for 6 days	Extended spectrum	I and II Schizonts
3	Sulphaquinoxaline	0.5 per cent in feed, 0.043 per cent in drinking water for 2 days with 3-5 days interval.	*E. tenella, E. necatrix* and *E. acervulina*	II Schizonts
4	Sulphaquinoxaline + Pyrimethamine	Synergistic; 14 ppm + 45ppm in feed/water	*E. tenella, E. necatrix* and *E. acervulina*	I and II Schizonts
5	Nitrofurazone + Furazolidone	55 mg/kg + 55 mg/kg	*E. tenella* and *E. necatrix*	II Schizonts

Sl.No.	Drug	Dose	Coccidia	Stage of Coccidia
6	Ionophore compounds			
	a) Monensin	0.121 per cent in feed	Superior to amprolium	
	b) Lasolacid	0.005 - 0.0075 per cent in feed	High degree of activity	
	c) Salinomycin	0.01 per cent in feed	Significant activity	
		Coccidiocidals		
1	Robenidine	0.0066 per cent in feed	-	I Schizonts

Control: Primary prophylaxis in vaccination.

Coccivac - vaccine with live attenuated oocysts of *E. tenella, E. maxima, E. acervulina, E.mivati* and chicken isolates.

Route - Eye spray/cabinet spray/in feed.

Age - Day old healthy chicken.

Precaution - Vaccine sensitive to anticoccidials.

Other vaccines are Livacox - Q (attenuated quadrivalent vaccine), Immunocox, Coccivac-D (8 species) for breeders and layers, Initial infection of 100-700 oocysts/ each species followed by repeated daily doses of 1-5 oocysts for 20 days produces immunity by trickle infection which is reinforced by reinfection of oocysts in the litter. Selective breeding of domestic fowl is effective control method to increase the genetic resistance of the host. Nutritional supplement/antagonism- Vitamin- A for recovery of the host; Vitamin-K to reduce the mortality due to haemorrhage and a high protein diet. Isolation of sick birds. Reduced drug rate to older birds allows limited exposure to developing coccidia so that it leads to acquired immunity. Recommendation of Switch programme where drugs are switched between batches of broilers and Shuttle programme where drugs are switched within life-span of each batch. Good ventilation to reduce humidity in the house to keep the litter dry. Heaping the litter for 24 hours to reach a temperature of 50°C and forking for destruction of oocysts. Avoidance of contamination of feeders and waterers with droppings. Continuation of anticoccidials in water for 5 days. Burning the infected materials and sprinkling the quick lime @2-3 kg/10 sq.feet over the litter. Avoidance of overcrowding in poultry houses. Isolation of young chicks from adults. Keep the waterers and feeders at higher level. Feeding chicks with coccidiostat in chick mash. Thorough disinfection and fumigation (Ammonia + Potassium permanganate) in the premises before the entry of newly hatched chicks.

5.6. Ceonorosis

Taenia multiceps multiceps is an intestinal parasite of canids (especially dogs, foxes, and jackals) and occasionally people. Its intermediate hosts include sheep, goats, deer, antelope, chamois, rabbits, hares, horses, and less commonly cattle, which acquire this tapeworm's eggs while grazing. After ingestion, some oncospheres hatch and reach the brain, developing by endogenous budding into a metacestode (larval) stage known as *Coenurus cerebralis*. Initial invasion and development of the oncospheres may be responsible for acute suppurative meningoencephalitis. The fully developed coenurus may be 5–6 cm in diameter and cause increased intracranial pressure, which results in ataxia, hypermetria, blindness, head deviation, stumbling, and paralysis. This clinical condition is colloquially known as gid, sturdy, or staggers. In sheep, palpation of the skull caudal to the horn buds may reveal refraction; surgery to remove the cyst, including its wall, has a reasonable chance of success and is justified in valuable animals. Dogs associated with sheep and other livestock should not be fed the brain or spinal cord from infected animals and should be dewormed regularly.

Coenurosis in Sheep

Caused by metacestode stage (*Coenurus cerebralis*) of dog tape worm - *Taenia multiceps, Coenurosis in goat* – caused by metacestode stage (*Coenurus cerebralis*) of dog tape worm - *Taenia gaigeri, Coenurosis in rabbits* – caused by metacestode stage (*Coenurus serialis*) of dog tape worm - *Taenia serialis.*

Taenia gaigeri

Definitive Host: Dog and fox

Location: Small intestine

Intermediate Host: Goat

Metacestode stage: *Coenurus cerebralis*

Location: Brain, spinal cord and intermuscular and subcutaneous connective tissue.

Taenia serialis

Definitive Host: Dog and fox

Location: Small intestine

Intermediate Host: Lagoamorphs

Metacestode stage: *Coenurus serialis*

Location: Intermuscular and subcutaneous connective tissue.

Taenia hydatigena

Definitive Host: Dog, wolves and other carnivores

Location: Small intestine

Intermediate Host: Sheep (Mainly) and pig (Domestic and wild ruminants are also affected)

Metacestode stage: *Cysticercus tenuicollis* (6 cm in size and containing single scolex invaginated into a long neck).

Location: Peritoneal cavity

Life cycle and epidemiology: Similar to *T. ovis*

Pathogenesis

Clinical Signs

In lambs – unthriftiness, immature cysticercus– liver – traumatic hepatitis – death (Hepatic cysticercosis), mature cysticercus – peritoneal cavity – no harm.

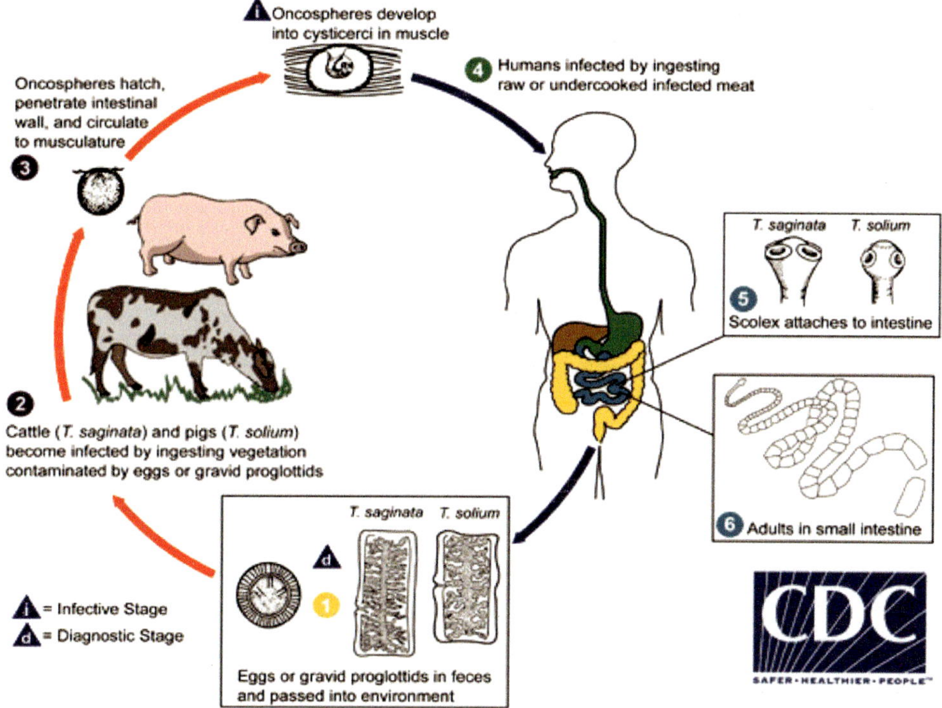

Figure 5.6

Taeniasis is the infection of humans with the adult tapeworm of *Taenia saginata* or *Taenia solium*. Humans are the only definitive hosts for *T. saginata* **and** *T. solium*. **Eggs or gravid proglottids are passed with feces–1; the eggs can survive for days to months in the environment. Cattle (*T. saginata*) and pigs (*T. solium*) become infected by ingesting vegetation contaminated with eggs or gravid proglottids–2. In the animal's intestine, the oncospheres hatch–3, invade the intestinal wall, and migrate to the striated muscles, where they develop into cysticerci. A cysticercus can survive for several years in the animal. Humans become infected by ingesting raw or undercooked infected meat–4. In the human intestine, the cysticercus develops over 2 months into an adult tapeworm, which can survive for years. The adult tapeworms attach to the small intestine by their scolex–5 and reside in the small intestine–6. Length of adult worms is usually 5 m or less for *T. saginata* (however it may reach up to 25 m) and 2 to 7 m for *T. solium*. The adults produce proglottids which mature, become gravid, detach from the tapeworm, and migrate to the anus or are passed in the stool (approximately 6 per day). *T. saginata* adults usually have 1,000 to 2,000 proglottids, while *T. solium* adults have an average of 1,000 proglottids. The eggs contained in the gravid proglottids are released after the proglottids are passed with the feces. *T. saginata* may produce up to 100,000 and *T. solium* may produce 50,000 eggs per proglottid respectively.**

Diagnosis

Intermediate Host: similar to *T. ovis*

Differential diagnosis – Differentiated from acute fascioliasis

Treatment: No valuable

Control: Similar to *T. ovis*

Taenia multiceps

Definitive Host: Dog and fox

Location: Small intestine

Intermediate Host: Sheep

Metacestode stage: *Coenurus cerebralis*

Location: Brain and spinal cord

Coenurus cerebralis - Large fluid filled cyst about 5 cm or more in diameter, the cyst wall containing several hundred scolices in clusters.

Life cycle and Epidemiology: Similar to *T. ovis.*

In addition: In IH: older lambs and adults are high risk group

Pathogenesis: The developing larval stages of metacestode reaches brain and spinal cord. Large numbers of immature metacestode migrate in the brain and spinal tissues and produces yellowish to reddish migratory tracts. It leads to acute meningioencephalitis especially in adult lambs. The immature metacestodes develop into mature fluid filled cyst. The cyst produces space occupying lesions and exerts pressure on tissues of brain and spinal cord. Some cases it causes softening of skull bone and finally leads to perforation.

Taenia ovis

Definitive Host: Dog

Location: Small intestine

Intermediate Host: Sheep

Metacestode stage: *Cysticercus ovis*

Location: Massetors, heart and diaphragm

Life cycle: Similar to *T. saginata*

Epidemiology: Infected dogs - passes gravid proglottids through faeces, Pasture contamination

Entry of stray dogs into pasture land. Using of untreated shepherd dog (that are not dewormed against tape worms) for shepherding of sheep on pasture land. Dissemination of eggs in the pasture land through wind and insects.

Intermediate Host: Passive ingestion of egg along with pasture grass.

Definitive Host - Passive ingestion of meat containing cysticercus possibly by stray dogs stands around unauthorized slaughter houses on road side, they eat the throwaway inedible portion of meat which containing *cysticercus ovis*. Feeding of infected offal to house hold dogs.

Pathogenesis: Similar to *T. saginata*

Clinical Signs

Intermediate Host: No clinical signs, unaesthetic that decrease meat value.

Diagnosis

Intermediate Host: Only by meat inspection and serology no value.

Definitive Host: Characteristic egg

Treatment: Intermediate Host: no value

Control: Control of epidemiological factors.

Taenia pisiformis

Definitive Host: dog (mainly) and other carnivores

Location: Small Intestine

Intermediate Host: Lagomorphs, primarly: Rabbit, hares and rodents, *Metacestode stage: C. pisiformis*

Location: Peritoneal cavity attached to viscera

Taenia taeniaformis

Definitive Host: dog (mainly) and other carnivores

Location: Small Intestine

Intermediate Host: Rodents

Metacestode stage: *C. fasciolaris*

Location: Liver

Clinical Signs

Based on the location the clinical signs may varies

In brain: Staggers or Gid or Sturdy

Parietal region - surface of cerebral hemisphere – left side.

Animals held its head in affected side (left) and moves in circle – left direction and right eye may be blind. Parietal region - surface of cerebral hemisphere – right side. Animals held its head in affected side (right) and move in circle – right direction and left eye may be blind. Anterior part of the brain- head lowered and held against chest, walk in straight line until to hit on hard objects and remain motionless for some time. Ventricle of the brain – opposite to above condition.

Cerebellum – animal become hyperaesthetic – animal walks in jerky or staggering gait.

In spinal cord: Progressive paresis of one or both hind limbs.

Due to mature: Ataxia, hyper excitability, is varying degree of blindness, muscle tremor, nystagmus and occasionally found dead.

Diagnosis

Live animals: Through antemortem – difficult to detect. Opthalmoscopic examination of the eye prior to development of clinical signs.

Dead animals: postmortem examination.

Treatment: Generally useless, high doses of albendazole may be tried. Surgical removal of cyst, if it present in the surface of brain.

Control: Control of epidemiological factors.

5.7. Echinococcosis

Echinococcus granulosus is a tapeworm found in the small intestine of the canid definitive host. Its eggs are ingested by the intermediate hosts, wild and domestic herbivores, *e.g.*, sheep, cattle, and moose. People can also serve as intermediate hosts. After hatching in the intestine of the intermediate host, the oncospheres invade the circulatory system and lodge in various organs (the liver and lungs), where they develop into large, thick-walled, unilocular hydatid cysts that bud protoscolices endogenously. Hydatids have been rarely reported in the CNS of domestic animals and are rare in people, in which they produce symptoms similar to those of a brain tumor. Foxes are the definitive host for a related species, *Echinococcus multilocularis*. Microtine rodents (such as voles) are the intermediate hosts. This parasite has been rarely found in the brain of people, in which the invasive, thin-walled multilocular hydatid cysts produce innumerable exogenous daughter cysts that bud protoscolices. Surgical intervention is more successful in removing unilocular hydatid cysts of *E. granulosus*.

Echinococcus granulosus granulosus

Pastoral cycle: Oncosphere contaminated pasture → sheep → feeding of offals with fertile cyst to dog. Camel and reindeer act as reservoir. Pastoral cycle – primary source of hydatidosis for man.

Sylvatic cycle: Wild ruminants → wild canids, Less important source for human beings.

Epidemiology

Agent: Strain variation occurs (mentioned earlier). Strains differ in morphologically and chemically. Horse strain – host specific – not infective for human. Sheep strain – not host specific – infective for human.

Pasture contamination: Similar to *T. ovis*.

Infection rate: less when compare to other Taeniids, Infected dog shed – one gravid proglottid per week. Egg containing oncosphere – viable in pasture for 2 years.

Infection of Intermediate Host and Definitive Host: Similar to *T.ovis*.

Infection of man: Accidental ingestion of egg, when childrens playing with infected dogs. Consumption of infected dog faeces contaminated feed and water.

Echinococcus granulosus

Strain	*E. granulosus granulosus*	*E. granulosus equinus*
Distribution	Worldwide	Europe
Definitive host	Dog and carnivores	Dog and carnivores
Intermediate host	Domestic and wild ruminants, pig and man	Horses and donkey

Metacestode stage: Hydatid stage.

Location: Visceral organs – lung and liver.

Sheep: 70 per cent in lung and 25 per cent in liver.

Horse and cattle: 90 per cent in liver.

Morphology

Adult worm: Smallest cestode of domestic animals (6mm), consist of 3 or 4 segments, Gravid segment is half the length of rest of segment.

Hydatid Cyst

Types of cyst

(a) **Sterile cyst:** Not infective for dog. In horse – 27 per cent of cysts are sterile, in sheep - 51 per cent of cyst are sterile and in cattle and pig most of cysts are sterile.

(b) **Fertile cyst:** Infective for dog.

Size: 5 – 10 cm in size (maximum of 50cm)

Cyst Wall

Outer layer: Thick and made up of concentrically arranged laminated membrane

Inner layer: Germinal layer and granular in nature.

Cyst fluid - Pale yellow in colour - contains 17 to 200 mg of protein per ml.

Brood capsule – Protoscolices attached on the inner granular layer or detached and float free in the hydatid fluid – "Hydatid sand".

Daughter cyst: Develops within the mother cyst. If mother cyst rupture – protoscolices and brood capsules – develops external daughter cyst.

Life cycle: Proglottids/egg → Intermediate host (6 - 12 months) → Definitive host (40 - 50 days).

Echinococcus multilocularis

Definitive Host: Wild canids, domestic dog and cat

Location: Small intestine

Intermediate Host: Rodents, Large mammals and man

Metacestode stage: Hydatid cyst – liver – mostly multilocule

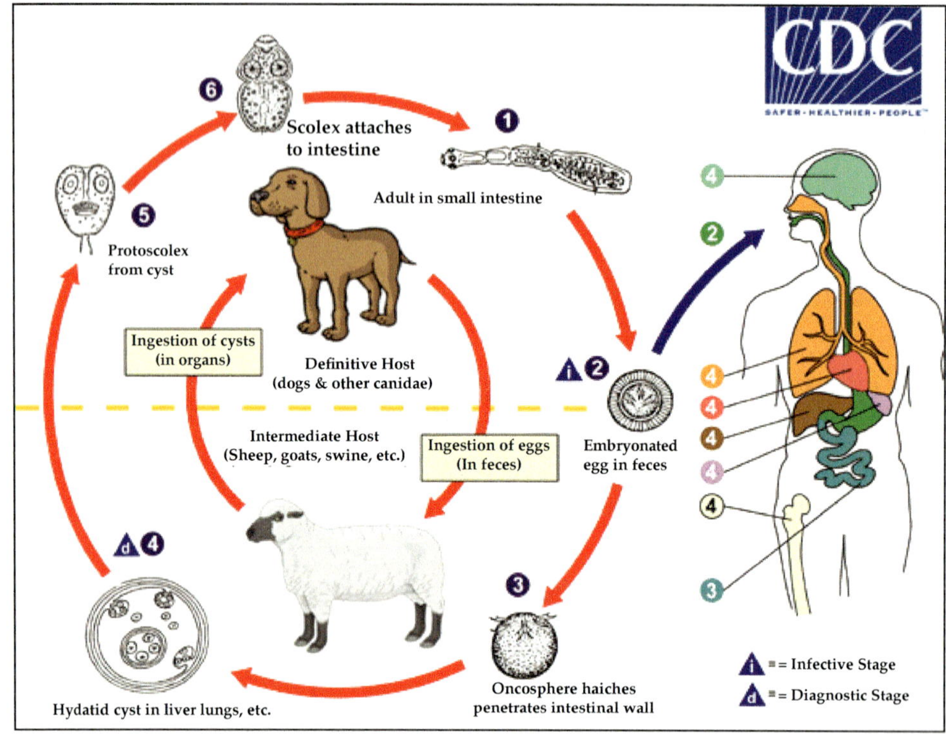

Figure 5.7

The adult *Echinococcus granulosus* (3 to 6 mm long)–1 resides in the small bowel of the definitive hosts, dogs or other canids. Gravid proglottids release eggs–2 that are passed in the feces. After ingestion by a suitable intermediate host (under natural conditions: sheep, goat, swine, cattle, horses, camel), the egg hatches in the small bowel and releases an oncosphere–3 that penetrates the intestinal wall and migrates through the circulatory system into various organs, especially the liver and lungs. In these organs, the oncosphere develops into a cyst–4 that enlarges gradually, producing protoscolices and daughter cysts that fill the cyst interior. The definitive host becomes infected by ingesting the cyst-containing organs of the infected intermediate host. After ingestion, the protoscolices–5 evaginate, attach to the intestinal mucosa–6, and develop into adult stages–1 in 32 to 80 days. The same life cycle occurs with *E. multilocularis* (1.2 to 3.7 mm), with the following differences: the definitive hosts are foxes, and to a lesser extent dogs, cats, coyotes and wolves; the intermediate host are small rodents; and larval growth (in the liver) remains indefinitely in the proliferative stage, resulting in invasion of the surrounding tissues. With *E. vogeli* (up to 5.6 mm long), the definitive hosts are bush dogs and dogs; the intermediate hosts are rodents; and the larval stage (in the liver, lungs and other organs) develops both externally and internally, resulting in multiple vesicles. *E. oligarthrus* (up to 2.9 mm long) has a life cycle that involves wild felids as definitive hosts and rodents as intermediate hosts. Humans become infected by ingesting eggs–2, with resulting release of oncospheres–3 in the intestine and the development of cysts–4 in various organs.

Pathogenesis

Intermediate Host: Egg →IMH →small intestine → Release of oncosphere → Development of adult metacestode stage → Liver and lung → systemic circulation

Clinical Signs

Intermediate Host: Clinical signs based on severity of infection and location of cyst, heavy infection – affected organs function impaired, rupture of cyst – anaphylatic shock. Alveolar hydatidosis: it is due to *E. multilocularis* – malignant tumor and metastasis.

Diagnosis

Intermediate Host

Animals: Rare only by postmortem examination.

Man: Serology: CFT and CIE.

Treatment

Intermediate Host: man.

Aspiration of cyst fluid and irrigated of cyst cavity with 2.5 per cent - 10 per cent formalin (not commonly used) or own serum. Care should be taken to avoid spillage of cyst fluid while aspiration. Surgical removal of cyst. Higher doses of mebandazloe, albendazole and praziquantel.

Control: Similar to *T. ovis.*

Epidemiology of metacestode infections in the intermediate host

Following factors influences incidence and prevalence of infection in IMH

level of environmental contamination:

Infected Definitive Host: Infected direct host passes proglottids through faeces which contain numbers of infective eggs, which acts as source of infection, and contaminate feed, water and pasture land.

Pasture contamination: *T. saginata* and *T. solium* – night soiling habit of infected human beings. Other Taeniids – entry of stray dogs into pasture land and using of untreated dogs for shepherding of animals in pasture land.

Presence of suitable susceptible host: If suitable susceptible IH are exposed to infective egg and pickup the infection harbour the metacestode stage which is infective for DH.

Dispersion of egg on pasture land: Taeniid eggs travel upto 80 m under suitable environmental conditions. Movement of wind.

Invertebrate host: flies (blow flies), beetles and earth worm.

Egg survival: Normal condition survive upto 6 months, senescent oncosphere – unable to penetrate the intestinal wall if it is ingested by the suitable intermediate. These type of oncospheres are used for immunization.

Age of the Intermediate Host

Sheep: Unweaned lambs are under high risk because of infected lambed ewes acts as a potential reservoir of infection for this. Lambs less than 5 weeks old – maternal immunity - protection: Lambs greater than 5 weeks old – depletion of maternal immunity and at this time lambs starts nibbling of grasses. Lambs reared on contaminated pasture land from birth onwards - develops strong immunity to reinfection.

Calves: In endemic area – neonatal infection occur with oncosphere of *T. saginata* – calf not able to develop protective immunity – infection throughout their life.

Immune response of host (Definitive Host): Animal develops a marked protective immunity to reinfection with metacestodes. The duration of immunity is about one year in the absence of reinfection.

Heterologus infection: Cross protection observed between *Taenia* species.

Pathogenesis of Dog and Cat Tapeworm

General: Heavy infection – non specific abdominal symptoms, diarrhoea of constipation, unthriftiness and pot bellied appearance.

D. caninum: Due to irritation of anal spincter, to drag its anus over the ground or other objects, Gravid proglottids drop off from infected animals and migrate over chair, floor or clothes for some minutes – aesthetically unpleasing to owner.

D. latum

Man: Abdominal discomfort, Pernicious anaemia – Vit B_{12} - Macrocytic hypochromic anaemia.

Diagnosis

Characteristic egg:

D. caninum – egg pockets

D. latum – operculated egg

E. granulosus – for identification of small gravid segments – dog should be treated with vermifuge to expel whole worm as such and screening for worms in faeces for subsequent two days.

Treatment: Arecoline hydrobromide – 1 to 2 mg/kg (contraindicated for cats), Bithionol – 200 mg/kg, Hexachlorophen – 15 mg/kg, Niclosamide – 100 to 150 mg/kg, Nitroscanate – 50 mg/kg, Praziquantel – 5 mg/kg, Dichlorphen – Dog: 0.3 mg/kg and cat: 0.1 to 0.2 mg/kg, Micronized mebendazole, Body weight less than 2 kg – 100 mg/kg twice a day for five days, Body weight greater than 2 kg – 200 mg/kg twice a day for five days, Drug dichlorophen and micronized mebendazole are not effective against Echinococcus infection in dogs.

Control: Control of IH + regular deworming of dog, dogs should not fed raw meat, freezing of fish below – 20°C for 24 hours. Prevent capturing of small wild animals (rat, mice and hares)which act as a IH. *D. caninum* – flea control. *D. latum* – avoid feeding of raw fish

5.8. Fasioliasis (Liver fluke disease or liver rot)

Fascioliasis is an infectious disease caused by *Fasciola* parasites, which are flat worms referred to as liver flukes. The adult (mature) flukes are found in the bile ducts and liver of infected people and animals, such as sheep and cattle. In general, fascioliasis is more common in livestock and other animals than in people. Two *Fasciola* species (types) infect people. The main species is *Fasciola hepatica*, which is also known as "the common liver fluke" and "the sheep liver fluke." A related species, *Fasciola gigantica*, also can infect people.

Fasciola hepatica: Mostly found in temperate and cooler area of high altitude in tropical and subtropical countries.

Fasciola gigantica: Mostly in tropical countries.

Morphology: Broad-leaf like body

Host Affected

Natural host: Cattle, Buffalo, Sheep, Goat and other ruminants

Unusual host: Horse and Man

Location

Immature flukes: Small intestine, peritoneal cavity and liver parenchyma

Mature flukes: Bile duct

Intermediate host (Amphibious snail)

Fasciola hepatica: *Lymnaea truncatula*

Fasciola gigantica

L. auricularia

L. acuminata and L.rufescens (India and Pakistan)

Epidemiology

Hatching of eggs: Optimum temperature - 10 – 26°C and Relative humidity – 70 per cent. Summer – 21 days and winter – 90 days.

Snail: Optimum temperature for breeding: 10– 28°C. Increasing in environmental temperature: Mortality of snail occurs (Infectivity falls). Size of snail: Size directly related with release of Metacercariae. Moist and warm condition (mud) grow well. Under unfavorable condition goes to hibernation.

Ecology of Lymnea: Permanent habitat – poorly drained soils, ditches, area of seepage and spring. Temporary habitat – Hoof marking of animals (clay soil). pH- slight acid pH favour growth.

Clinical Signs

Sheep

Acute: Sudden death without showing clinical signs. Blood stained frothy exudate from nostrils and anus – Resembles Anthrax.

Sub acute/chronic: Sub-acute severity is more but duration is less, Chronic – severity is less with long course, Intermittent soft faeces, occasionally diarrhoea, Progressive weight loss, Inter-mandibular oedema – Bottle Jaw, Pale mucous membrane, skin become dry and Brittle, falling out in punches.

Cattle: Similar to sheep, Reinfection of adult pregnant cow – migration to foetus (prenatal infection). Experimental infection of fascioliasis increase susceptibility of cattle to *Salmonella dublin* infection. Fascioliasis / Ostertagiasis complex. Diarrhoea is not feature of fascioliasis unless it is complicated by the presence of *Ostertagia* larva.

Chronic Fascioliasis: Most common form (ingestion of few metacercariae). Morbidity – 30 per cent and Mortality – 10 per cent.

Hepatic Fibrosis - Immature flukes

Life Cycle of *Fasciola*

See Figure 5.8a.

Pathogenesis: Presence of worms and eggs in the intestine and peritoneal cavity: not much pathogenic changes. Presence of worms and eggs in the liver and bile ducts: principle lesions encountered.

Sheep

Acute fascioliasis: Morbidity and Mortality High, 6–8 weeks old sheep are highly affected. Severity of disease is directly related to number. of metacercariae ingested (10,000), Traumatic hepatitis – migration of immature fluke aided by suckers. Extensive destruction of liver parenchyma and marked haemorrhage, If number. of immature flukes entered in to liver is so high – rupture of liver capsule - haemorrhage falls into peritoneal cavity.

Post - mortem Examination: Liver enlarged in size, pale, friable and fibrinous clot observed on surface, while incision extensive - haemorrhage tracts with immature flukes, If liver capsule is ruptured the blood clots observed in the abdominal cavity.

Sub-acute fascioliasis: If number. of metacercariae ingested is less (<10,000), liver is covered by migratory tracts – infiltration of inflammatory cells. Inflammatory cells mount immune response (not upto protective level) Early fibrosis, Majority of fluke reaches bile ducts and become mature fluke – Cholangitis.

Complication: Anaerobic condition created by migratory flukes favours multiplication of *Clostridium novyi* – Black disease

Infection of Snail: Longevity of Metacercariae.

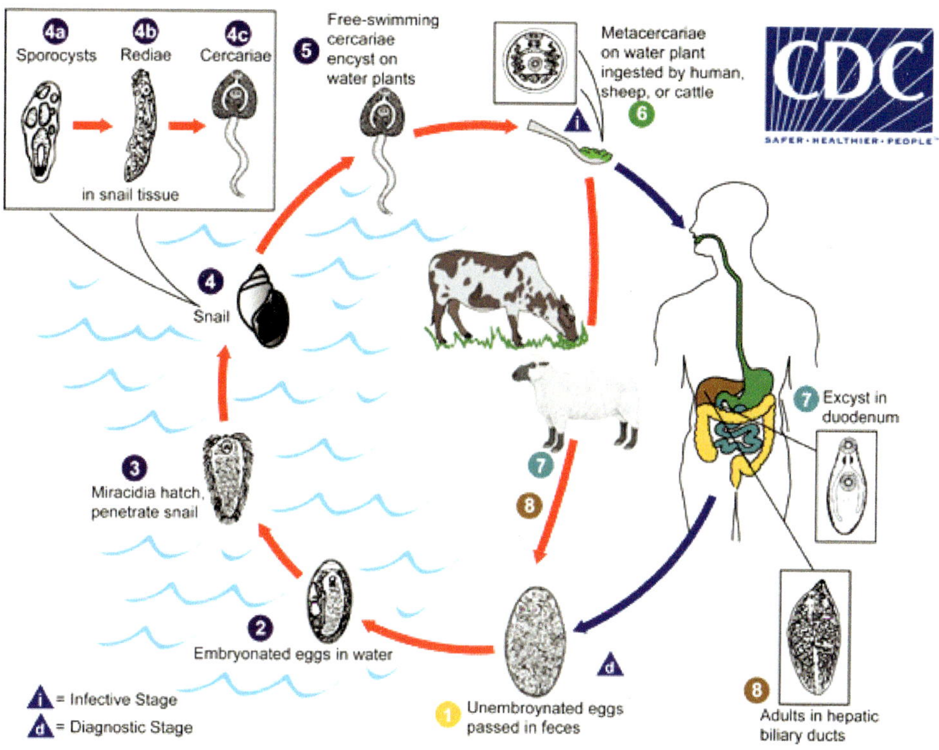

Figure 5.8a

Immature *Fasciola* eggs are discharged in the biliary ducts and in the stool–1. Eggs become embryonated in water–2, eggs release miracidia–3, which invade a suitable snail intermediate host–4, including the genera *Galba, Fossaria* and *Pseudosuccinea*. In the snail the parasites undergo several developmental stages (sporocysts–4a, rediae–4b, and cercariae–4c). The cercariae are released from the snail–5 and encyst as metacercariae on aquatic vegetation or other surfaces. Mammals acquire the infection by eating vegetation containing metacercariae. Humans can become infected by ingesting metacercariae-containing freshwater plants, especially watercress–6. After ingestion, the metacercariae excyst in the duodenum–7 and migrate through the intestinal wall, the peritoneal cavity, and the liver parenchyma into the biliary ducts, where they develop into adult flukes–8. In humans, maturation from metacercariae into adult flukes takes approximately 3 to 4 months. The adult flukes (*Fasciola hepatica*: up to 30 mm by 13 mm; *F. gigantica*: up to 75 mm) reside in the large biliary ducts of the mammalian host. *Fasciola hepatica* infect various animal species, mostly herbivores (plant-eating animals).

Natural condition: 4-6 weeks, *Experimental Condition:* 9 – 11 months, *Relative Humidity:* > 70 per cent - increases the survivability, *Good hay making:* infectivity retained considerable period, *Ensilage:* Survive not more than 35 – 57 days

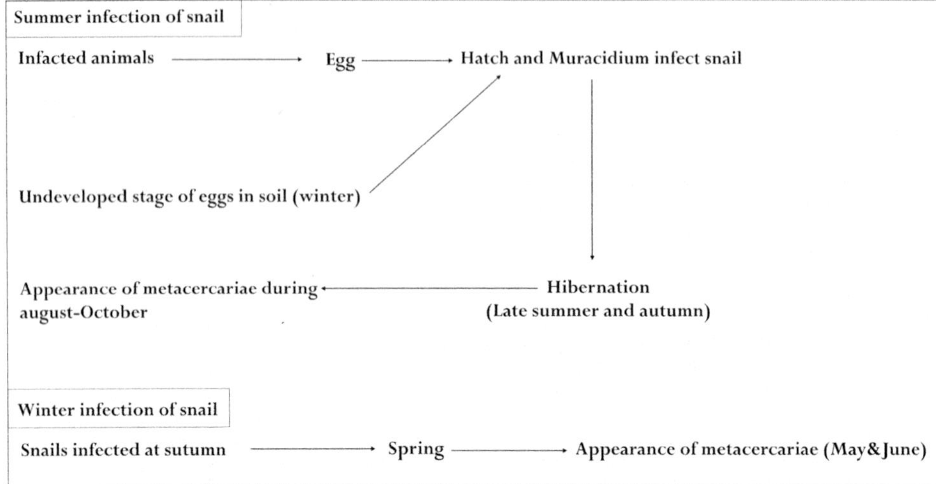

Figure 5.8b. Infection of Snail.

Immunity and Immunization

Natural immunity

Cattle - Reinfection of *F. hepatica* - moderate to high immunity, Sheep - fails to develop protective immunity

Active immunity

Cattle – Three doses of irradiated metacercariae of *F. hepatica*, Age - 6 – 9 months, Sheep – Not effective. Sheep infected with *Taenia hydatigena* give immunity to *F. hepatica* but reverse not possible

Postmortem Changes

Acute: Blood stained exudate – stained and rule out for Anthrax. Liver enlarged in size, pale, friable and fibrinous clot observed on surface. While incision extensive - haemorrhage tracts with immature flukes. If liver capsule is ruptured the blood clots observed in the abdominal cavity

Subacute and Chronic: Calcification of bile ducts and enlargement of gall bladder, Cattle - Lungs – Hazel-nut sized cysts containing brownish gelatinous material in which a live/dead and calcified flukes are observed.

Diagnosis

Based on clinical signs and history, identification of characteristic egg in faeces.

Amphistome Egg (Paramphistomum cervi)	*Fasciola Egg (Fasciola hepatica)*
Large size	Smaller in size
Transparent shell	Yellow coloured shell
Distinct operculum	Indistinct operculum
Embryonic cells are clear	Embryonic cells are not clear

Treatment: Older drug (mostly effective against mature flukes), Carbon tetrachloride (oldest – 50 years), Recommended for adult fluke of sheep only (not for Cattle). Hexachorethane – 90 per cent is effective against mature flukes. Cattle – 220 to 400 mg/kg in divided doses (3-4). Sheep – 20 to 30 grams/animal. Hexachlorophene - 90 per cent is effective against mature flukes. Cattle – 10 to 20 mg/kg, Sheep – 15 to 20 mg/kg, hetol – against adult flukes. Cattle – 125mg/kg, Sheep – 150 mg/kg, Bithionol. Cattle – 30 –35 mg/kg (66 to 68 per cent). Sheep - 40 mg/kg (90 to 100 per cent -chronic fasioliasis)

Recent drugs (Active against mature and immature flukes): Diamphenethide – 100 to 150 mg/kg (90 to 100 per cent for Adult), Drug of choice for acute fascioliasis in sheep. Oxyclozanide, Cattle – 10 to 15 mg/kg (mature -100 per cent), Sheep – mature - 15 to 20 mg/kg and Immature - 45 mg/kg, Rafoxanide, Sheep and Cattle – 7.5 mg/kg, Mature - more than 90 per cent and Immature – 50 to 90 per cent, Nitroxynil

Sheep and Cattle: Mature (100 per cent)- 10 mg/kg and Immature (90 per cent) – 15 mg/kg, Benzimidazole (Albendazole and Oxfendazole), Albendazole – Sheep - 7.5 mg/kg and Cattle – 15 mg/kg.

Latest drug (Active against mature and highly effective against immature flukes): Triclabendazole – 10 mg/kg body, highly effective against immature flukes, Sheep – single dose remove all stages (over one week old). Cattle – two doses remove over 4 weeks aged flukes, Movement of stock from the infected pasture, Closantel - 7.5 mg/kg.

Deworming Schedule

Sheep: Deworming schedule for sheep in endemic areas to reduce pasture contamination. In late April/May – adult sheep – treated for adult and late immature flukes (Triclabendazole). In October – entire flock with triclabendazole. In January – entire flock drug off mature flukes (Albendazole). In areas having high rain fall - additional dose on June (4-6 weeks after early April/May dose). In October/November (4 weeks after early October dose).

Cattle: Every December and May to prevent pasture contamination on spring and winter.

Control: Control similar to Amphistomes.

Control of Snail

Physical – Improving drainages.

Chemical - Applying molluscicides, Copper sulphate - 1 in 1,00,000 solution for water reservoir. Copper sulphate powder - 10 – 35 kg/hectare should be, applied along with sand for easy apply and sheep are not allowed to graze until rainfall occurs, N-tritylomorpholine – 0.45 kg/680 liters/hectare is introduced, Time of application - Spring or mid summer. Biological – rearing of ducks, geese and frog - infected water sources.

5.9. Leishmaniosis

Leishmaniosis is a disease caused by protozoan parasites of the genus *Leishmania* and transmitted through the bites of female phlebotomine sand flies. More than

23 species of *Leishmania* have been described, most of which are zoonotic. The most important *Leishmania* parasite to affect domestic animals is *L. infantum*, also known as *L. chagasi* in Latin America. Dogs are the main reservoir host for human visceral leishmaniosis caused by *L. infantum*, and the disease is potentially fatal in dogs and people. Because the internal organs and skin of the dog are affected, the canine disease is termed viscerocutaneous or canine leishmaniosis. Cats, horses, and other mammals can be infected by *L. infantum* or other *Leishmania* species. The disease in cats is rarer than in dogs and may manifest in cutaneous or visceral organs. *L. braziliensis*, the cause of tegumentary canine leishmaniosis, is widespread in regions of South America and may geographically overlap with *L. chagasi*. Canine leishmaniosis is a major zoonosis endemic in >70 countries. It is prevalent in southern Europe, Africa, Asia, South and Central America, and sporadically in the USA. It is also of concern in nonendemic countries where imported disease constitutes a veterinary and public health problem.

Leishmania

Members of this genus primarily occur in mammals and other hosts like lizards and bats. They cause disease in man, dogs and various rodents. The parasite, Leishmania is heteroxenous, transmitted by sand flies. It is found amastigote stage in the cells of its vertebrate host and in the promastigote stage in the intestine of sand fly and in culture. They undergo morphological transformation and multiplication in vectors. It is major importance as a disease in man. In human, 3 types are reported, Visceral; Cutaneous; Muco-cutaneous.

Leishmania sp. of Domestic Animals

Leishmania spp	*Host*	*IMH/Vectors*	*Location*	*Disease*
L. tropica *L.major* *L. aethiopica* (India)	Man, Dogs, Gebrils and other wild rodents	Blood sucking Phlebotamine sand flies - *P.argentipes* (Promastigote)	Macrophages and other cells of RES (amastigote)	Cutaneous Leishmaniasis, Oriental Sore, Delhi boil, Muco - Cutaneous Leishmaniasis, Old World Leishmaniasis, Aleppo Button
L.donovani *L. infantum* (India)	Man, Dogs, and other wild Carnivores	Blood sucking Phlebotamine sand flies - *P.argentipes* (Promastigote)	Macrophages and other cells of RES of Spleen, Liver, Bone marrow and other sites (amastigote)	Visceral Leishmaniasis, Kala-azar, Black Fever, Dum Dum Fever, Asia Fever.
L. braziliense	Man and Lower animals	Blood sucking Phlebotamine sand flies - *P.argentipes* (Promastigote)	Macrophages and other cells of RES (amastigote)	Muco - Cutaneous Leishmaniasis

Location

Vertebrate host: Amastigote form in macrophages and other cells of RES in skin, spleen, bone marrow, lymph nodes, muscles and other sites or also in large mononuclear cells in blood.

Invertebrate host: Promastigote form in gut.

Morphology: Amastigote in vertebrate host is ovoid/round; only nucleus and kinetoplasts are seen in stained preparation. Romanowsky staining - Cytoplasm appears as blue, nucleus as red and kinetoplast as purple. Promastigotes in vectors are spindle shaped (3.5 µm).

Life Cycle

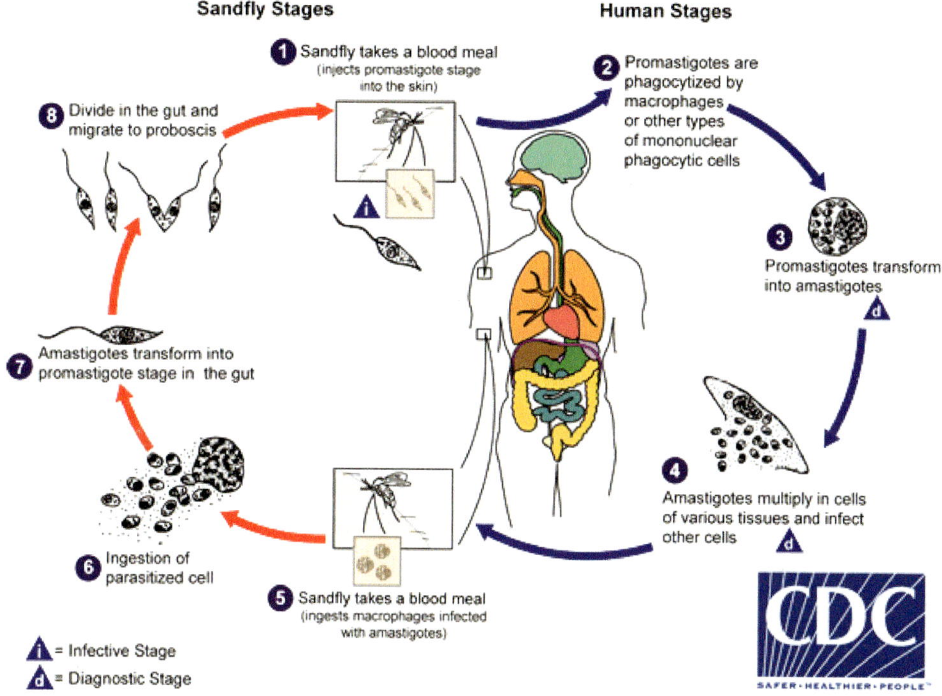

Figure 5.9

Leishmaniasis is transmitted by the bite of infected female phlebotomine sandflies. The sandflies inject the infective stage (*i.e.*, promastigotes) from their proboscis during blood meals–1. Promastigotes that reach the puncture wound are phagocytized by macrophages–2 and other types of mononuclear phagocytic cells. Progmastigotes transform in these cells into the tissue stage of the parasite (*i.e.*, amastigotes)–3, which multiply by simple division and proceed to infect other mononuclear phagocytic cells–4. Parasite, host, and other factors affect whether the infection becomes symptomatic and whether cutaneous or visceral leishmaniasis results. Sandflies become infected by ingesting infected cells during blood meals (5, 6). In sandflies, amastigotes transform into promastigotes, develop in the gut–7 (in the hindgut for leishmanial organisms in the *Viannia* subgenus; in the midgut for organisms in the *Leishmania* subgenus), and migrate to the proboscis.

Epidemiology

Transmission: By feeding or inoculation on infected host by sand flies. Infection also occurs when infected sand flies are crushed on the skin, *e.g,* Kala-azar fever. Mechanical transmission by biting flies. By needle passage as a possible method Visceral leishmaniasis-Direct infection by means of excretion of infected individuals.

Reservoir status: Dogs, cats, opossums and rodents are reservoirs.

Season: Countries with hot and dry climate.

Immunity: In cutaneous form, spontaneous cure is followed by immunity for up to 20 years. In visceral form, Infection persists in the animal.

Pathogenesis

Cutaneous Leishmaniosis: Differentiated as dry or moist or mildly erthymatous encountered in Old World and the muco-cutaneous form is encountered in New world. Dry form is more common and is urban in dogs; moist form is prevalent in rodents and gebrils.

Incubation period: 3 to 4 weeks after bite.

Man-Dry form: Promastigotes in macrophages of skin undergo maturity and resultant amastigotes are released after rupture of cells and infect other cells. The first detectable lesion occurs. The first detectable lesion occurs after 3-4 weeks after bite by the fly as a reddish papule, developing into a crust, forming a shallow ulcer which enlarges gradually and reach several centimeters in diameter. Coalescence of ulcers occurs and spread over large areas. In uncomplicated cases, healing occurs in 2-12 months leaving a deeply pigmented and depressed scar. Infection is rarely fatal.

Dogs: Similar to man; Ulcers on different parts of the body - lips and eyelids.

Visceral Leishmaniasis: Indian Kala–azar fever is important and is highly fatal in man. Incubation period: 10 days to more than year.

Man: Clinical signs appear usually after 3-6 months beginning with irregular fever; malaise, head ache, occasional abdominal pain, dysentery or diarrhea and bleeding of mucons membrane of mouth and nostrils; Darkening of the skin and hairs become brittle; Progressive enlargement of the spleen and liver fills almost entire abdomen which is striking feature of the disease. In advanced cases, there is ulceration of the digestive tract and great emaciation. In untreated cases, mortality is 70- 90 per cent, higher in adults than infants due to intercurrent disease. Post Kala-azar dermal Leishmaniasis: Following recovery after treatment, whitish spots develop into lentil- sized nodules in the skin on the face and neck.

Disease in RES: Increase in RES cells and the most affected organs are spleen, liver, bone marrow and lymph nodes; enlargement of malphigian corpuscles in spleen and fatty infiltration of Kupffer cells in liver; Macrophages, myelocytes and neutrophils of the bone marrow are filled with parasites; enlargement of lymph nodes, progressive leucopenia, monocytosis and anaemia.

Dogs: Naturally, no involvement of dogs with Indian Kala- azar and otherwise pathogenesis is similar to man, either cutaneous or visceral lesions. Anaemia, emaciation and diarrhea resulting in death. In chronic cases - Cutaneous lesions like eczema, scurfy degeneration and loss of hair are characteristics of the disease, moreover cutaneous ulcers in some cases around lips, eyelid and nostrils; spectacles due to depilation of hair around the eyes.

Diagnosis: Clinical signs, Lesions in living condition, Demonstration of parasites in peripheral blood smears, thick blood smears and centrifuged citrated blood for visceral form. In Cutaneous form- examination of skin scrapings from the edge of the lesion by Romanowsky staining is the method of choice in dogs. Examination of biopsy material from lymph nodes, spleen, and sternal/iliac crest puncture of bone marrow in visceral form. Culture of blood in NNN media for promastigotes.

Immunodiagnostic tests: CFT, IFA, IHA and Indirect agglutination tes, Napier's aldehyde test, Chopra's antimony test, formal gel test and Urea stilbamide test.

Treatment: In man, successful with organic antimony compounds and less effective in dogs.

Cutaneous form: Anthiomaline (lithium antimony thiomalate) - 1 ml rising by 0.5 to 2.5 ml on alternate days, 4-6 times; I/M.

Both forms: Pentavalent sodium stilbo gluconate (Pentastam) and trivalent sodium antimonyl gluconate (Triostan) are widely used.

Visceral form: Diamidines- Pentamide isothiocyanate – 2 mg/kg- 6 injections; 3 mg/kg - 7 injections; 4 mg/kg 13 injections at 2-3 hrs interval. I/V; very effective against *L. donovani* infection.

Control: Control of sand flies by various CHC and OPC. Measures against breeding places of flies by removal of dense and decaying vegetation around houses, fine mosquito nets in square should be used for human beings. Dogs with dermal lesions should be treated or destroyed. Control of stray dogs.

5.10. Nematodirus

The species of *Nematodirus* found in the small intestine of sheep are similar in morphology and life cycle to *N. helvetianus*. Clinical infections are of considerable importance in the UK, New Zealand, and Australia, where lamb mortality may reach 20 per cent in affected flocks if animals are untreated. The parasites are also endemic in some parts of the Rocky Mountain States of the USA, where they occasionally cause clinical disease in lambs.

In areas where clinical infections are common, the disease has a characteristic seasonal pattern. Many of the eggs passed by affected lambs lie dormant through the remainder of the grazing season and the winter, with large numbers of larvae appearing during the early grazing period of the following year. Thus, the lambs of one season contaminate the pastures for the next season's lambs; fortunately, the life cycle can be broken if the same area is not used for lambing each year. Most clinical infections are seen in lambs 6–12 wk old.

N. battus is seen in the UK and other parts of Europe and also in North America. Eggs hatch after a period of chill and then a rise in ambient temperature to a day/night mean of 10°C (50°F). This occurs in late spring in temperate areas. The hatching requirements mean that there is generally one generation of *N. battus* per year, although in the UK, occasional outbreaks in the autumn have been reported. The parasite can be highly pathogenic, because large numbers of larvae hatch over a short period at a time when young lambs are beginning to take in significant quantities of grass. Disease may be associated with developing larval stages and may be seen within 2 wk of challenge, *i.e.* during the prepatent period (15 days). Other *Nematodirus* spp often are found in low-rainfall regions (*e.g.*, the Karroo in South Africa and inland Australia) where other parasites are rarely seen.

Nematodirosis is characterized by sudden onset, "loss of bloom," unthriftiness, profuse diarrhea, and marked dehydration, with death as early as 2–3 days after an outbreak begins. Nematodirosis is commonly confined to lambs or weaner sheep, but in low-rainfall country where outbreaks are sporadic, older sheep may have heavy infections. The lesions usually consist of dehydration and mild catarrhal enteritis, but acute inflammation of the entire small intestine may develop. Counts of dikhuaaa10,000 worms, together with characteristic signs and history, are indicative of clinical infections. Affected lambs may pass large numbers of eggs, which can be identified easily; however, because the onset of disease may precede the maturation of the female worms, this is not a constant finding.

Nematodirus helvetianus is generally recognized as the most common bovine species, although other species, *e.g.*, *N. spathiger* and *N. battus*, can also infect cattle. The adult males of *N. helvetianus* are ~12 mm long and the females 18–25 mm. The eggs develop slowly; the infective third stage is reached within the egg in 2–4 wk and may remain within the egg for several months. Eggs may accumulate on pasture and hatch in large numbers after rain to produce heavy infections over a short period. The eggs are highly resistant, and those passed by calves in one season may remain viable and infect calves the next season. After ingestion of infective larvae, the adult stage is reached in ~3 wk. Worms are most numerous 10–20 ft (3–6 m) from the pylorus.

Signs, which include diarrhea and anorexia, usually develop during the third week of infection before the worms are sexually mature; clinical infections may be seen in dairy calves from 6 wk onward. Diagnosis is difficult during the prepatent period, but during the patent period it is easily made on the basis of the characteristic eggs. Relatively small numbers of eggs are produced. Fecal sampling of both healthy and sick calves in an affected group will increase the chance of making a diagnosis. Immunity to reinfection develops rapidly. Necropsy may show only a thickened, edematous mucosa.

Location: Small intestine

Morphology: Adult large sized – 10 to 15 mm

Egg: Larger in size (8 cell stage)

Species

N. spathiger – Sheep, goat, cattle and other ruminants. *N. battus* – Sheep. *N. abnormarlis* - Sheep, goat and camels.

Epidemiology

Embryonation: Similar to Strongyles

Hatching: Larvae inside the egg become sensitized to hatch by prolonged exposure to cold conditions (2- 3°C) and the stimulus to hatching is the raise of soil temperature (21°C).

Survivability: Only few weeks. Level of infection in lambs depends upon hatching date and lambing date

Host: Young animals (grazing) are highly susceptible. In older animals and in adults the infection is very milder and become source for pasture contamination.

Life cycle: Similar to *Trichostrongylus* spp.

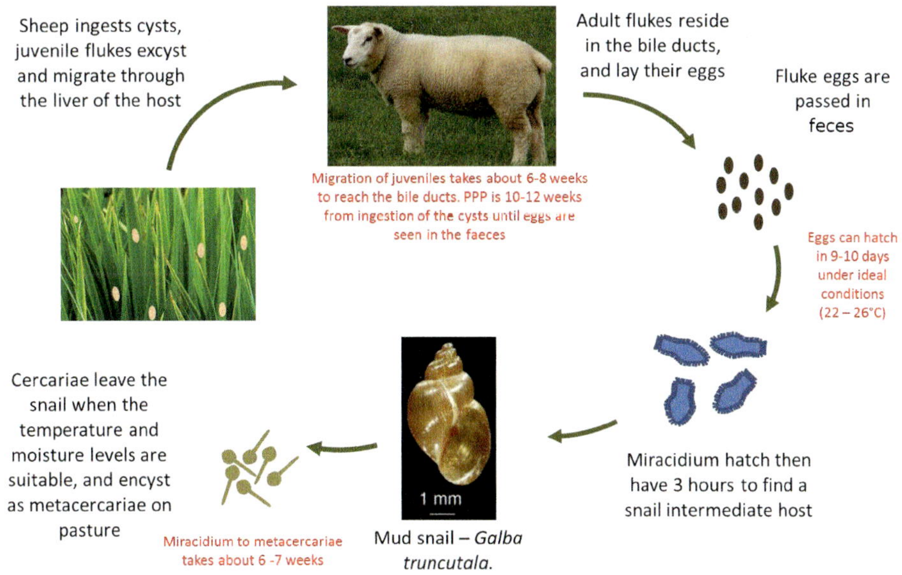

Figure 5.10.Life cycle of *Nematodirus.*

Pathogenesis: L3 penetrate tunneling and extensive destruction of mucosa villous atrophy.

Clinical Signs

Acute enteritis: Excessive mucus secretion and larvae is enclosed by mucus material. Severe diarrhea.

Nature of diarrhoea: Blackish- green followed by yellowish in colour, Anorexia, Inappetance, dehydration, prostration and finally death.

Mortality: 30 per cent (in 10 weeks old)

Immunity: Surviving lambs (3 weeks after recovery) – Drop in EPG and become resistant to infection.

Diagnosis: Based on clinical signs, fecal examination.

Control: Predict time of occurrence and prevent exposure of lambs to infected pasture grass. Prophylatic deworming – two to three time at an interval of 3 weeks.

5.11. Parascaris

Adult *Parascaris equorum* are stout, whitish worms, up to 30 cm long, with three prominent lips. The life cycle is similar to that of *Ascaris suum*, with a prepatent period of 10–12 wk. Large numbers of infective eggs can remain viable for years in contaminated soil. Adult animals usually harbor very few if any worms. The principal sources of infection for young foals are pastures, paddocks, or stalls contaminated with eggs from foals of the previous year.

In heavy infections, the migrating larvae may produce respiratory signs ("summer colds"). In heavy intestinal infections, foals show unthriftiness, loss of energy, and occasionally colic. Intestinal obstruction and perforation have been reported. Intestinal stages compete for absorption of essential amino acids. Diagnosis is based on demonstration of eggs in the feces. If disease due to prepatent infection is suspected, diagnosis may be confirmed by administration of an anthelmintic, after which large numbers of immature worms may be seen in the feces.

On farms where the infection is common, most foals become infected soon after birth. As a result, most of the worms are maturing when the foals are ~4–5 month old. Treatment should be started when foals are ~8 wk old and repeated at 6- to 8-wk intervals until they are yearlings. All broad-spectrum equine anthelmintics are effective against the adult and immature worms in the small intestine and, therefore, ascarids are readily controlled by routine anthelmintic administration. However, there have been reports of resistance of *P. equorum* to ivermectin and moxidectin in North America and Europe. Efficacy on any given farm should be monitored using a fecal egg count reduction test. In cases in which verminous pneumonia due to *Parascaris* migration has developed, therapeutic benefit may be achieved by treatment with ivermectin or fenbendazole (the latter at 10 mg/kg/day for 5 consecutive days) concurrent with appropriate antimicrobial therapy. *Parascaris* infection can be effectively prevented by daily administration of pyrantel tartrate once foals are eating grain regularly.

Parascaris equorum (*P. equorum*)

Host: Equines (Mainly), Zebra and cattle.

Location: Small intestine.

Morphology

Adult: 50cm long.

Egg: Subglobular with a thick coarsely pitted albuminous layer.

Life cycle: Similar to *A. suum*, Prepatent period: 80 days.

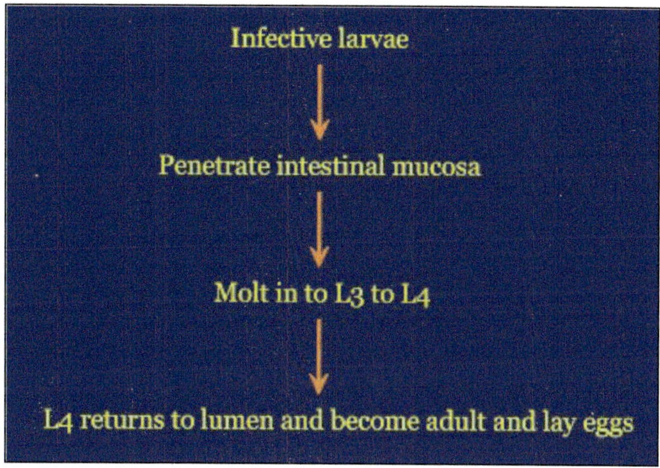

Figure 5.11. Life cycle of *Parascaris equorum*.

Epidemiology: Similar to *A. suum*

Host: Foals: 3- 9 months old are highly susceptible.

Pathogenesis and clinical signs

Immature: *Heavy infection* - coughing and circulating eosinophilia.

Adult: Catarrhal enteritis - diarrhoea - fetid in odour, pale in colour – flatulence, General malaise and debility, rough hair coat and pot bellied appearance.

Summer cold: Fever, pneumonia, coughing and whitish nasal discharge. Liver damage and bile duct obstruction is seen.

Complication: Due to migratory adult worms - bile ducts, Penetrate bowel wall and cause localized or generalized peritonitis, Adults worms twisted and balled up - cause an obstruction.

Diagnosis: Similar to *A. suum*

Treatment: Thiabendazole - 44 mg/kg; Mebendazole - 10 mg/kg; Fenbendazole - 7.5 mg/kg; Cambendazole - 20 mg/kg; Dichlorvos - 26 -52 mg/kg; Haloxon - 50 -70 mg/kg.

Prophylactic Schedule: First dose - first month of age, Second dose - 4 - 6 weeks after the first dose.

Prophylaxis: Brood mares should be treated for Ascarids before foaling. Boxes in which mares foal should be thoroughly cleaned before the event. Stables should be cleaned such a way that contamination is not likely to occur. Proper manure disposal. Foal should be run with its mother in a clean paddock.

5.12. Schistosomiasis

Schistosomiasis is a common parasitic infection in cattle and rarely in other domestic animals in Africa and Asia. Although schistosomes may act as important pathogens under rare conditions favoring intensive transmission, most infections in endemic areas are subclinical. However, high prevalence rates of subclinical infections cause significant losses due to longterm effects on growth and productivity and increased susceptibility to other parasitic or bacterial diseases.

Schistosomes are members of the genus *Schistosoma*, family Schistosomatidae. Adult worms are obligate parasites of the vascular system of vertebrates. Schistosomes are dioecious. The mature female is more slender than the male and normally is carried in a ventral groove, the gynaecophoric canal that is formed by ventrally flexed lateral outgrowths of the male body.

Of the 19 species reported to naturally infect animals, 8—are parasites of ruminants—have received particular attention, mainly because of their recognized veterinary significance: *S. mattheei, S. bovis, S. curassoni, S. spindale, S. indicum, S. nasale, S. incognitum*, and *S. japonicum*. *S. mattheei* is found in southeastern Africa, from the Cape Province in South Africa northward to Tanzania and Zambia. *S. bovis* is found in the Mediterranean region and Middle East, and is common in northern, western, and eastern Africa (except Egypt) extending southward to Central Angola, southern Congo, and possibly northern Zambia. *S. curassoni* has been found in ruminants in Senegal, Mauritania, Mali, Niger, and Nigeria. *S. spindale* has been recorded from India, Sri Lanka, Indonesia, Malaysia, Thailand, and Vietnam. The distribution of *S. indicum* appears confined to the Indian subcontinent. *S nasale* is found in India, Sri Lanka, Bangladesh, and Myanmar. *S. incognitum* has been reported from India, Thailand, and Indonesia. *S. japonicum* is endemic in several countries of the Far East. Some of these species are known to interact in areas where they coexist, and instances of interspecific hybridization have been reported, *e.g.*, the cattle parasites *S. bovis* and *S. curassoni*. Novel molecular tools have also provided evidence for the natural hybridization between *S. haematobium*, a parasite of people, and *S mattheei, S. bovis*, and *S. curassoni*. The hybridization between human and ruminant schistosomes is of particular interest, because for this to occur, host switching must have taken place of *S mattheei, S. bovis*, or *S. curassoni* into people or of *S. haematobium* into domestic livestock.

To differentiate the different *Schistosoma* spp., egg morphology (size, shape) can be used. The species can also be differentiated through such taxonomic features as morphologic (adult worms), life-cycle, or behavioral characteristics; chromosomes; host specificity; or enzyme and DNA studies.

Epidemilogy

Skin penetration: Horses and cattle may get infection while standing in the infected water sources. Buffaloes get infection while wallowing in the infected water sources. Slow moving water favour – entry of cercariae into body of animal. Consumption of water contaminated with cercariae. Highest rainfall (Season – Sepember to October)

Species affected: Sheep and goat, Cattle >buffalo

Age: Older bovines (>3 years). Infection also occurs 5- 6 months old calves.

Sex: both sexes are equally affected.

Life Cycle of Schistosomes

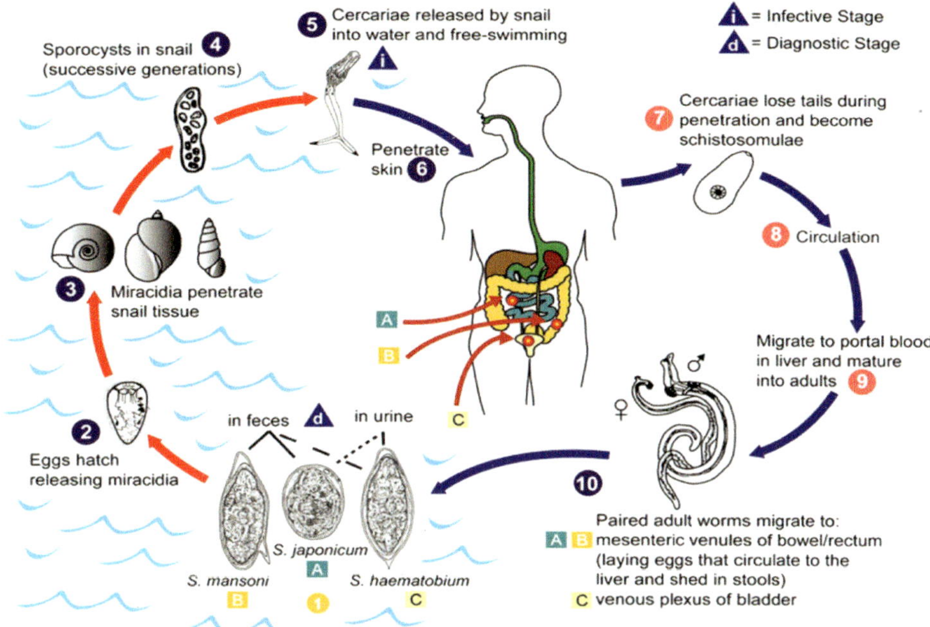

Figure 5.12a

Eggs are eliminated with feces or urine–1. Under optimal conditions the eggs hatch and release miracidia–2, which swim and penetrate specific snail intermediate hosts–3. The stages in the snail include 2 generations of sporocysts–4, and the production of cercariae–5. Upon release from the snail, the infective cercariae swim, penetrate the skin of the human host–6, and shed their forked tail, becoming schistosomulae–7. The schistosomulae migrate through several tissues and stages to their residence in the veins (8, 9). Adult worms in humans reside in the mesenteric venules in various locations, which at times seem to be specific for each species–10. For instance, *S. japonicum* is more frequently found in the superior mesenteric veins draining the small intestine–A, and *S. mansoni* occurs more often in the superior mesenteric veins draining the large intestine–B. However, both species can occupy either location, and they are capable of moving between sites, so it is not possible to state unequivocally that one species only occurs in one location. *S. haematobium* most often occurs in the venous plexus of bladder–C, but it can also be found in the rectal venules. The females (size 7 to 20 mm; males slightly smaller) deposit eggs in the small venules of the portal and perivesical systems. The eggs are moved progressively toward the lumen of the intestine (*S. mansoni* and *S. japonicum*) and of the bladder and ureters (*S. haematobium*), and are eliminated with feces or urine, respectively–1. Pathology of *S. mansoni* and *S. japonicum* schistosomiasis includes: Katayama fever, hepatic perisinusoidal egg granulomas, Symmers' pipe stem periportal fibrosis, portal hypertension, and occasional embolic egg granulomas in brain or spinal cord. Pathology of *S. haematobium* schistosomiasis includes: hematuria, scarring, calcification, squamous cell carcinoma, and occasional embolic egg granulomas in brain or spinal cord. Human contact with water is thus necessary for infection by schistosomes. Various animals, such as dogs, cats, rodents, pigs, hourse and goats, serve as reservoirs for *S. japonicum*, and dogs for *S. mekongi*.

Intermediate host

Name of the Snail	*Name of Trematode*
Indoplanorbis exustus	*S. nasalis, S. indicum* and *S. spindale*
Lymnaea luteola	*S. nasalis* and *S. incognitum*
Lymnaea acuminate	S. spindale

Developmental stages: Redia and metacercariae stages are absent. Two generation of sporocysts (I and II). Immature schistosomes – Schistosomula.

Morphology: Schistosomes are called as blood flukes. *Unisexual* – dimorphic trematode.

Female - Long (12 –28 mm) and slender.

Male - Comparatively small in length (9-22 mm) and having gutter-like groove (Gynaecophoric canal) in which female lodges at the time of copulation.

Cercariae - Tail forked - *Furcocercous cercariae.*

Egg - 100 –500 μm long, spindle in shape without operculum. Some species having lateral spines.

Nasal Schistosomiasis-Snoring, Disease/Pseudotubercle/Actinobody Formation: Cattle and buffalo (infection rate – 40 –50 per cent) and Horses. *S. nasalis* - nasal mucosal vein – induction of inflammatory and granulomatous response.

Clinical Signs

Cattle: Rhinitis – mucoprulent discharge, sneezing and dyspnoea. Adult parasite – dilation of vein and thrombosis of vein. Nasal mucosa studded with small granulomas and small abscess containing eggs. Chronic cases – proliferation of nasal epithelium. Space occupying lesion - breathing difficulties – snoring.

Buffalo: Pin sized eruption and congestion of nasal mucosa – Actinobodies, Diarrhoea, sometimes blood stained and contains mucus, Anorexia, thrust and emaciation.

Clinical pathology: Anemia, Eosinophilia, hypoalbuminemia, hypergamma-globulinemia, Dyshaemopoisis and expansion of plasma volume.

Diagnosis

Based on history, clinical signs and clinical pathology, demonstration of characteristic eggs, measuring cell mediated immune response.

Human Schistosomiasis-Bilharziasis: *S. mattheei, S. japonicum, S. mekongi, S. mansoni and S. haematobium.* Swimmers itch/Clay-diggers itch/Hunters itch/ Cercarial dermatitis/Rice-Paddy itch. Skin penetration of cercariae of non-human Schistosomes – Avian (*Trichobilharzia* spp. and *Austrobilharzia* spp) and animal Schistosomes (*Heterobilharzia* spp.). Form of Cutaneous larva migration, Initial mild erythema, oedema will appear

Chronic cases – Severe pruritis and a papular or pustular eruption

Treatment - Application of benzyl benzoate over the body and Antihistaminic therapy.

Prevention - Wearing protective clothing while working in the infected water sources.

List of Schistosomes

Schistosome sp.	*Host*	*Location*
S. bovis	Cattle, sheep and goat	Portal and mesenteric veins
S. spindale	Ruminants, pig and dog	Mesenteric veins
S. indicum	Ruminants, equines and camels	Portal and mesenteric veins
S. haematobium	Pig, monkeys and man	Veins of mesenteric, bladder, urethra and ureter
S. nasalis	Buffalo, cattle, goat, sheep and horse	Nasal vein
S. incognitum	Pig and dog	Mesenteric vein

Pathogenesis

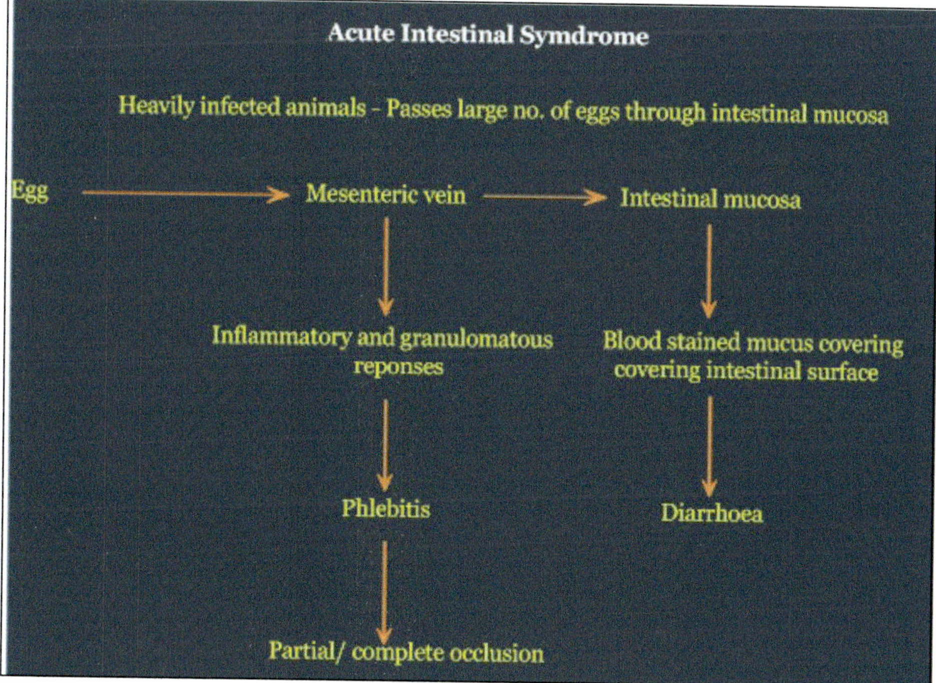

Figure 5.12b. Pathogenesis of Schistosomes.

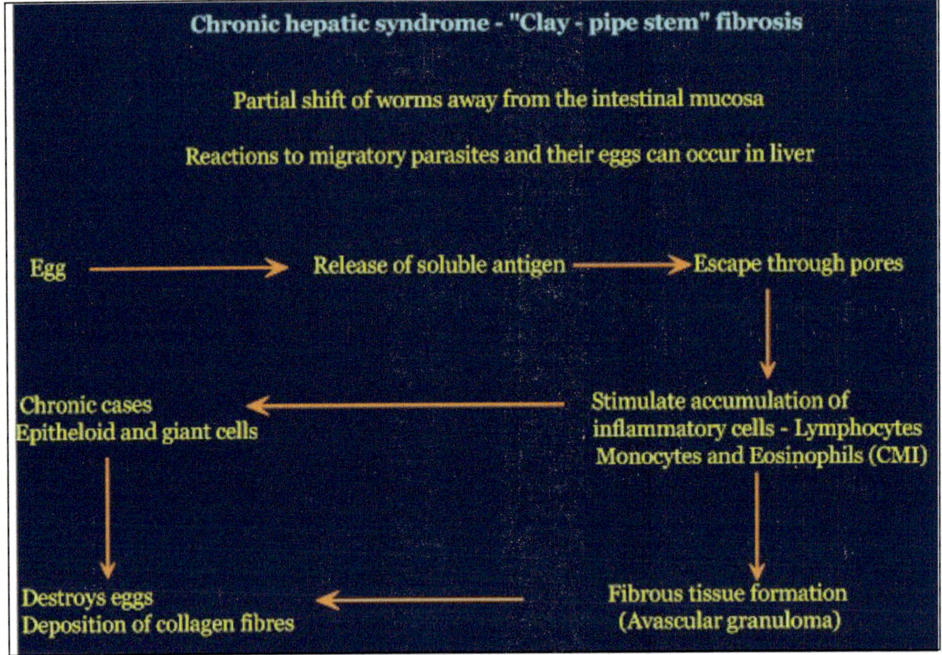

Figure 5.12c. Pathogenesis of Schistosomes.

Immunity

Natural immunity – cattle.

Artificial immunity: Irradiated Schistosomula of *S. mattheei* and *S. bovis.*

Route - S/C or I/M

Cattle and sheep - Induce greater than 60 per cent protection.

Treatment and Control

Human Schistosomiasis: Praziquantel – 60 mg/kg single dose or in divided doses (drug of choice)**:** Niridazole, Hycanthone, Lucanthone and Furapromidium.

Stibophen: Cattle - 7.5 mg/kg for 6 days

Lucanthone: Cattle – 30 mg/kg; Sheep - 30 –50 mg/kg for 3 days

Hycanthone: Sheep – 3 –6 mg/kg

Trichlorophon: Cattle – 50 –7 0 mg/kg orally 4 – 6 doses

Niridazole: Sheep – 100 mg/kg for 3 days

Praziquantel: Sheep and goat – 60 mg/kg

Nasal Schistosomiasis: Tartar emetic - 2 mg/kg. Sodium antimony tartrate – 1.5 mg/kg twice a day for 2 days. Trichlorophon - 30 –40 mg/kg three doses.

Control: Management practices and snail control similar to that of Amphistomiasis and Fascioliasis, Biological control *Schistosomes* larvae. Larval stages of *Echinostoma* spp. – used as predatory on schistosome larvae within the snail intermediate host, Microsporidial protozoa – *Nosema eurytremae*. Avoid contact of infected water sources.

5.13. Strongylidae

More than 40 species of small strongyles in several genera have been found in the cecum and colon of domestic equids, each with its own site of preference. They have been referred to as trichonemes, cyathostomes, and currently cyathostomins. They belong to the subfamily Cyathostominae of the family Strongylidae, and ~10 species are particularly prevalent. Most are appreciably smaller than the "large strongyles," but *Triodontophorus* spp (sometimes classified as nonmigratory large strongyles) are almost as long as *Strongylus vulgaris*.

Unlike the large strongyles, small strongyles do not migrate extraintestinally, because early development is confined to the wall of the intestine. Third-stage larvae may progress to the fourth stage without interruption, or they may undergo hypobiosis and resume development only after prolonged periods of dormancy or hypobiosis. When L_4 emerge from the gut wall, they feed superficially on the mucosa and may rupture capillaries but are less pathogenic than the large strongyles. They molt to the adult stage. An exception is *T. tenuicollis*, which is found in clusters and can produce severe ulcers in the wall of the colon. Generally, however, the resulting erosions of the mucosa are slight and hard to visualize. Consequently, it is common to recover thousands of adult worms from apparently healthy horses that have received limited anthelmintic treatment. In heavier infections, however, disruption may be extensive enough to disturb digestive and absorptive function, resulting in loss of condition and even catarrhal enteritis of the large intestine.

Strongylus

Species: *S. equinus* - Caecum and colon of equines, zebra. *S. vulgaris* – Large intestine – equines. *S. edentatus* - Large intestine – equines.

Morphology: Adult - Robust, dark red worm, Female - 32 – 40 mm and males – 26 – 35 mm long. Well developed buccal capsule (*S. edentatus* – buccal capsule – no teeth).

Egg*:* Oval, thin shelled enclosing segmented yolk when laid.

Coverings: Outer chitinous shell, Inner delicate vitelline membrane, Fluid cavity yolk and inner membrane.

Epidemiology

Host: Infection is more severe in foals, adults resistant to reinfection.

Bionomics: Embryonation, Hatching, Survivability of larvae in environment, Infection of definite host and exsheathment

Embryonation: Temperature: optimal temperature 26°C (Embryonation also occur at 7.2°C and arrested at 0°C), O_2 tension: Increased O_2 tension favours

Embryonation, Moisture (Relative humidity): 70 per cent (Desiccation unfavourable for embryonation).

Hatching: Optimum temperature - 26°C (below 9°C it is affected), Relative humidity: 70 per cent

Survivability of larvae in environment, Ensheathed larvae – protected from adverse weather conditions, L1 and L2 feed on soil bacteria and L3 doesn't fed and utilise stored nutrient, if L3 not found suitable host leads to exhaustment of stored food reserves – leads to death. Larvae does not actively enter the host. It is passively swallow along with feed and water. Environmental stimuli: possibility of finding the host through crawl up grass blades.

Soil*:* Negatively geotrophic - crawl up blades of grasses or other herbages from soil

Light*:* Positively phototrophic to mild light and negatively phototrophic to strong light and darkness. Larvae crawl up grass blades only in the early morning, towards evening and other times of the day in dull weather at night and during strong light hours larvae descend to soil.

Moisture*:* Flim of water is necessary for crawl up on grass blades.

Temperature*:* Migration is more and active during warm weather than cold.

Survivability of Larvae in the Environment

In Soil: Some larvae penetrate into soil where they survive more readily than on the surface. Loose sandy soil – penetrate more deeper than clay soil. In water - larvae sink on bottom of the pond and survive for a month or more.

In pasture grass: Conditions favorable for migration (warm and daily fluctuation of light and loose soil) – Larvae more active and utilize all stored nutrient – death is faster. In dry seasons - not more than three months, in cooler climate - even year or more.

Infection of Definite Host and Exsheathment

Infection of definitive host: Passive ingestion of infective larvae along with grass blades or water

Exsheathment in small intestine: Host stimulus are as follows - unionized bicarbonates - undisassociated Co2 - Dissolved gas Co2 - 70 per cent - Intestinal pH – 7.3 - Intestinal temperature (37°C). By the host stimuli the larvae secrete "Exsheathing fluid" which contains leucine aminopectidase - LAP. These enzymes breaks sheath along with larval movement.

Order: Strongylida

Super family: Strongyloidea

Family: Strongylidae

Genus Strongylus

Strongyles worm

Oesophagostomum - Strongyles worm

Super family: Ancylostomatoidea

Family: Ancylostomatidae

Genus: *Ancylostomum* -Hook worms; *Bunostomum* - Hook worms

Epidemiology of *Oesophagostomum columbianum* in Host

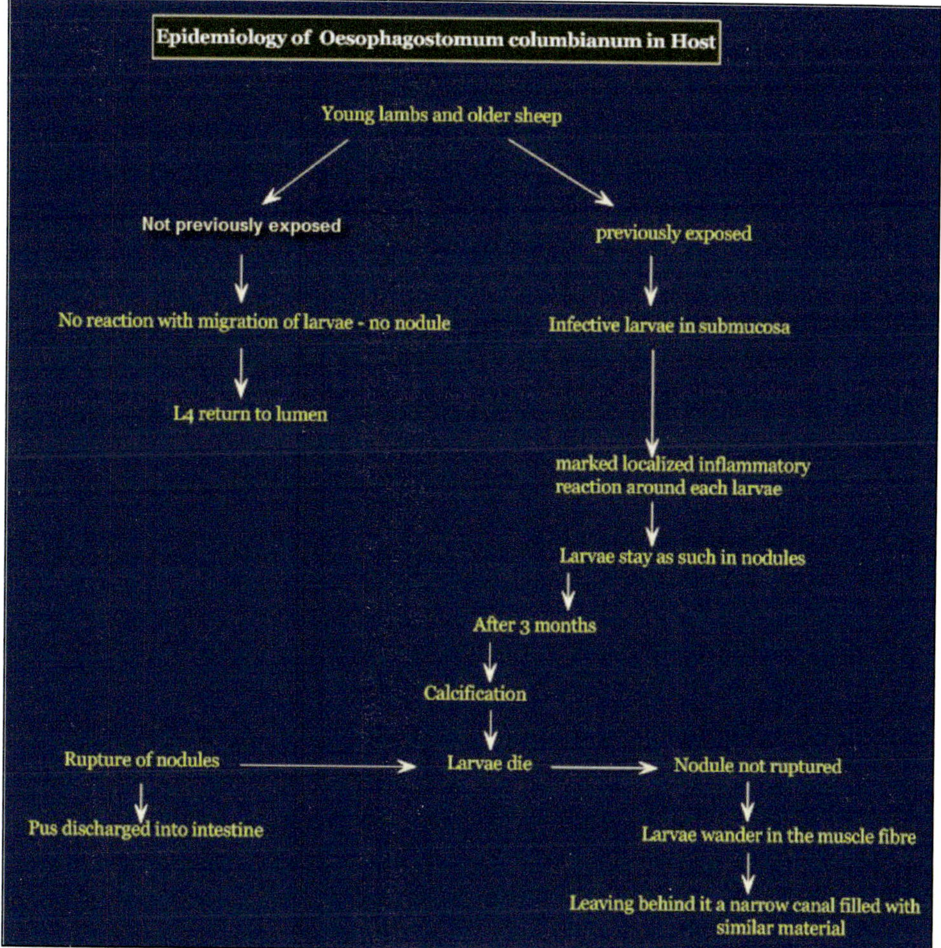

Figure 5.13a. Epidemiology of *Oesophagostomum columbianum* in host.

Life Cycle of *Strongylus* Sp.

See Figure 5.13b.

Nodular Worm of Pigs

Species: *O. dentatum* – Large intestine, *O. brevicaudum* - Large intestine, *O. mapelstonei* - Large intestine.

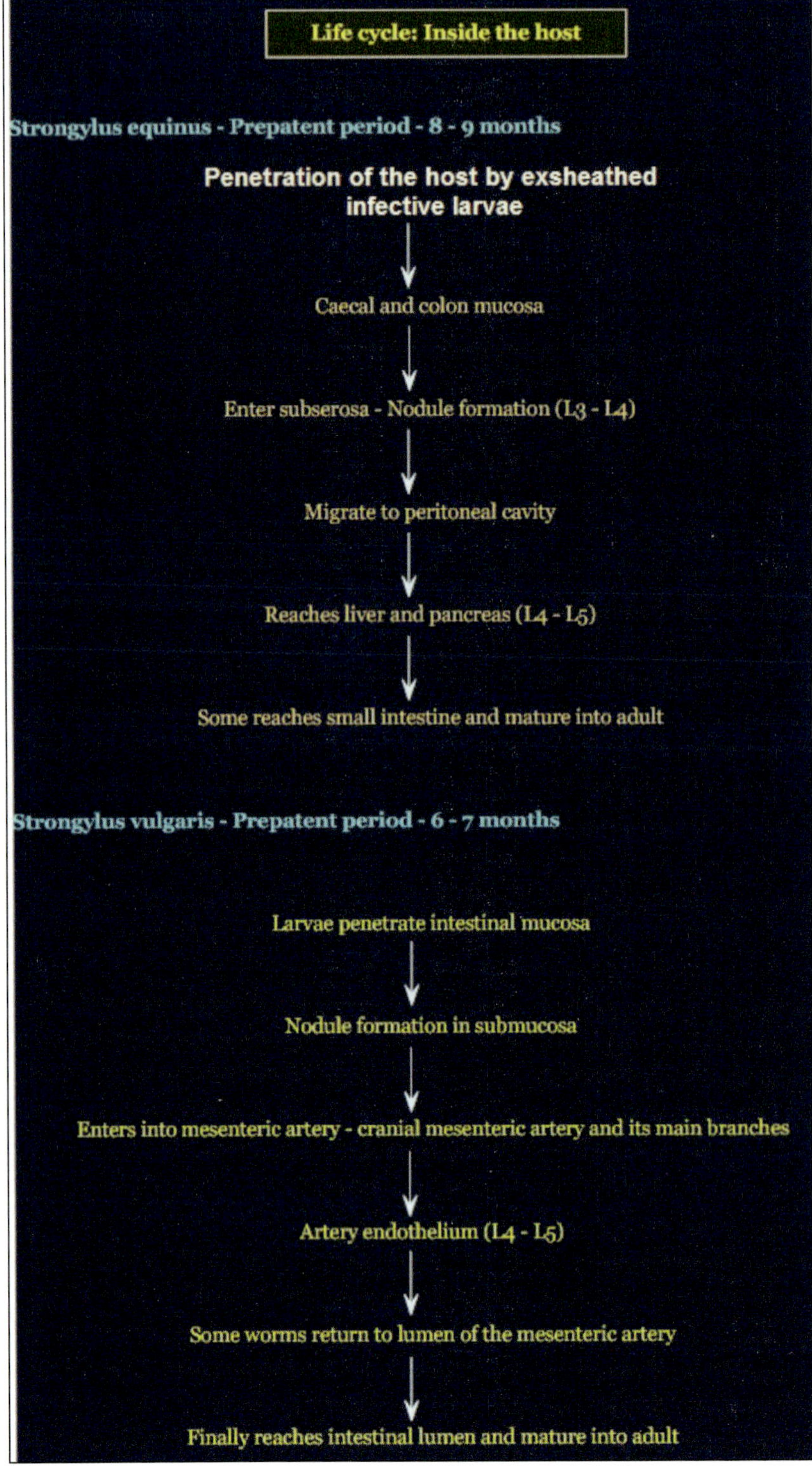
Life cycle: Inside the host
Strongylus equinus - Prepatent period - 8 - 9 months
Penetration of the host by exsheathed infective larvae
Caecal and colon mucosa
Enter subserosa - Nodule formation (L3 - L4)
Migrate to peritoneal cavity
Reaches liver and pancreas (L4 - L5)
Some reaches small intestine and mature into adult
Strongylus vulgaris - Prepatent period - 6 - 7 months
Larvae penetrate intestinal mucosa
Nodule formation in submucosa
Enters into mesenteric artery - cranial mesenteric artery and its main branches
Artery endothelium (L4 - L5)
Some worms return to lumen of the mesenteric artery
Finally reaches intestinal lumen and mature into adult

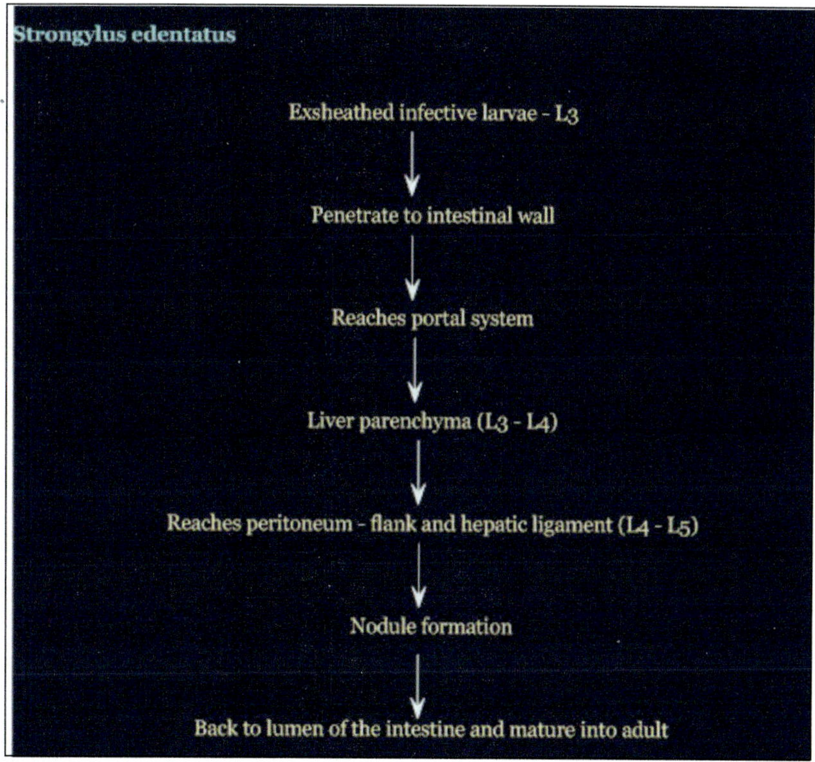

Figure 5.13b. Life Cycle of *Strongylus* sp.

Life cycle, epidemiology, pathogenesis, clinical signs are similar to *O. columbianum:* Thin sow syndrome, Adult female - chronic infection with periodic acute flare-up, Spring farrowing sows - Resumption of development of hypobiotic larvae, Weight loss after farrowing reduced milk yield and adverse affect of growth of litter.

Control: Similar to A. suum

Oesophagostomum columbianum

Common name: Nodular worm (causes formation nodules on the intestine wall)

Host: Sheep, goat, camel and wild antelopes

Location: Colon

Morphology: Adult worm Length: 1 – 2 cm

Egg: Thin shelled embryonated eggs (Blastomere 8 – 16 cell stage)

Life Cycle

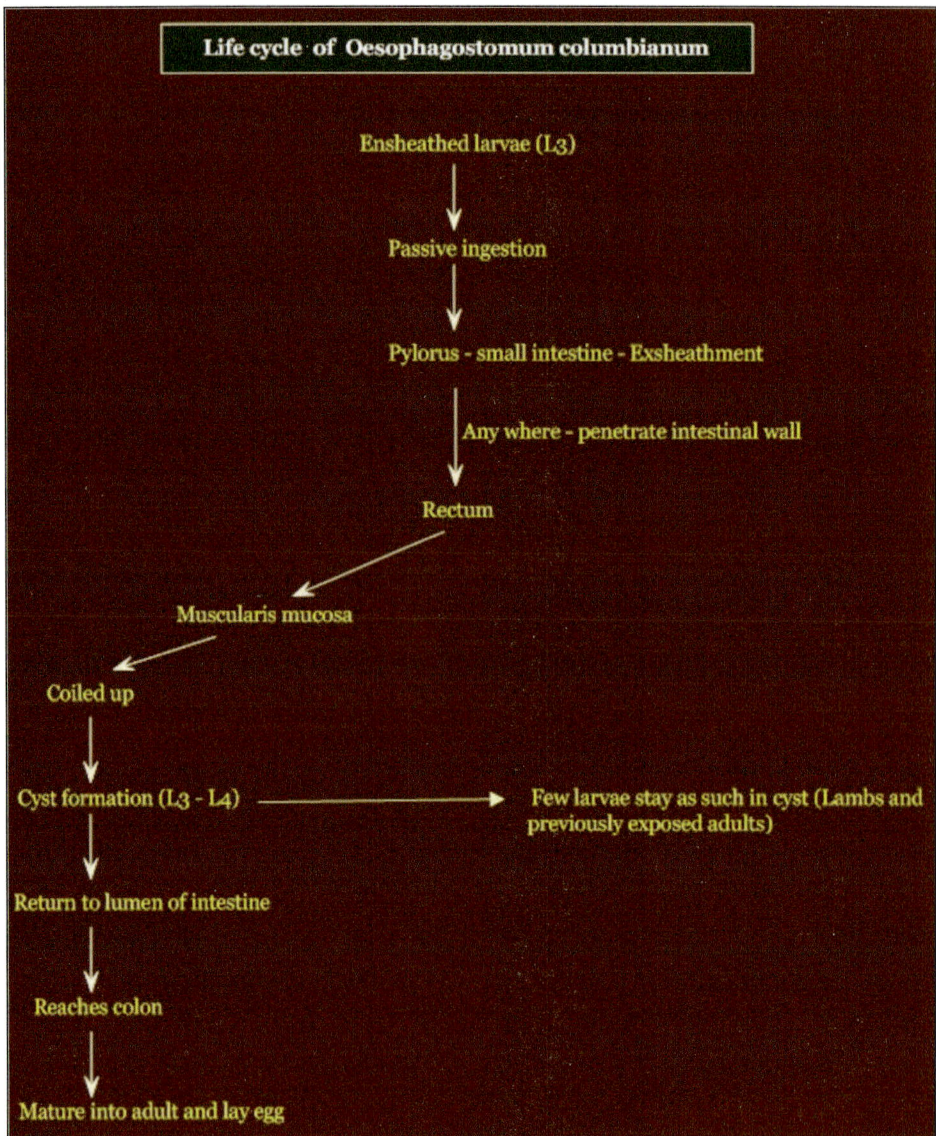

Figure 5.13c. Life Cycle of *Oesophagostomum* sp.

Oesophagostomum sp. *other than O. colombianum*

Species: *O. venulosum* - similar to *O. colombianum* - harmless – nodule seldom seen, *O. indicum* - similar to *O. colombianum*, *O. radiatum*

Host: Cattle, zebu, water buffalo

Location: Large intestine

Life cycle and epidemiology: Similar to *O. colombianum*

Pathogenesis

Acute*:* Infection of small and large intestine - black fetid diarrhoea.

Chronic*:* Young stock – extensive nodule - Pimply gut, Intermittent diarrhoea followed by continous purging, resulting in emaciation, prostration and often death. Nodule size - 5 cm.

Clinical Signs: Anorexia, Anemia (Normocytic and Normochromic), Hypoproteinemia (protein loosing gastroenteropathy)

Immunity: Good immunity to *O. radiatum*, partially due to age and partially due to previous exposure (unweaned calves having problem)

Treatment: Benzimidazole compound, Levamisole and piperazine

Pathogenesis of Strongylus

See Figure 5.13d.

Strongylus edentates

Larvae migration in liver: More than 4,000 larvae - haemorrhagic and fluid filled nodules, Less than 500 larvae - no clinical signs

Adult: Plug feeder - ingestion of plugs of intestinal mucosa. Damage to blood vessels. Blood suckers - Loss of blood - anemia (Normochromic and Normocytic)

Pathogenesis: Young sheep (200 –300 adult worm - severe infection). Extensive nodule formation (2 cm) - Pimply gut, Interfere digestion, absorption and bowel movement, Superlative nodule - ruptured into peritoneal cavity – peritonitis and multiple adhesions, Congestion and thickening of intestinal of wall.

Clinical signs (dose dependant): 500 larvae – depressed feed intake and utilization, 500 - 2000 larvae. Marked persistent diarrhoea associated with loss of weight. Exhaustion and death (if animal is not removed from source). Faeces - dark green in colour, contains mucus (rarely blood). In chronic cases – initially diarrhoea followed by constipation. Progressive emaciation and general weakness, skin dry and wool is unthrifty. Hypoalbumineamia - submandibular oedema. Chronic oesophagostomiasis in sheep – extreme emaciation and cachexia with atrophy of muscles, ending in complete prostration for 1- 3 days and finally death.

Immunity: Prolonged survival of L4 on nodules in the gut wall and the lack of an effective immunity - control difficult.

Diagnosis: Examination of faeces – L4 larvae in acute cases and egg in chronic cases, fecal culture - differentiation from other GI nematode, Identification of adult worm by autopsy.

Treatment: Benzimidazole compound, Levamisole and morental.

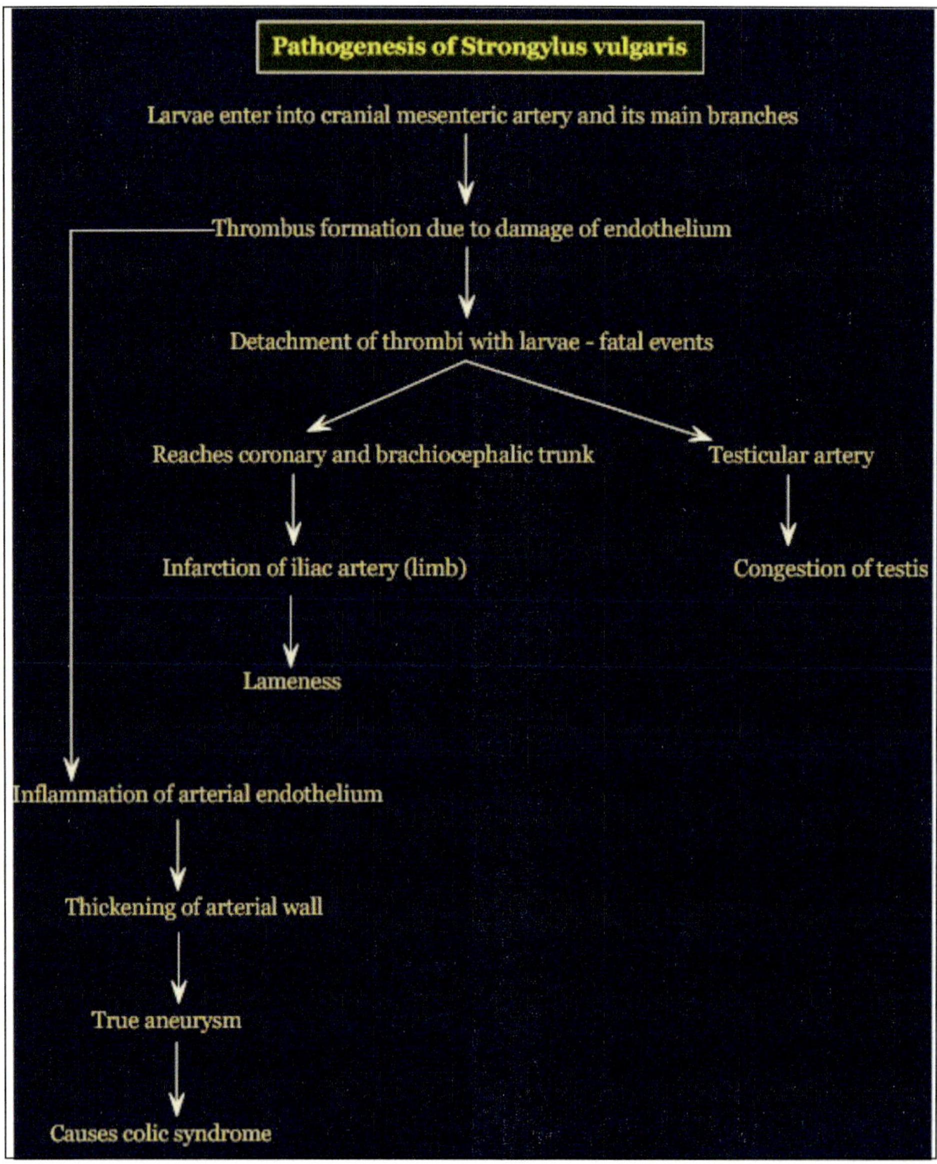

Figure 5.13d. Pathogenesis of *Strongylus*.

Clinical signs: Slow development: Diarrhoea - Soft faeces with bad odour. Reduced appetite, emaciation, rough coat, Anemia, edematous swelling on abdomen and legs.

Diagnosis: Based on EPG - 1,000, Fecal culture - Identification of L3 larvae, Based on clinical signs, Aneurysm in cranial mesenteric artery – palpated through rectal examination (Large pulsating bodies - 6 –7 cm), Aneurysm and colic - abdominal auscultation - hyper motility of intestine. Vertebral percussion - lumbar and sacral region - pain evinced. Paracentesis - peritoneal fluid – Differential count of WBC - neutrophilia and esinophila.

Treatment: Piperazine at 220 mg/kg - effective various when combined with other compounds. Thiabendazole at 44 mg/kg - effective against intestinal Strongyles. Thiabendazole at 440 mg/kg- twice - effective against migratory larvae. Mebendazole at 10 mg/kg - effective against adult worm. Fenbendazole at 7.5 mg/kg - effective against adult worm. Fenbendazole at 60 mg/kg - effective against adult worm and Migratory larvae. Cambendazole at 20 mg/kg - effective against adult worm. Oxbendazole at 5- 10 mg/kg. Pyrental at 90 mg/kg. Dichlorvas at 26 – 32 mg/kg through feed. Holoxon at 50 – 70 mg/kg. Ivermectin - larvae present in anterior mesenteric artery.

Prophylactic Schedule: High stocking density and favorable environmental condition - once in six weeks. High stocking density and unfavorable environmental condition (winter) - once in two weeks). Low stocking density - once in three months.

Treatment for colic: Verminous aneurysm - 6 per cent iron dextran and 5 per cent dextrin through I/V – antithrombin activity.

Prophylaxis: Routine anthelmintics - all grazing animals over two moths of age treated with broad spectrum anthelmintics (change of drugs once in 6 months). Pasture and Grazing management - not over grazed or over stocked. Alternative grazing: Horse + Sheep; Horse + Cattle (cattle will assist reduction of larvae burden pasture; horse Strongyles do not infect ruminants). Rotational grazing: nourishing mares and their foals, don't graze the same area for successive year, Special attention for foals - fed only wholesome fodder. Proper disposal of manure - heaping - generation of heat - destroy eggs, Any new animals introduced - treat and quarantine for 48 – 72 hours.

5.14. Strongylideaea

Family Strongyloididae comprises of free living, parasitic and both forms. Parasitic forms are parthenogenetic in nature.

Species

S. papillosus - Sheep, goat, cattle, rabbit and wild ruminants.

Location: Small intestine

S. westeri - Horses, pig and zebra

Location: Small intestine

S. stercoralis - Dog, cat and man

Location: Small intestine

S. cati – Cat

Location: Small intestine

S. ransomi - Pig

Location: Small intestine

S. avium - Poultry

Location: Small intestine

Morphology: Egg: Blunt ends and thin shells, contain fully developed embryos when passed in the faeces of host.

Epidemiology

Agent: Parasitic form (Infective larvae) - having Triploid chromosome. Free living female - having diploid chromosome. Free living male - having haploid chromosome. Parthenogenic female produces following type of eggs. Egg with triploid chromosome - give rise to parasitic female. Egg with diploid chromosome - infective female larvae and free living female. Egg with haploid chromosome - free living male. Infection rate: In heterogony (under worm and moist condition) – each parasitic female produces 35 egg per copulation (during its life time produce, 180 eggs).

Host: Piglets, foals, calves, lambs - neonatal infection (through colostrum) after birth - mobilization of arrested larvae in tissues of ventral abdominal wall of the dam which are subsequently mobilized and excreted through milk. For very young animal reservoir of larvae is a tissue of dam - clinical strongyloidosis in foals and pigs - successive progeny from same dam - give heavy infection. *S. ramsoni* – Prenatal infection in pigs.

Environment: Larvae are not ensheathed and susceptible to adverse environmental condition. Warm and moisture - favours accumulation of infective larvae.

Clinical signs: Skin lesion. Severe diarrhoea which may be blood stained, dehydration, anorexia, loss of weight and finally death (especially piglets mortality - 50 per cent). Foals - acute diarrhea.

Life Cycle of Strongyloides

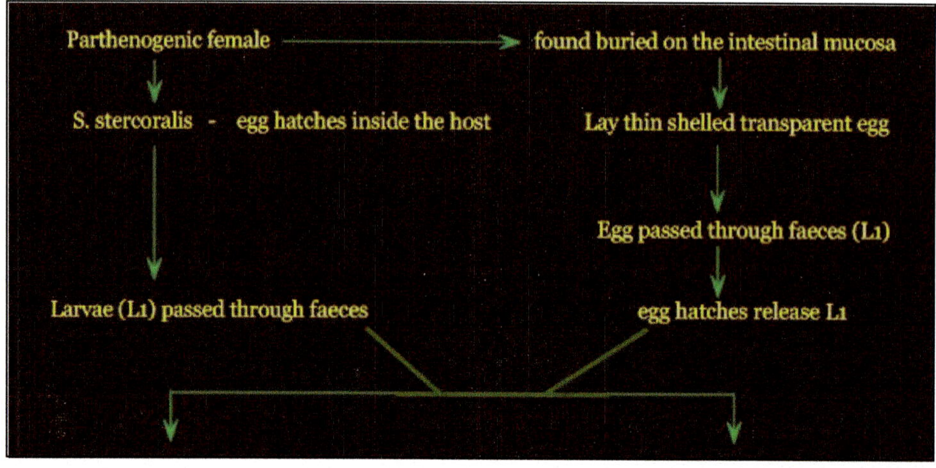

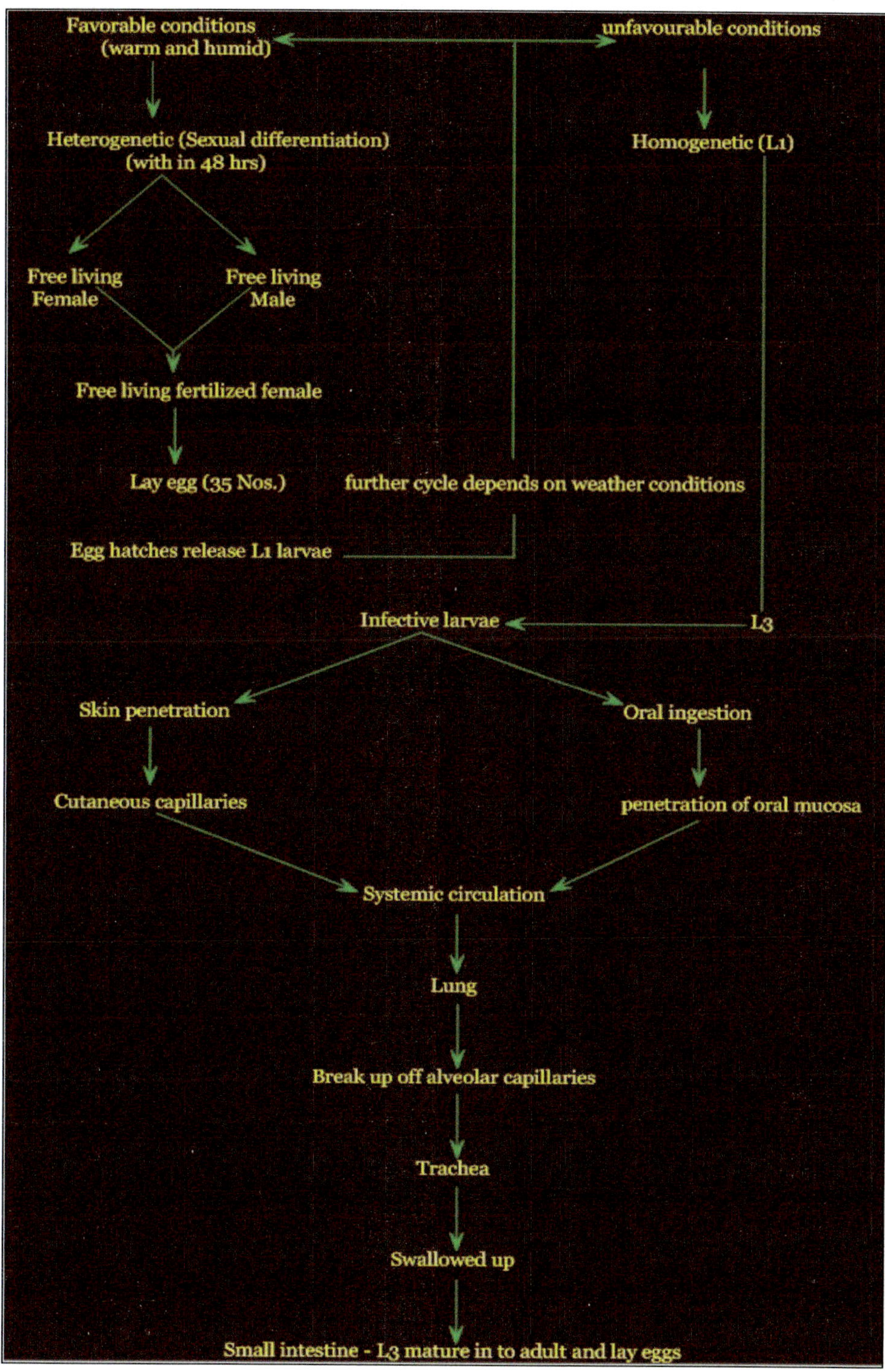

Figure 5.14. Life Cycle of Strongyloides.

Immunity: Infection with few infected larvae - in young animals - marked immunity. Foals - satisfactory immunity -15 to 23 weeks after birth.

Diagnosis: Based on clinical signs. Demonstration of eggs, larvae in faeces.

Treatment

In sheep: Thiabendazole - 75 mg/kg orally.

In pigs: Thiabendazole - 50 mg/kg through feed, Levamisole – 5 - 10mg/kg.

In dog: Diethylcarbomazine – 100 mg/kg, Dithiazanine – 5 mg/kg (10 daily doses), Pyvinium pamoate – 20 mg/kg (5 days), Thiabendazole - 50 -75 mg/kg – highly effective.

In foals: Cambendazole - 20 mg/kg, Fenbendazole – 50 mg/kg.

Prophylaxis: Infected larvae susceptible to desiccation - providing clean quarter. For prenatal and transclostral infection - in anticipated cases and treat before manifestation of clinical signs.

In pigs: Mebendazole @ 72 – 104 mg/kg for daily 12 – 14 days prior to furrowing. Levamisole @ 140 mg/kg - total dose. Ivermectin -Single dose - 4 –16 days prior to furrowing.

Pathogenesis

***S. papillosus*:** Catarrhal enteritis - duodenum and proximal jejunum. Skin penetration by infective larvae - erythematous reaction – which favours introduction of foot rot organism into skin around feet.

***S. stercoralis*:** Especially puppies - summer months - catarrhal enteritis of small intestine - necrosis and sloughing of mucosa

***S. ransomi*:** Especially suckling piglets

Epidemiology: Oral infection – through infected larvae - adhere on udder and teats, from dam through skin penetration - from soil and litter, colostral infection - patent infection – very short (4 days). Protein losing gastroenteropathy. Erythematous skin lesion may be seen - pulmonary disorder is not frequent in natural outbreaks – verminous pneumonia in all animals, petechial/ecchymotic haemorrhagic in lungs.

5.15. Tape Worm Infection

Taenia solium

Egg - Spherical in shape

Definitive Host - Man

Location - Small intestine

Intermediate Host - Pigs (including wild boars), dog – rarely susceptible and Human being (acts as both Definitive and Iintermediate Hosts)

Metacestode stage - *Cysticercus cellulosae*

Location - Skeletal and cardiac muscles

Life cycle - Similar to *T. saginata*

Taenia saginata

Egg - Oval in shape

Definitive Host - Man

Location - Small intestine

Intermediate Host: Cattle, other ruminants, Wild animals - Llama and reindeer are also susceptible.

Wildbeast, Giraffe and antelope – not susceptible.

Metacestode - Cysticercus bovis

Location - Cardiac, skeletal and masseter muscles (also tongue and diaphragm).

Life Cycle

Infected human beings → proglottids → IH (10 weeks) → DH (100 days).

Epidemiology

Infection rate

Infected person actively sheds about 10 proglottids per day. Rate of egg shedding - 10 × 2,50,000 eggs/proglottids = 25, 00, 000 eggs per day. Proglottids eliminated either passively through faeces or actively migrate out of the anus due to its motility. If proglottids migrate out off anus, which contaminate the body surface of infected human beings and his belongings or fall on the ground. The survival of the eggs is strongly influenced by climatic conditions. Under wet and moist conditions, eggs may survive over a month, and increases risk to cattle. Eggs are very susceptible to dry conditions and are rapidly destroyed during the drier months. Eggs are released due to disintegration of proglottids, which may remain viable for several weeks or months in environment.

- Infected liquid manure - 71 days
- Sewage – 16 days
- River – 33 days
- Contaminated pastures – 159 days
- Sludge – 210 days

Poor standards of personal hygiene of infected human population is responsible for the spread of cysticercosis. In some societies such as nomadic pastoral people there is a high risk of animals becoming exposed to infected faeces. Abnormal eating habits of cattle due to certain mineral deficiencies (pica) may result in cravings that increase the exposure through the ingestion of faeces. Sewage water is an important route of dissemination of infection. Sewage water treatment has no effect on infectivity of eggs. Birds that consume infected sewage water and disseminate the infection.

Infection of Intermediate Host

Passive ingestion of contaminated pasture. Neonatal calves may be infected when they are handled by infected person (with motile proglottids). Prenatal infection has been recorded.

Survivability of Metacestode in Intermediate Host

- Degree of infection and age of animals. Normally 4- 6 months (maximum of 9 months).
- Neonatal infection – long periods

Infection of Definitive Host

- Ingestion of raw or under cooked beef (Measely beef).
- Changing of food habits – fast foods
- If cattle slaughtered 9 months after infection (without reinfection) - infection rate in human beings is very less.

Cysticercosis

Muscular cysticercosis

Bovine cysticercosis – caused by metacestode stages (*C. bovis*) of human tape worm – *T. saginata*. Porcine cysticercosis - caused by metacestode stages (*C. cellulosae*) of human tape worm – *T. solium*. Ovine cysticercosis - caused by metacestode stages (*C. ovis*) of dog tape worm – *T. ovis*.

Abdominal cysticercosis

Caused by metacestode stages (*C. teunicollis*) of dog tape worm – *T. hydatigena.*

Other cysticercosis

Cysticercosis of lagomorphs - caused by metacestode stages (*C. pisiformis*) of dog tape worm – *T. pisiformis*. Cysticercosis of rodents - caused by metacestode stages (*C. fasciolaris*) of dog and cat tape worm – *T. taeniaformis.*

Neurocysticercosis or Cerebralcysticercosis

- If human beings infected with metacestode stage of *T. solium*.
- The *C. cellulosae* secondarily present in the ventricle of brain and in affected persons, becomes racemose and proliferate in nature.
- They are clinically characteised by neuralgia, paralysis, epileptic seizures and ends in fatal.

Clinical signs: *T. saginata* and *T. solium*

Definitive Host

- Non-specific abdominal pain (epigastric pain).
- Diarrhoea or constipation.

Intermediate Host

- ☆ Asymptomatic.
- ☆ Heavy infection causes myositis, myocarditis, muscular stiffness and weakness.

Pathogenesis of *T. saginata* and *T. solium*

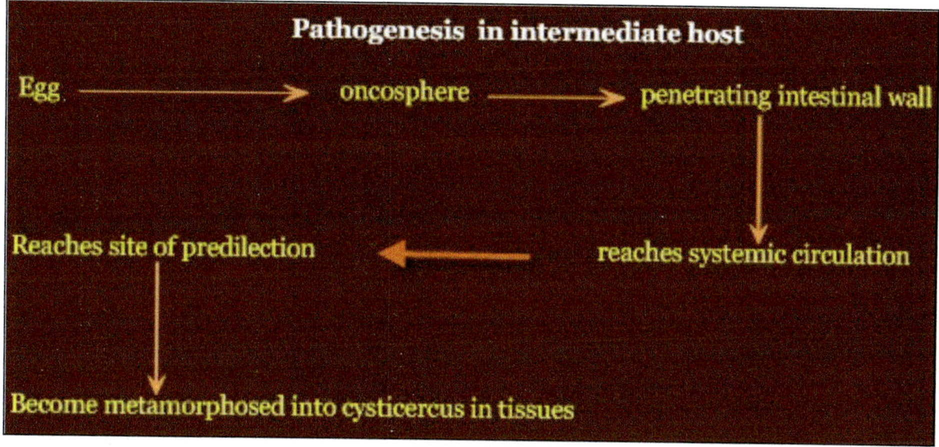

Figure 5.15. Pathogenesis of *T. saginata* and *T. solium.*

Definitive Host

Cysticercus reaches small intestine and become changed in to adult worm. Adult worm lay the eggs (prepatent period –100 days) – no much pathogenic changes.

Intermediate Host

Passive ingestion gastric and intestinal juice.

- ☆ *Cattle* – *C. bovis* – masseters, heart, tongue and diaphragm (**measely beef).**
  - ☆– *C. cellulosae* - masseters, heart, tongue and skeletal muscles **(measely pork).**
- ☆ *Man* - *C. cellulosae* - primarily on subcutaneous tissues and secondarily on brain and ocular cavity.

Diagnosis and Treatment

Diagnosis of T.saginata and T. solium

Definitive Host

- ☆ *T. saginata* - perianal swab.
- ☆ Identification of characteristic egg/proglottids.

Intermediate Host

- ✰ Post mortem examination of carcasses.
- ✰ Serological test – ELISA, CIEP and Western blotting.

Treatment of T. saginata and T. solium

Human Beings

- ✰ Praziquantel – 10 mg/kg.
- ✰ Niclosamide – 2 g (total dose).
- ✰ Paromomycin - 5 mg/kg.
- ✰ Quinacrine – 7- 10 mg/kg.
- ✰ Inorganic tin compounds.

Animals

- ✰ Albendazloe – 50 mg/kg – effective against mature metacestode.
- ✰ Praziquantel – 50 mg/kg – highly effective against both mature and immature metacestodes.

Prevention and Control

Prevention of T. saginata and T. solium

- ✰ Treating of infected persons (especially animal handlers).
- ✰ Public education and hygiene.
- ✰ Proper meat inspection – made multiple incisions of suspected carcasses.
- ✰ Freezing of carcasses.
  - ❒ – 5°C for 15 days
  - ❒ – 10°C for 9 days
  - ❒ – 15 to – 30°C for 6 days
- ✰ Insist through cooking of meat (> 56°C for 5 mts.)

Immunoprophylaxis against *T. saginata*

Homologous vaccine - *In vitro* culturing of oncosphere of *T. saginata* releases secretory and excretory antigen

Active immunization in calves: Secretory and excretory antigen administered in calves before infection (after infection there is no useful).

Passive immunization in calves: Secretory and excretory antigen administered to periparturient cows either through intramuscularly or intramammary route. Calves are immunized while consuming colostrum/milk from immunized dam.

Disadvantage of Homologous vaccine: *Invitro* culturing of oncosphere – zoonotic significance.

Heterologus vaccine: *In vitro* culturing of oncospheres of *T. taeniaformis* releases secretory and excretory antigen, which capable of inducing high level protective immunity against heterologus parasite – *T. saginata.* Intramuscular injection of eggs of *T. hydatigena* in cattle – induces partial immunity against heterologus parasite.

5.16. Theleriosis

Theileriases are a group of tickborne diseases caused by *Theileria* spp. A large number of *Theileria* spp are found in domestic and wild animals in tick-infested areas of the Old World. The most important species affecting cattle are *T. parva* and *T. annulata,* which cause widespread death in tropical and subtropical areas of the Old World. *T. lestoquardi, T. luwenshuni,* and *T. uilenbergi* are important causes of mortality in sheep.

Both *Theileria* and *Babesia* are members of the suborder Piroplasmorina. Although *Babesia* are primarily parasites of RBCs, *Theileria* use, successively, WBCs and RBCs for completion of their life cycle in mammalian hosts. The infective sporozoite stage of the parasite is transmitted in the saliva of infected ticks as they feed. Sporozoites invade leukocytes and, within a few days, develop to schizonts. In the most pathogenic species of *Theileria* (*e.g., T. parva* and *T. annulata*), parasite multiplication occurs predominantly within the host WBCs, whereas less pathogenic species multiply mainly in RBCs. Development of the schizont stage of pathogenic *Theileria* causes the host WBC to divide; at each cell division, the parasite also divides. Thus, the parasitized cell population expands and, through migration, becomes disseminated throughout the lymphoid system. Later in the infection, some of the schizonts undergo merogony, releasing merozoites that infect RBCs, giving rise to piroplasms. Uptake of piroplasm-infected RBCs by vector ticks feeding on infected animals is the prelude to a complex cycle of development, culminating in transmission of infection by ticks feeding in their next instar (trans-stadial transmission). There is no transovarial transmission as occurs in *Babesia*. Occurrence of disease is limited to the geographic distribution of the appropriate tick vectors. In some endemic areas, indigenous cattle have a degree of innate resistance. Mortality in such stock is relatively low, but introduced cattle are particularly vulnerable. Unlike in babesiosis, in theileriasis there is no evidence of increased resistance in calves <6 moths old.

Theileriosis in Sheep and Goat

Theileria lestoquardi (formerly *T. hirci*) causes a disease in sheep and goats similar to that produced in cattle by *T. annulata*, with which it is closely related. *T. lestoquardi* is transmitted by ticks of the genus *Hyalomma*. The limited available epidemiologic data indicate that *T. lestoquardi* has a more restricted geographic distribution than that of *T. annulata,* being particularly prevalent in the Middle East and northeast Africa. Mortality can approach 100 per cent. Schizonts can readily be demonstrated in Giemsa-stained smears of needle biopsies from swollen superficial lymph nodes.

Recently, two species of *Theileria, T. luwenshuni* and *T. uilenbergi,* have been identified as the causal agents of a severe disease in sheep in China. These species are morphologically indistinguishable and cause similar disease but can be distinguished by DNA typing methods. They are transmitted by ticks of the genus *Haemaphysalis*. Schizonts are detected in a range of tissues, but later and in smaller numbers than in other pathogenic *Theileria* spp. Piroplasms are consistently detected in RBCs. Morbidity and mortality rates of up to 65 per cent (*T. luwenshuni*) and 75 per cent (*T. uilenbergi*) have been seen in susceptible animals introduced into endemic areas. Affected animals show sustained fever and anemia.

Several other nonpathogenic *Theileria* spp (*e.g., T. ovis*) are also widely distributed. Piroplasms of these species are polymorphic.

- **Morphology**: Oval and rod shaped.
- **Life cycle**: Similar to cattle.
- **Pathogenesis**: Similar to Bovine Tropical theileriosis.

Acute: High fever, listlessness, nasal discharge, anaemia, jaundice, atony of rumen, weakness, transitory haemoglobinuria, petechial haemorrhage on abomasal mucosa, edematous lungs, enlargement of lymph nodes, No cross immunity between *T. hirci* and *T. ovis*.

Diagnosis: Examination of stained blood, lymph nodes or spleen.

Theileria sp. of Domestic Animals

The *Theileria orientalis* group, consisting of the closely related parasites *T. orientalis, T. buffeli,* and *T. sergenti,* has a worldwide distribution. These parasites are transmitted by ticks of the genus *Haemaphysalis*. The piroplasms are larger than those of *T. parva* and *T. annulata*, and they multiply principally by intraerythrocytic division. Mortality, particularly in indigenous cattle, is rare, but infection can sometimes result in progressive chronic anemia.

T. mutans and *T. velifera* are found in Africa, where they are transmitted by ticks of the genus *Amblyomma*. Multiplication occurs mainly by intraerythrocytic division. The piroplasms are morphologically indistinguishable from those of *T. orientalis* and *T. taurotragi* (an African parasite of eland and cattle), but the parasites can be differentiated by serologic tests such as indirect fluorescent antibody and by DNA typing. Some strains of *T. mutans* are pathogenic as well. In addition, concurrent infection may add to the pathogenicity of *T. parva*.

Sl.No.	*Theileria*	*Vectors*	*Disease*	*Pathogenicity*
		Cattle and Buffalo		
1	*T.annulata* (India)	Hyalomma marginatum Hyalomma anatolicum (Transtadial transmission)	Tropical Theileriosis, Mediterranean coast fever, Tropical Piroplasmosis, Egyptian Fever	Highly pathogenic
2	*T. parva*	Rhiphicephalus appendiculatus Hyalomma anatolicum (Transtadial transmission)	Bovine Theileriosis, East Coast fever, Turning Sickness, African Coast Fever, Corridor disease, Rhodesian tick Fever, Rhodesian Red Water disease	Highly pathogenic

Sl.No.	Theileria	Vectors	Disease	Pathogenicity
3	*T. mutans* (India)	*Rhiphicephalus appendiculatus* *Haemophysalis bispinosa* *Haemophysalis punctata* (Transtadial transmission)	Benign Bovine Theileriosis, Turning Sickness African Coast Fever	Non-fatal/ Slightly pathogenic
Sheep and Goat				
1	*T. hirci* (India)	*Rhiphicephalus bursa* *Hyalomma anatolicum anatolicum* (Transtadial transmission)	Malignant Theileriosis	Highly pathogenic
2	*T. ovis*	*Rhiphicephalus bursa* *Haemophysalis* spp (Transtadial transmission)	Benign Theileriosis	Non -pathogenic

Members of this family occur in mammals. They have small, round, ovoid, irregular or bacilli form merozoites, as the parasites are pleomorphic and occur in lymphocytes, histocytes and erythrocytes of vertebrate host. Ixodid ticks are vectors in their life cycle transmitting the parasites to animals. The species are of great economic importance to dairy animals. Theileriosis is characterized by fever and lymphoproliferative disorders which may be associated with leukopenia/anaemia.

Location: Lymphocytes and erythrocytes (sometimes in monocytes).

Epidemiology

Age: Both young calves (even 2-3 days old) and adults are affected.

Breed: Highly virulent in European breeds of cattle, but all breeds are susceptible, especially in dairy animals and crossbred animals and less virulent in local zebu breeds; Mortality in exotic cattle is up to 70 per cent. In endemic areas, all animals are virtually infected but the case- fatality is 10 -20 per cent and is confined to calves.

Transmision: Transtadial transmission (stage to stage) by ticks of *Hyalomma* spp. Infection from tick larvae to nymph or nymph to adult occurs. Sporogony and gamogony takes place in salivary gland if the tick. Schizogony takes place in the host – lymphocytes and RBCs- erythrocytic stages. Congenital transmission occasional in calves.

Carrier status: Indigenous cattle without clinical signs remain as a constant source of infection to susceptible animals; Buffaloes, may act as carriers; Recovered animals with long lasting immunity act as carriers; Wild animals may also transmit the disease.

Immunity: Cell-mediated immunity is proved by leucocyte migration inhibition test. No cross immunity occurs between *T. parva* and *T. mutans*. Immunity is developed by all 3 stages- sporozoites, schizonts and erythrocytic stages; each developmental stage elicits a homologous immune response and may provide a partial protection against infection with all other stages.

Season: In India, mostly animals suffer during summer and rainy seasons (May - Oct) which is attributable to high incidence of tick vectors. In tropical areas, ticks are active through out the year. Incidence due to stress of hot and humid weather.

Mixed infection: Mixed infection with *Anaplasma/Babesia spp* is common.

Theileriosis, East Coast Fever: East Coast fever, an acute disease of cattle, is usually characterized by high fever, swelling of the lymph nodes, dyspnea, and high mortality. Caused by *Theileria parva*, and transmitted by the tick vector *Rhipicephalus appendiculatus*, it is a serious problem in east and southern Africa.

Life cycle: Similar to *T. parva.*

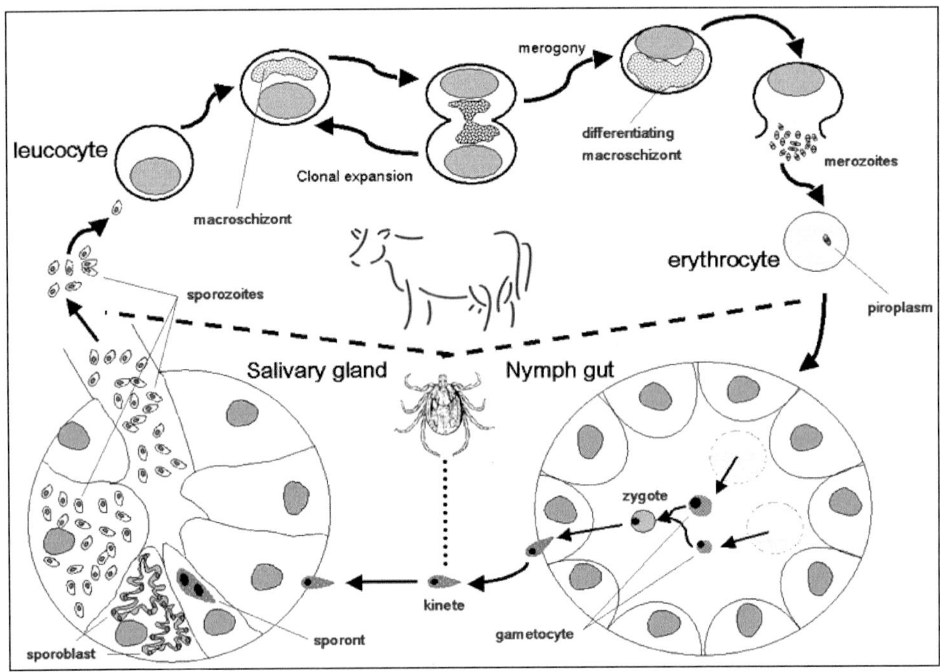

Figure 5.16. Life cycle of *Theileria*.

Pathogenesis: Serious disease in cattle; High rate of mortality.

Acute form: More common; fever (41. 7 °C), enlargement of superficial lymph nodes, swelling of eyelids and ears, diarrhoea with blood and mucus, marked emaciation. Edema of lungs causes death immediately.

Sub acute: Frequent in calves; less pronounced symptoms.

Turning Sickness: In east and Central Africa, signs are circling movements and abduction of limbs; immunity is solid and specific.

Diagnosis: Demonstration of Schizonts in lymph node biopsy. Demonstration of erythrocytic forms is difficult.

Theileriosis, Pathogenesis and Lesions

Pathogenesis: Mortality varies from 10- 90 per cent. Incubation period: 9 to 25 days.

(a) **Per acute form:** Common one lasting for 3 - 4 days or upto 20 days. First sign is fever (40.5 –41.5°C), continuous or intermittent persisting for 3- 20 days. The other signs after few days appear including inappetence, cessation of rumination, rapid heart beat, weakness, reduced milk production, enlargement of superficial lymph nodes and odema of the eyelids. Marked anaemia, haemoglobinuria, bilirubinuria and bilirubinaemia, icterus of conjunctiva with petechial haemorrhage, jaundice, high colored urine, prostration and death. Laboured breathing, serous nasal discharge, coughing, restlessness and starry coat. Diarrhoea with blood and mucus in faeces, greatly emaciated (RBCs < 1 million/cmm); Death after 15 days.

(b) **Sub acute form:** Fever is irregularly intermittent for 15 days, then the animal recovers.

(c) **Chronic form:** Intermittent fever, in-appetence, marked emaciation, some degree of anaemia, icterus for 4 weeks or longer, in some cases, sudden death may occur within 1-2 days.

(d) **Mild form:** Little is seen, but mild fever, in appetence, listlessness, slight digestive disturbances, lachrymation for few days and moderate anaemia.

Cerebral theileriosis: Nervous signs predominate and brain impression smears reveal Koch's Blue bodies.

(e) **Cutaneous form:** Some cases reveal urticarial type of skin lesions and haemoglobinuria.

Lesions: Emaciated body of the carcass, pale mucous membrane, enlargement of the superficial lymph nodes, spleen and liver. Distension of the gall bladder with thick bile; Congestion and petechial haemorrhages on the kidney and lungs. in few cases, necrotic infarcts of brain. Punched necrotic ulcers in the abomasum are pathognomonic; in young calves, abomasum is full of undigested clots of milk. Haematological changes, fall of haemoglobin (< 2 gm/ml), reduced PCV, reduced RBC count (1.5-2 million/Cmm), leukocytosis followed by leukopenia.

Diagnosis: Based on clinical signs. Demonstration of erythrocytic forms (piroplasms) in pheripheral blood smears. Demonstration of Koch's blue bodies (schizonts) in lymphocytes from lymph nodes. For latent cases, serological tests can be employed CFT, capillary tube agglutination test, IFA.

Others: IHA, AGID, Dot-ELISA, LMI test, Conglutination Complement Absorption test (CCA), Gel agglutination test, immunoelctrophoresis. By autopsy, examination for lesions.

Differential diagnosis: Anaplasmosis, Babesiosis, Trypanosomosis, Ehrlichiosis.

Treatment

Different drugs respond differently with schizonts and erythrocytic stages of the parasite and none of the drugs are fully effective; but buparvaquone is fully effective in clinical cases.

To combat the anaemic changes, haematinics as supportive therapy.

- Buparvaquone (Butalex) - Naphthaquinone drug and drug of choice.
  - @ 2.5 mg/kg, deep I/M against different stages of T. annulata, it is effective.
  - 2nd dose at 48 hours intervals.
- Parvaquone - 10 mg/kg, deep I/M, effective against piroplasmic stage.
- Berenil (Diminazene aceturate) – 2.5 to 5 mg/kg, deep I/M; Doubtful against erythrocytic stage.
- Oxytetracycline - 20 mg/kg for 7 days; I/M; effective against of schizogony.
- Halofuginone (stenorol*) – Potent against schizont stage but toxic.
  - 1 to 2 mg/kg as 2 doses, as tablets.

Others

Methohexate, 3 per cent Tryphan blue solution, Sulpha drugs, Diethyl carbamazine citrate, Babesan, Chloramphenicol, Sulphadimidine+ chloroquine phosphate, Nivaquin and Famaquin.

Theileriosis, Prophylaxis and Control

By Chemoprophylaxis + Immunoprophylaxis + Tick control.

- Wide spread and strict application of acaricides.
- Use of genetically resistant breeds.
- Immunoprophylaxis.

Tissue culture vaccines (Rakshavac-T*)

Attenuated Schizonts of *T. annulata* developed by *in vitro* cultivation of bovine lymphocytes infected with *T. annulata* schizonts. A dose of 2 x 10^6 infected cells suspended in serum free tissue culture remains viable at 4 °C for 1 week and used to vaccinate cattle.

Age: Cross–bred and exotic cattle of 2 months/above.

Dose: 3 ml, S/c, annually.

Infection and Treatment method: A potentially lethal known dose of stabilate of ground up infected ticks together with a long acting formulation of OTC or Buparvaquone is developed. It suppresses the development of the parasite and allows the effective CMI response with minimal disease response.

Subunit vaccines: Antigen to be included is sporozoites and Schizonts that induce CD^4 + T cells and antigen stimulating specific response like cytotoxic cells.

Recombinant antigens: Immunization with recombinant sporozoites/ merozoites surface antigen partially protect against sporozoite which are poorly immunogenic. For *T. annulata,* it induces the innate immune response.

5.17. Toxocariasis

Toxocariasis is an infection transmitted from animals to humans (zoonosis) caused by the parasitic roundworms commonly found in the intestine of dogs (*Toxocara canis*) and cats (*T. cati*).

Toxocara vitulorum, Epidemiology

Host

- ☆ Cattle, Zebu and Indian buffalo, sheep, and goat are also susceptible.
- ☆ Buffalo calves are highly susceptible, due to prenatal and neonatal infection.
- ☆ Larvae present in dams milk up to 30 days after parturition.
- ☆ If no tissue migration - prepatent period: 3 - 4 weeks.
- ☆ Pregnant cows body tissues acts as a reservoir of larvae for its offspring (features is the reservoir of larvae in the tissues of cows with subsequent milk borne transmission, ensuring that calves are exposed to infection from the first day of life).
  - ❒ Agent: Similar *to A. suum*
  - ❒ Environment: Similar to *A. suum*
- ☆ *Infection rate:* adult worm lay 80,00,000/day.

Toxocariasis, Species, Host and Location

Species	*T. canis*	*T. cati*	*T. vitulorum*
Host	Dog and fox	Cat and wild felids	Cattle, Zebu and Indian buffalo
Location	Small intestine	Small intestine	Small intestine

Toxascaris leonina

Host: Dog and cat

Location: Small Intestine

Paratenic host: Mice

Morphology

Male – 7 cm and female – 10 cm

Egg: Slightly oval with stomach thick shell

Life cycle: Direct – but not complex

Egg (L2) → Passive ingestion → Small intestine → L2 → Adult → eggs

Pathogenesis and Clinical Signs

Pot bellied, intermittent diarrhoea and possibly anemia.

Diagnosis and treatment: Similar to *T. canis*

Control

- ☆ Hygienic maintenance
- ☆ Prevent the exposure
- ☆ Prevent capturing of paratenic host.

Toxocara canis

Species: Toxocara canis

Host: Dog and fox

Location: Small intestine

Morphology

Adult: male – 10 cm and female –18 cm.

Egg: Similar to *T. vitulorum* (egg is dark brown and thick pitted in albuminous layer).

Life cycle: Direct – complex in nature.

Toxocara cati

Host: Cat and wild felids

Location: Small intestine

Morphology

Male - 6 cm and female - 10 cm long

Egg: Similar to *T. canis* (Colour less thick pitted albuminous layer).

Life cycle: Direct

Prenatal infection does not occur. Paratenic host involves in the life cycle – Earth worm, cockroaches, chicken, sheep and other animals fed with infective eggs. Transmammary only occurs.

Paratenic host: Rodents with L2.

Transmammary: Infection in kittens is derived from the milk of infected queens. Larvae occur in the milk throughout lactation when queens infected with eggs and transported to the mammary gland after on extended period in other tissues before lactation commences.

Pathogenesis and clinical signs

Pot belly, diarrhoea and poor hair coat

Diagnosis and treatment: Similar to *T. canis*

Control

Removal of kitten from infected dams. Similar schedule as that of *T. canis*.

Toxocara vitulorum

Morphology

Adult: 30 cm in length, body does not tapers much towards extremities.

Egg: Subglobular in shape, finely pitted albuminous layer.

Life cycle and Transmission: Direct and complex in nature

Male	Age less than 4- Month-Old	Horizontal transmission	No vertical transmission
	Age greater than 4-month- Old	Infection - not completion of life cycle	No vertical transmission
Female	Age less than 4- month- old	Horizontal transmission	No vertical transmission
	Age greater than 4-month -old	No horizontal transmission	Vertical transmission

Life Cycle of *Toxocara canis*

See Figure 5.17a.

Life Cycle of *Toxocara vitulorum*

Direct and complex in nature

See Figure 5.17b.

Pathogenesis

- Light infection - less than 70 larvae/calf - infection unnoticed.
- Heavy infection - 70 -500 larvae/calf - clinical disease.
- Lung: Verminous pneumonia – haemorrhagic and necrotic foci.

Clinical Signs

Calf hood mortality

- Diarrhoea - steatorrhoea - mud coloured evil smelling faeces.
- Colic - signs resembling intestinal obstruction.

Diagnosis

- Based on history and clinical signs.
- Identification of characteristic eggs.

Treatment

- Benzimidazole compounds
- Morantel citrate - 10 mg/kg -mature and immature
- Levamisole - 7.5 mg/kg - mature and immature
- Piperazine - 250 mg/kg

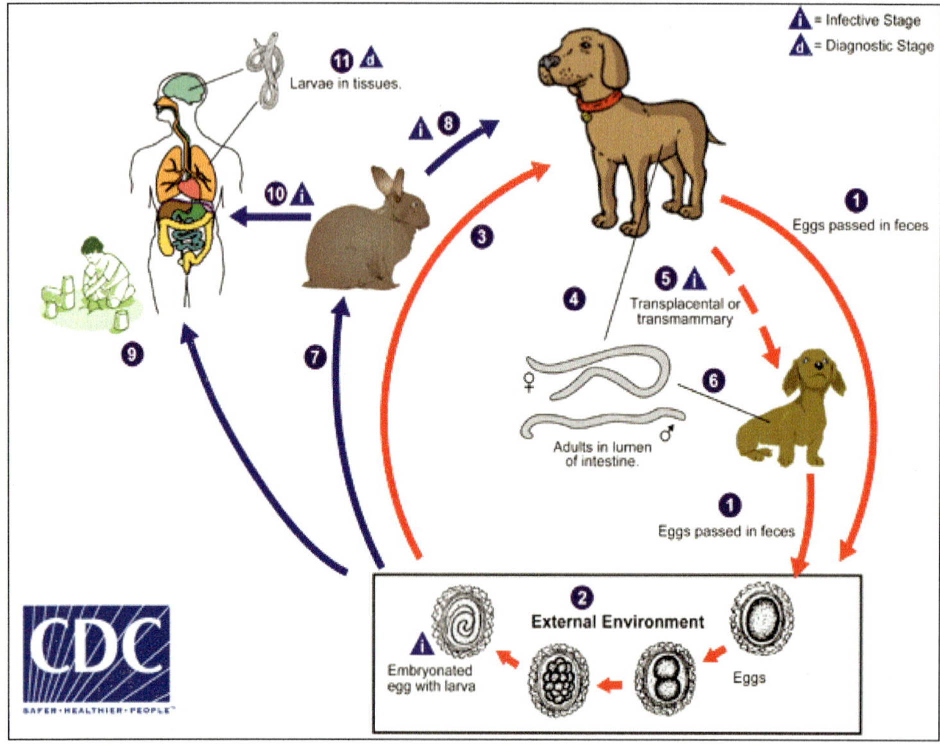

Figure 5.17a.

Toxocara canis **accomplishes its life cycle in dogs, with humans acquiring the infection as accidental hosts. Unembryonated eggs are shed in the feces of the definitive host–1. Eggs embryonate and become infective in the environment–2. Following ingestion by dogs–3, the infective eggs hatch and larvae penetrate the gut wall. In younger dogs, the larvae migrate through the lungs, bronchial tree, and esophagus; adult worms develop and oviposit in the small intestine–4. In older dogs, patent infections can also occur, but larval encystment in tissues is more common. Encysted stages are reactivated in female dogs during late pregnancy and infect by the transplacental and transmammary routes the puppies–5, in whose small intestine adult worms become established–6. Puppies are a major source of environmental egg contamination. *Toxocara canis* can also be transmitted through ingestion of paratenic hosts: eggs ingested by small mammals (*e.g.* rabbits) hatch and larvae penetrate the gut wall and migrate into various tissues where they encyst–7. The life cycle is completed when dogs eat these hosts–8 and the larvae develop into egg-laying adult worms in the small intestine. Humans are accidental hosts who become infected by ingesting infective eggs in contaminated soil–9 or infected paratenic hosts–10. After ingestion, the eggs hatch and larvae penetrate the intestinal wall and are carried by the circulation to a wide variety of tissues (liver, heart, lungs, brain, muscle, eyes)–11. While the larvae do not undergo any further development in these sites, they can cause severe local reactions that are the basis of toxocariasis. The two main clinical presentations of toxocariasis are visceral larva migrans and ocular larva migrans. Diagnosis is usually made by serology or the finding of larvae in biopsy or autopsy specimens.**

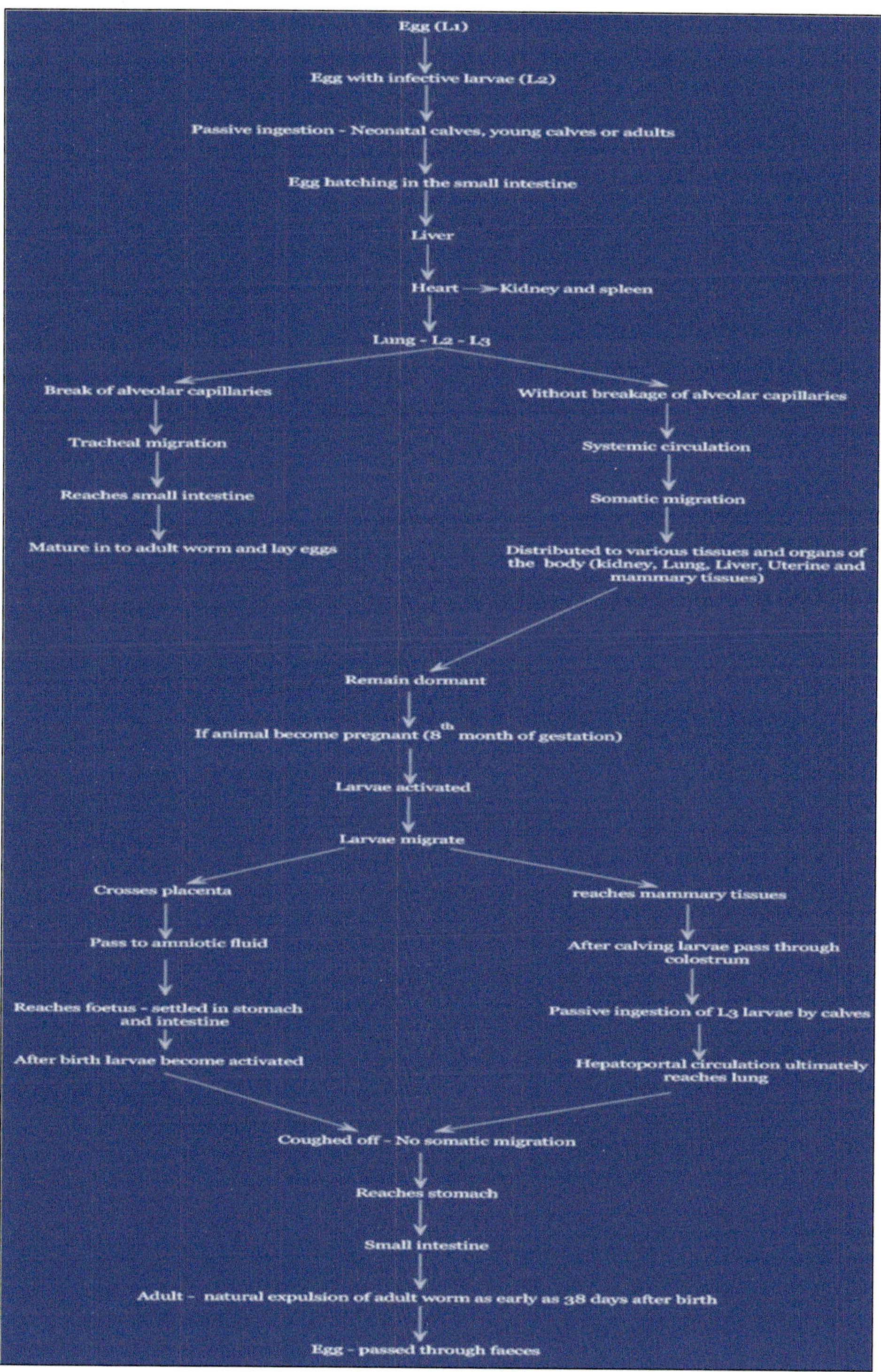

Figure 5.17b. Life cycle of *Toxocara vitulorum*.

Control

- The prevalence of infection can be drastically reduced by treating of calves at 3 and 6 weeks of age preventing developing worms reaching patency.

Prophylactic Schedule: (Buffalo calf)

- First dose - 15th days of age
- Second dose - 30th days of age
- Third dose - 3rd month of age
- Fourth dose - 6th month of age
- Fifth dose - one year of age

Pathogenesis

Puppies

- Heavy infection in puppies - death of whole litters.
- Migration of larvae through lung in new born puppies - pneumonia (uncommon) and pulmonary oedema, haemorrhage and eosinophilia.
- In infected puppies fed with milk of food, causes vomition and leads to inhalation pneumonia.
- Death occur in 2- 3 weeks old puppies.
- Mucoid enteritis, intestinal ulcers, perforation of intestine and peritonitis.
- Occlusion of gut - perforation – peritonitis.

Aberrant Site

- Bile duct – inflammatory changes - occlusion.
- CNS – nervous disorder.

In Adult

- Progressive malaise associated with vomition and diarrhoea as worm mature it.
- Stomach and small intestine.

Clinical Signs

- Migratory larvae - pneumonic signs - coughing, increased respiratory rate, frothy nasal discharge.
- Adult – diarrhoea, pot bellied and tucked up abdomen and rough hair coat.
- Aberrant site CNS - nervous conclusion.
- Death due to intestinal obstruction.
- Most fatalities from *T. canis* infection occur during pulmonary phase and pups which have been heavily infected transplacentally and may die with in a few days of birth.

Prophylactic Schedule

Puppies		Bitches	
Time Schedule	*Purpose*	*Time Schedule*	*Purpose*
—	—	Pregnant bitches 3 weeks before whelping to 2 days after whelping - daily high doses of fenbendazole	To eliminate transplacental and transmammary infection
2nd weeks of age (I dose)	To eliminate prenatal infection	Same time when pups are treated	To eliminate transmammary infection
4th to 5th week of age (II dose)	To eliminate prenatal infection	Same time	To eliminate transmammary infection
2nd month of age (III dose)	Neonatal infection through milk or from environment	—	—
Once in every 3 – 6 months	Routine prophylatic	Once in every 3-6 months	Routine prophylatic

Weakening of Immunity (PPR)

- Occurrence of eggs in faeces of bitches after whelping as a result of weakening of immunity and contaminated environment.
- Lactogenic hormone (prolactin), which permits mobilization of larvae from somatic tissues to small intestine through lung, larvae under go maturation and become adult.
- Habit of whelped bitches to eat faeces of puppies, which may contains immature worms. The immature worms enter small intestine of bitches and become adult.
- Post parturient infection are eliminated within a few weeks of the termination of lactation.
- Not all larvae are mobilized during pregnancy and some may remain under in the tissues and eliminated through subsequent pregnancies.
- The duration of larvae in bitches may be long and animals infected for upto 385 days and is being capable of transmitting infection to puppies.
- Factors which induce mobilization and migration are unclear but probably there is a hormonal basis involved.

Diagnosis

- Based on history and clinical signs.
- Demonstration of eggs on direct smear method.

Treatment

- Piperazine - mature worm - 100 mg/kg and immature worm - 200 mg/kg.

- ☆ Diethycarbamazine (DEC) - 50 mg/kg (contraindicated for dogs with patent infection of *D. immitis*).
- ☆ Dichlorvos – 12 – 15 mg/kg body weight.
- ☆ Trichlorophan - 75 mg/kg.
- ☆ Pyrental pamoate – 5 mg/kg.
- ☆ Nitroscanate - 50 mg/kg.
- ☆ Mebendazole - 10 mg/kg (twice a day for 2 days).
- ☆ Fenbendazole - 100 mg/kg (As single dose or divided doses) (useful for pregnant bitches).

Control

- ☆ Good hygienic maintenance in kennels.
- ☆ More over long-term control consist of regular treatments for adult worm to lower or to eliminate environmental contamination.
- ☆ Kennels should be made up of impervious surfaces and floor should be thoroughly cleaned.
- ☆ To control entry of rodents in kennels.
- ☆ Prenatal and neonatal infection of young puppies are controlled by treating of pregnant bitches and her litter with suitable prophylactic schedule as follows.

5.18. Tricomoniasis

Trichomonosis, Introduction

- ☆ Members of this family have 3 anterior flagella and no pelta.
- ☆ They are found in the digestive tract and genital organs as commensals.

Tritrichomonas foetus

- ☆ A sexually transmitted organism causing a specific venereal disease, bovine trichomonosis or bovine trichomonad abortion in cattle and is charecterized by infertility, early abortion, pyometra and inapparent infection in bulls.

***Trichomonosis fetus*, Epidemiology**

Strain of the parasite

- ☆ Three serological distinct strains: a) Belfast b) Manley c) Brisbane.
- ☆ Outbreaks due to Manley strains are few.

Incidence

- ☆ Highest in those countries where bulls are kept for natural service.

Susceptible age group

All age groups.

Transmission

- By coitus under natural conditions.
- By teaser bulls.
- By artificial insemination is the most common of the other methods using infected semen.
- By gynecological examination, *i.e.*, use of speculum.

Survival of *Trichomonas*

- Does not survive when frozen in presence of glycerol at 37°C.
- Killed at ordinary refrigeration temperature.
- At lower temperature, organisms remain viable for up to 256 days.

Carrier Status

- Bulls are carrier and permanent sources of infection.
- In infected Cows, it is self-limiting, but untreated cows act as carriers for more than 1 year.

Immunity

- Little evidence as bulls become immuned to infection.
- Infected non-pregnant animals recover without treatment, but a small proportion of cows act as carriers and permanent sterility may occur despite immunity.
- Antibodies produced are
  - Humoral antibodies reaching systemic circulation from uterus, produced in when there is adequate infection with large number of organisms.
  - Uterine/vaginal antibodies developing locally and appear before humoral antibodies appear; The titre is high when organisms are numerous in uterine discharge and has a local control of parasites in vagina.
- Antibodies persist for 17 - 55 days and acquired through colostrum.

Trichomonosis fetus, Distribution, Host, Location and Morphology

Distribution

Worldwide, India - Reported in West Bengal, Bihar, Rajastan, Jammu and Kashmir and Odisha.

Host Affected

Cattle, also Zebu, buffalo, pigs, horses and deer but pathogenic only in cattle

Location

Cows: Uterus and internally the vagina.

Bulls: Preputial cavity.

Morphology

- ✰ Body is spindle to spear shaped (25um to 15 um).
- ✰ It has 3 anterior flagella and one posterior flagella which is free.

Trichomonosis fetus, Life Cycle

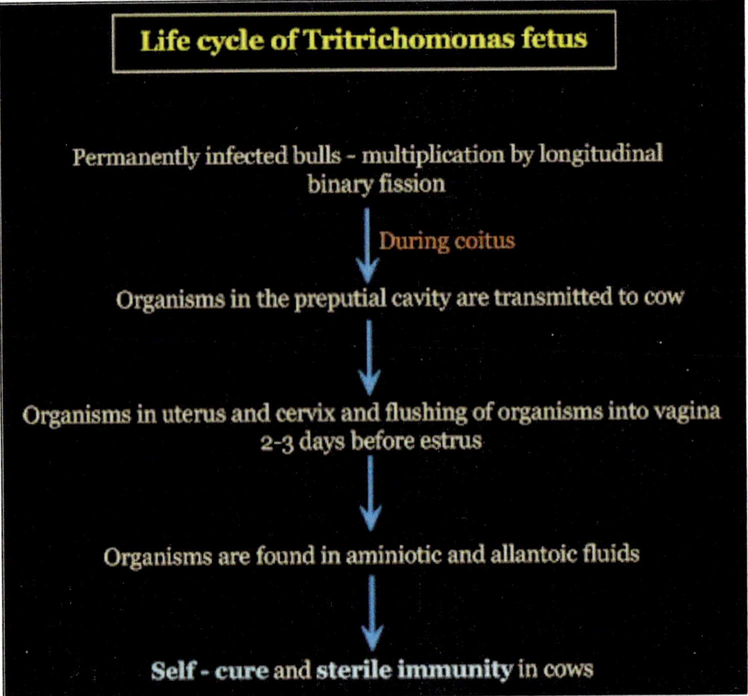

Figure 5.18a

Trichomonosis fetus, Pathogenesis and Clinical Signs

See Figure 5.18b.

Pathogenesis and Clinical Signs in Bulls

- ✰ Organisms are found in preputial cavity, most commonly; also in testes, epididymis and seminal vesicles.
- ✰ Spontaneous recovery is rare.
- ✰ Pain on micturition, disinclination to serve cows, mucopurulant discharge.
- ✰ Small red nodules in preputial mucus surface.

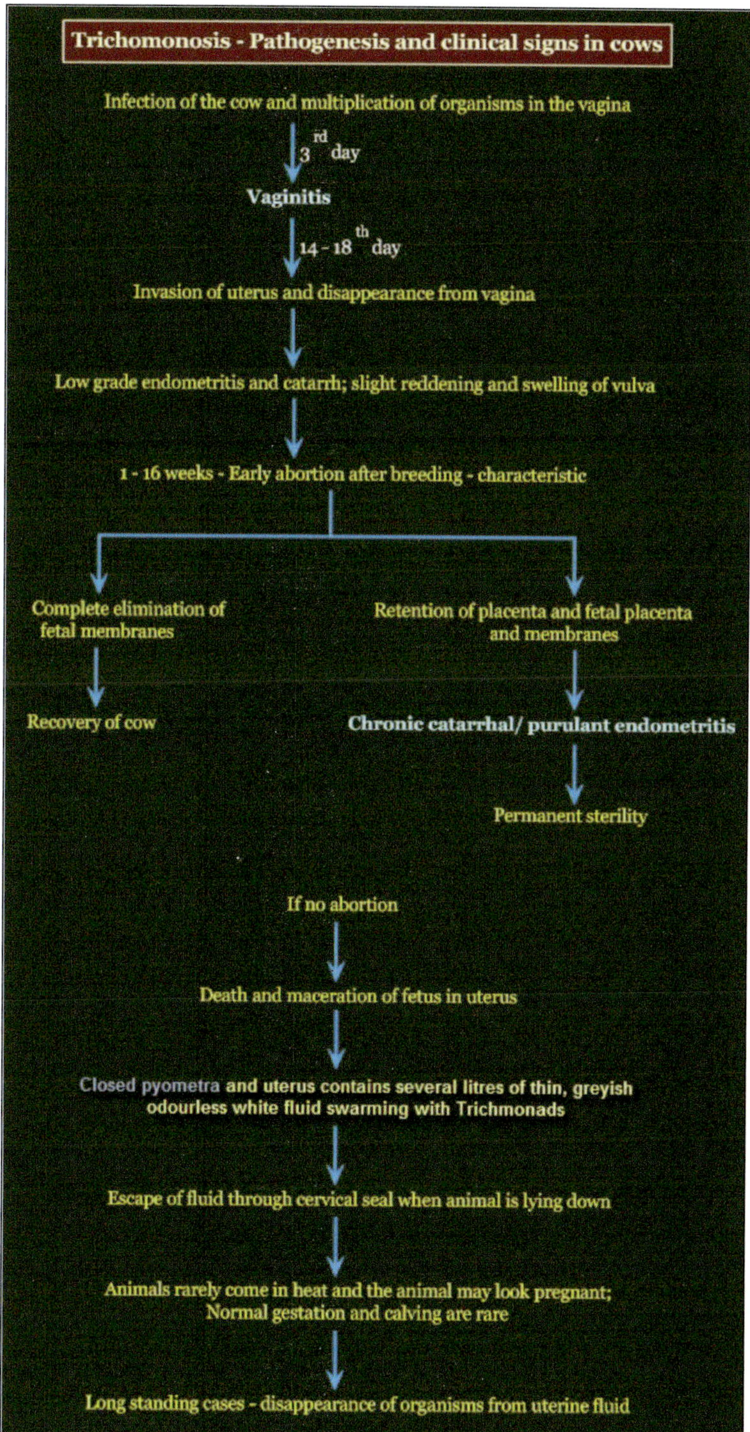
Trichomonosis - Pathogenesis and clinical signs in cows
Infection of the cow and multiplication of organisms in the vagina
3rd day
Vaginitis
14 - 18th day
Invasion of uterus and disappearance from vagina
Low grade endometritis and catarrh; slight reddening and swelling of vulva
1 - 16 weeks - Early abortion after breeding - characteristic
Complete elimination of fetal membranes
Recovery of cow
Retention of placenta and fetal placenta and membranes
Chronic catarrhal/ purulant endometritis
Permanent sterility
If no abortion
Death and maceration of fetus in uterus
Closed pyometra and uterus contains several litres of thin, greyish odourless white fluid swarming with Trichmonads
Escape of fluid through cervical seal when animal is lying down
Animals rarely come in heat and the animal may look pregnant; Normal gestation and calving are rare
Long standing cases - disappearance of organisms from uterine fluid

Figure 5.18b

- ✰ Signs disappear from1-2 weeks after infection.
- ✰ Clinical cases: Pain and swelling disappear.

Mechanism of Action

- ✰ Cell surface antigens by
  - ❒ Hydrolytic enzymes secreted by parasites which are involved in enzymatic alteration/destruction of host cells.
  - ❒ Lysosomal extracts containing neuraminidase which is cytotoxic to epithelial monocell layers.

***Trichomonosis fetus*, Diagnosis**

Case history

- ✰ Cases of early abortion; increased incidence of cows returning to sevice.
- ✰ Failure of animals to become pregnant except after repeated service.

Clinical signs: Increase in prevalence of vaginal discharge and pyometra in a herd.

- ✰ Confirmation by demonstration of organisms in the vagina/uterine discharges/fetus/amniotic fluid/allantoic fluid/fetal membranes/ placenta/fetal stomach contents or its mouth fluids.
  - ❒ Following abortion, organisms disappear within 48 hours.
  - ❒ In bulls: Preputial washings, rarely seminal fluid or semen.
  - ❒ The organisms will be observed as jerky movements and rotation of cells on their long axis, lashing flagella when examined in warm saline.
- ✰ Examination of the above preparations by Giemsa staining, if the organisms are too low to allow diagnosis.
- ✰ Culturing in CPLM (Cysteine-Peptone- Liver extract- Maltose serum) or Diamond's media.
- ✰ Serological tests
  - ❒ Cervical mucus agglutination tests-most satisfactory.
  - ❒ Vaginal mucus should be collected and atleast 3 negative examinations and 2 normal estrus periods confirm a cow as free from infection.
- ✰ Intradermal test
  - ❒ Not satisfactory
  - ❒ Inconsistent since animals maybe desensitized during acute uterine infection.

***Trichomonosis fetus*, Treatment and Control**

Treatment

Dimetridazole - effective systematically for cows and bulls @50 mg/kg, I.V or P.O.

Bulls: Difficult to treat, best to sell it for slaughter.

Injection of less than 1 per cent acriflavin solution into the prepuce and retained for 150 minutes with thorough massage and 2 courses with 5 successive treatments. 3 per cent hydrogen peroxide – partially effective.

Control

- ☆ Slaughtering/castration of infected bulls.
- ☆ Indescriminate breeding of untested bulls should be checked and only test authorized bulls should be permitted for breeding.
- ☆ Aborted cows should be given sexual rests for 3 consecutive estrus periods.
- ☆ Artificial insemination with proper care will reduce the incidence of disease.
- ☆ Maintenance of proper records of service date, calving *etc.*,at the farm helps in early diagnosis and control.
- ☆ Examination of breeding bulls for *T. fetus* before purchase.

5.19. Tricostrongylidae

Introduction

The family Trichostrongylidae includes the following genus:

- ☆ *Trichostrongylus*
- ☆ *Ostertagia*
- ☆ *Cooperia*
- ☆ *Nematodirus*
- ☆ *Haemonchus*
- ☆ *Mecistocirrus*
- ☆ *Paracooperia*

Ostertagia, Pathogenesis, Clinical Signs, Diagnosis and Treatment

Epidemiology

- ☆ Similar to *Trichostrongylus* (air temperature more than 10ºC).
  - ❒ Infection rate: adult worm lay - 100- 200 eggs/day.
  - ❒ Survivability of infective larvae in environment.
- ☆ Infective larvae resistant to cold and survive prolonged period in soil.
- ☆ Infective larvae not markedly resistant to desiccation.

Hypobiosis

- ☆ Out side the host (during unfavourable environmental conditions).
- ☆ Inside the host - depends upon age, previous exposure, reproductive status, proportion of challenge dose.

Pathogenesis

- Pathological changes occur in gastric gland and gastric mucosa.
  - Hyperplasia and thickening of mucosa and raised nodules.
  - Marked increase in abomasal pH – HCl production decreased.
  - Conversion of pepsinogen into pepsin is reduced.
  - Leakage of plasma protein into intestine - hypoalbuminaemia.

Clinical Signs

- Reduction of appetite, profuse watery diarrhoea – bright green in colour.
- Emaciation loss of weight.

Diagnosis

- EPG – 1,000 severe infection
- Larval count on pasture - 100/Kg of dried herbage - reduced growth rate - 1000/kg of dried herbage - leads to clinical diseases.

Clinical pathology – elevation of pepsinogen level. Response to treatment (indication of disease - Treatment with benzimidazole – animal return to normal).

Control

- Anthelmintics treatment and pasture management:
  - Feeding of uncontaminated pasture.
  - Alternative grazing and rotational grazing.

Haemonchus contortus

- *Embryonation and hatching:* Similar to Strongyles.
- *Development of infective larvae:* (Free living stage (L_1 and L_2) to parasitic stage (L_3).
  - High environmental temperature: 22°C to 27°C, development even occur at 5°C or 30°C but on lower rate.

Relative humidity: 85 per cent to 100 per cent

Rain fall: Precipitation of 5 cm/month (where the annual rainfall is less than 680 mm, development is delayed/arrested).

Dissemination of Larvae in the Environment

- By larvae itself - about 5- 10 cm
- Dung beetle
- Rainfall – flow of water
  - *Migration of larvae in grass blades:* Similar to Strongyles
  - *Survivability of egg/larvae in the environment*
- Egg (Prehatch stage): more resistant to adverse conditions – like freezing and desiccation.

- ☆ Infective larvae: resistant to desiccation and very low temperature.

Arrested Larval Development (Hypobiosis)

- ☆ The L_4 larvae in the host under go hypobiosis. Which is influenced by environmental condition (cold, hot and dry weather) and immunological component, *i.e.*, At the end of rainy season/beginning of dry season

Activation of Arrested Development

Influenced by:

- ☆ Season: Onset of rainy season
- ☆ Relaxation of immunity
- ☆ Not treated with anthelminthics

Infection rate: Adult worm lay 5,000 to 15,000 eggs/day.

H. placei

- ☆ Epidemiology is similar to *H. contortus*.
- ☆ In addition to that cattle fecal pad acts as a reservoir of infective larvae.
- ☆ In which the larvae survive for several months and ultimately released when fecal pad is sufficiently moistened by rain.

Host

H. contortus: Sheep

Age: Weaner age group (3 to 6 months) and lambed ewes are highly susceptible

Breed: Native breeds are highly resistant (Presence of anti-larval IgA antibodies) to infection than exotic and crossbred sheep.

Hemoglobin type: Sheep having homozygous Hb type AA resistant to infection than sheep having heterozygous Hb type AB.

H. placei: Cattle - less than 2 years old are highly susceptible.

Trichostrongylus (Black Scour Worms)

Morphology

Small, slender pale reddish brown.

Adult – 5 mm, infective larvae ensheathed larvae.

Egg: oval, thin shelled segmented yolk (32 cell stage when laid).

Species

T. colubriformis

- ☆ Host: Sheep, goat, cattle, camel and antelopes.
- ☆ Location: abomasum and anterior part of small intestine.

T. axei

- Host
  - Sheep, goat, cattle, deer and antelope Location: Abomasum.
  - Pig, horse, donkey and man Location: Stomach.

T. tenuis

- Host: Domestic and wild ducks, geese, fowl, G. fowl and turkey.
- Location: Caecum and small intestine.

Epidemiology

Bionomics

- Embryonation and hatching: similar to Strongyles

Development: (4 –6 days) L1 –L3 (Infective larvae)

- Temperature- 22 – 26°C (< 9°C no development)
- RH – 85 - 100 per cent.

Migration in Grass Blades

- Mild light – 62 foot candles (during early morning and late evening)
- Moisture - more than 0.12 ml/cm^2
  - Survivability of infective larvae in environment

T. axei

- Infective larvae more susceptible to cold and high temperature of the soil.
- Relative humidity – low detrimental to larvae.

T. colubriformis

- L3 resist desiccation, but L2 susceptible desiccation.

Dissemination of Larvae

- Larvae itself – migrate upto 5-10 cm
- Dung beetle and flow of water also play a role
- Infection rate
  - Adult worm lay – 100 – 200 eggs/day
  - Infection rate is influenced by
  - Number of adult worms
  - Level of host immunity
  - Age of the host
  - Species of parasite
  - Stage of infection

- ❐ Parturition
- ❐ Consistency of faeces

Ostertagia (Brown Stomach Worm)

Location: abomasum and rarely in small intestine

Morphology: Adult – 8 – 9 mm long

Species

- ✰ *O. ostertagi* – cattle, sheep and goat – rarely
- ✰ *O. circumcincta* - sheep and goat
- ✰ *O. trifurcata* – sheep and goat, cattle – rarely
- ✰ *O. pinnata* - sheep

Life cycle: Direct – prepatent period – 3 –4 weeks

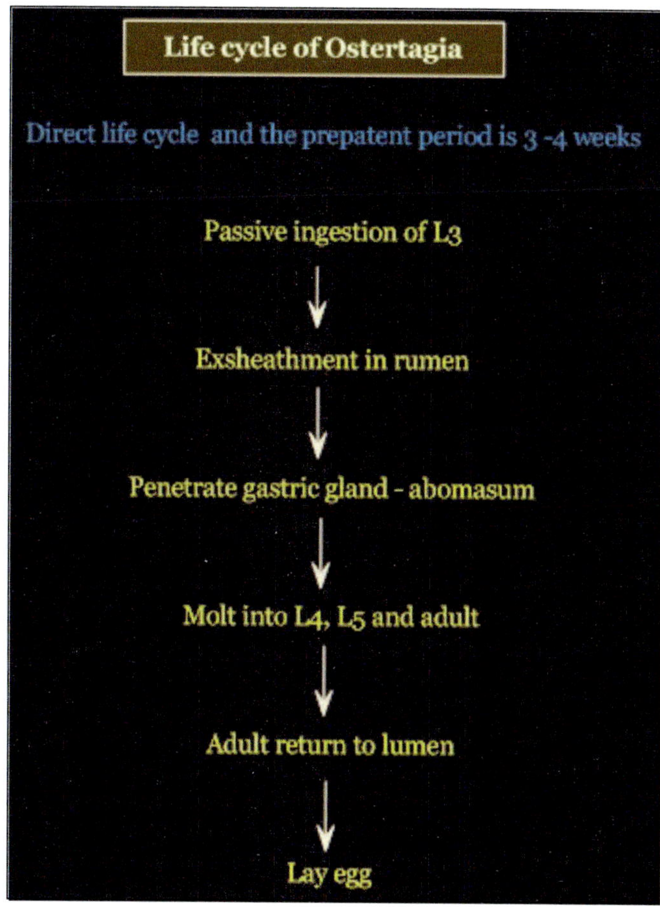

Figure 5.19a. Life cycle of *Ostertagia*.

Mecistocirrus, Cooperia* and *Paracooperia

Mecistocirrus

Species: *M. digitatus*

Host and Location

- ✰ Buffalo, Cattle, Sheep and goat - Abomasum
- ✰ Pig - Stomach

Morphology: similar to Haemonchus, size - 3-4 cm

- ✰ Epidemiology, life cycle, pathogenesis, clinical signs and diagnosis - Similar to *H. contortus*

Cooperia

Location: Small intestine, rarely on abomasum

Morphology

- ✰ Adult - Pale reddish in colour, Size: 5 mm
- ✰ Egg: Similar to *Trichostrongylus* spp.

Species

- ✰ *C. curticei* - sheep and goat; cattle –very rare
- ✰ *C. punctata* and *C. pectinata* - Cattle; Sheep – very rare
  - ❒ Epidemiology, life cycle, pathogenesis, clinical signs and diagnosis: Similar to *Trichostrongylus* spp.
  - ❒ Difference in Pathogenesis: less pathogenic

Paracooperia

Location: Small intestine, rarely on ceacum and colon

Species: *P. nodulosa*

Epidemiology, life cycle, pathogenesis, clinical signs and diagnosis: Similar to *Trichostrongylus* spp.

Difference in Pathogenesis: The larvae of this parasite occur in nodules of the intestinal wall.

P. nodulosa may be very pathogenic in young buffalo.

***Haemonchus*, Life Cycle**

Prepatent period

- ✰ *H. contortus*: 15 days
- ✰ *H. placei:* 30 days

Haemonchus

Morphology

Adult Worm

- ☆ Larger in size (1-3 cm) and visible under naked eye.
- ☆ Colour: Male: Even reddish in colour.
- ☆ Female: Uneven reddish in colour due to whitish ovaries twisted around reddish intestine.
- ☆ Having a small buccal capsule with slender tooth or lancet (Blood suckers).

Egg: Similar to *Trichostrongylus* spp (16 –32 cell stage)

Location: Abomasum

Species

- ☆ *H. contortus* - Sheep, goat, cattle and other ruminants (stomach worm or wire worm of ruminants)
- ☆ *H. placei* - Cattle, and sheep

Haemonchus, Clinical Signs and Post Mortem Changes

Clinical Signs

Sheep: Ovine haemonchosis

Cattle: Bovine haemonchosis

Hyper Acute

- ☆ Susceptible animal exposed to massive infection (> 10,000 infective larvae).
- ☆ EPG: > 1,00,000.
- ☆ Anemia, dark coloured faeces – sudden death due to rapid blood loss.

Acute

- ☆ Young animals exposed to heavy infection (1,000 - 10,000 infective larvae).
- ☆ EPG: 1,00,000.
- ☆ Anemia – fairly noticed – due to expansion of erythropoietic system.
- ☆ Anemia + Hypoproteinaemia – oedema on dependant part – submandibular region – bottle jaw.

Chronic

- ☆ Susceptible animal exposed to low infection (100 - 1,000 infective larvae).
- ☆ EPG: <2,000.
- ☆ Anemia and hypoproteinaemia are fairly noticed.
- ☆ Weakness, unthriftyness and emaciation.

Postmortem Changes

- Hydrothorax, hydropericardium and ascites.
- Watery blood.
- Abdominal fat – liquefied and become gelatinous in nature.
- Liver – light brown in colour – due to fatty changes.
- Abomasum: having reddish-brown fluid ingesta; worm present on the mucosal folds and bite marks noticed on the abomasal mucosa.

Clinical Signs, Immunity and Diagnosis of *Trichostrongylus* sp.

Clinical signs: Gastrointestinal disturbances – diarrhoea.

Acute Cases

- Sudden death, such animal neither emaciated nor anaemic
- Leg weakness – unable to stand

Chronic Cases

- Variable in appetite emaciation, rough and dry hair coat.
- Alternatively constipation and diarrhoea.
- Anemia is not well pronounced (mild one).
- Nature of faeces- dark diarrhoea – "Black scour worms".

Immunity

- Infection induces immunity to reinfection (intake of infective larvae or presence of adult worm).
- Cross immunity is observed between *Trichostrongylus* spp, not at generic level.

Diagnosis

- Demonstration of eggs in faeces.
- Faecal culture.
- Avian sp: Haemorrhagic typhilitis with diarrhoea – loss of appetite, emaciation and anemia - Grouse disease.

Immunity: Selfcure Phenomena

- Loss or expulsion of worm burden in the gastro-intestinal tract of the suitably infected and sensitized sheep can be induced by challenge dose of infective larvae.
- Self-cure and protection against infection are not necessarily interrelated - Immunity is not absolute.

Parasite Factors which induce Selfcure phenomena

- It is well noticed in *H. contortus* - sheep and *H. placei* – cattle
- Among the *H. contortus* subspecies – *H. contortus cayugensis* – self-cure was not recorded.
- Cross immunity was observed between species of *Haemonchus.*
- Cross immunity was observed between genus of *Haemonchus* and *Trichostrongylus*, but it is one way.
- *Haemonchus* induce immunity against Trichostrongylus and not vice versa.
- Exsheathed larvae induce good immunity than ensheathed larvae.
- Irradiated larvae induce good immunity.
- Size of the challenge dose is inversely related to the self-cure.

Other Factors which Induces Selfcure

- Feeding of lush pasture, which might due to presence of an allergic/ anthelmintic substance in the freshly growing grasses.
- Physiological alteration in the abomasum.
- Season: After rainfall it is well pronounced.

Host Factor which Induce Selfcure Phenomena

Species*:* Sheep – it is well pronounced

Breed*:* Native breed of sheep having good response than exotic and crossbred sheep (due to presence of anti-larval IgA antibodies in the native breed).

Age*:* Sheep greater than 6 months old having good response.

Hemoglobin type*:* Sheep with homozygous Hb type AA having good response than homozygous Hb type BB.

Stage of lactation*:* Relaxation of immunity – poor response.

Level of lymphocytes in peripheral blood*:* Sheep with low level of lymphocytes having low immune response.

Latent period for induction of Selfcure: 6-7 weeks

Postulated Mechanisms of Selfcure

Challenge dose of infective larvae (L_3) molt into L_4 inside the host.

- Developing larvae releases antigen, which induces immediate type of hypersensitivity reaction.
- Transient raise of blood histamines.
- Increase level of complement fixing antibodies.
- Intense mucosal oedema.
- Expulsion of worms.

Life Cycle and Pathogenesis of *Trichostrongylus* Sp.

Life Cycle

- ✰ Infection of definitive host: Through passive ingestion.
- ✰ Exsheathment (abomasum or small intestine).
  - ✰ Host stimulus
- ✰ Bicarbonate and Co_2 buffer
- ✰ Undisassociated Co_2 and dissolved Co_2
- ✰ Abomosal pH –7.3 and Temperature - 37 °C
  - ✰ Infective larvae secrete Leucine aminopectidase (LAP) and attack sheath.

Pathogenesis

T. axei

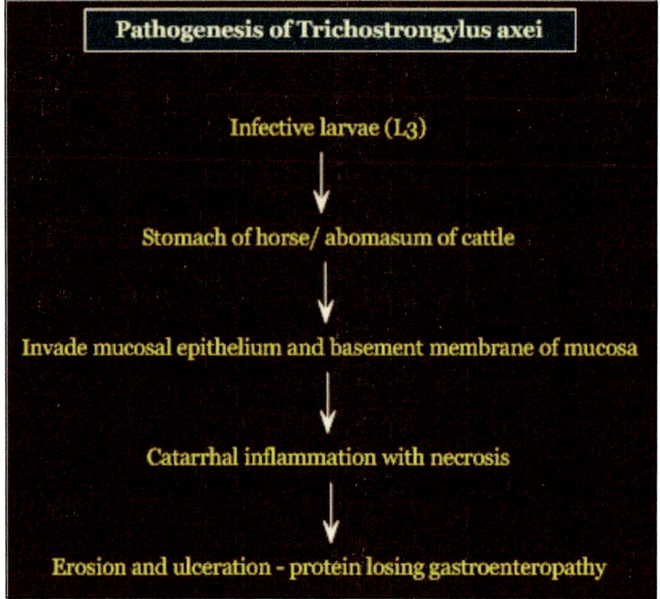

Figure 5.19b. Pathogenesis of *T. axei*.

T. colubriformis

Similar to *T. axei*

- ✰ It occurs in anterior part of small intestine.
- ✰ In mucosa - formation of tunnels between epithelium and basement membrane.
- ✰ Distortion and displacement of mucosal epithelium.
- ✰ Loss of plasma protein into intestine - hypoalbuminaemia.

In General Trichostrongylus spp.

- ✰ Loss of serum protein – anorexia - reduced feed intake – reduced food conversion ratio.
- ✰ Intestinal parasitism - increased gastric secretion of cholecystokinin – act on appetite centre in brain, leads to decreased appetite.
  - ❐ Absorption of calcium and phosphorus from intestine reduced – retarded bone growth and osteoporosis.

Haemonchus, Life Cycle

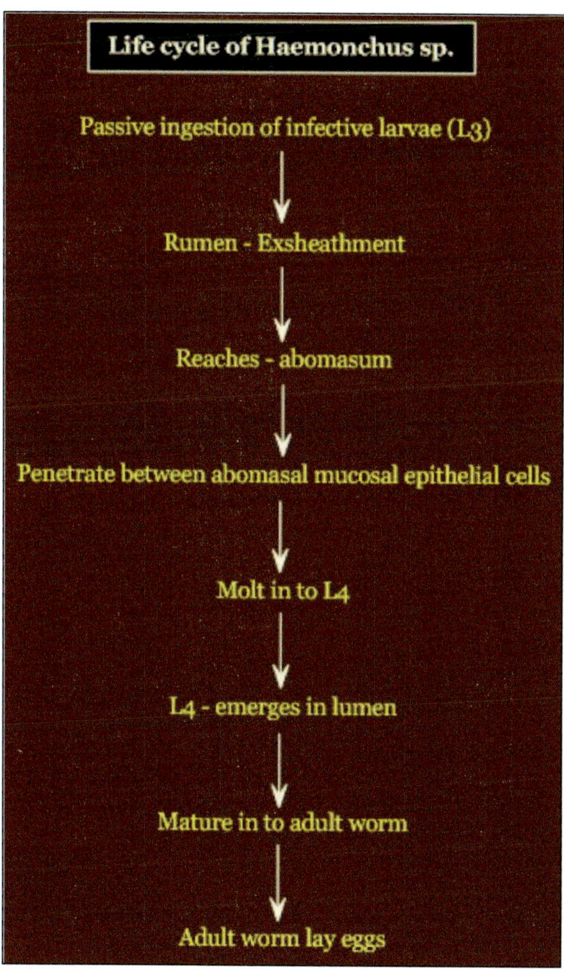

Figure 5.19c. Life cycle of *Haemonchus* spp.

Prepatent period

- ✰ *H. contortus*: 15 days
- ✰ *H. placei:* 30 days

Haemonchus, Pathogenesis

- ☆ Due penetration of infective larvae: Inflammation (haemorrhagic abomasitis) – protein losing gastroenteropathy – hypoproteinaemia (diarrhoea is not a characteristic feature).
- ☆ Anaemia: L4, L5 and adult worm suck: 0.05 ml/day. Anaemia occurs in following ways:
    - ❐ Blood sucker – blood sucking activity
    - ❐ Blood oozes – haemorrhagic – due to anti-coagulant secreted by the worm:
    - ❐ Hypoproteinaemia - reduced Haemoglobin synthesis.
- ☆ Anaemia is discussed in three phases based on PCV and serum iron level.

Phase I

- ☆ PCV: Reduced (22- 33 per cent) – Activation of erythropoietic system – compensatory loss.
- ☆ Serum iron level: Normal

Phase II

- ☆ PCV: level maintained, but less than normal level.
- ☆ Serum iron: decreased due to following factors.
- ☆ Marked loss of iron in the faeces (haemorrhagic).
- ☆ Limited capacity to reabsorp from intestine.
- ☆ Low level of bone marrow reserves.

Phase III

- ☆ PCV: rapid drop
- ☆ Serum iron: less than critical level (Dyshaemopoiesis)

Diagnosis

- ☆ Based on clinical signs
- ☆ Identification of eggs in faeces
- ☆ Fecal culture
- ☆ Autopsy of animal in the suspected flocks

Trichuris

Trichuris ovis

Host: Goat, sheep, cattle and other ruminants

Location: Caecum

Morphology

Adult: Anterior part of the body is long and slender while posterior part is much thicker.

Egg: Brown barrel - shaped, with a transparent plug at either pole.

Life Cycle

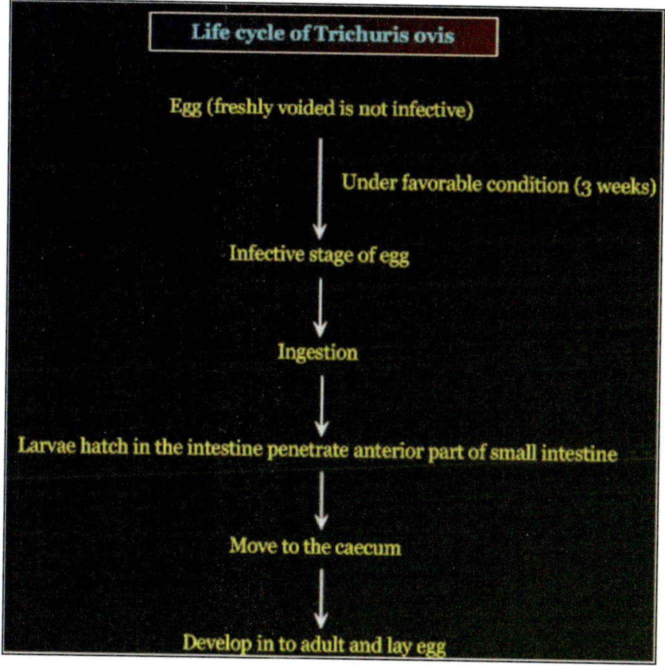

Figure 5.19d. Life cycle of *Trichuris* spp.

Epidemiology, Pathogenesis, Diagnosis, Treatment and Control

Epidemiology

- Development of infective stage depends on:
  - Prolonged lower temperature (6 – 20 °C)
  - Soil temperature and moisture
- Infective egg may remain viable for several years.
- Sheep over eight months of age show an age resistance to infection and a resistance to reinfection two to three weeks after primary infection.

Pathogenesis and clinical signs

- Blood feeder – cause anaemia, haemorrhage and some times cause jaundice and death.
- Adult forms a tunnel into the intestinal mucosa,
- Cause severe inflammation - diarrhoea.

Diagnosis

Presence of characteristic egg.

Treatment

- ✰ Methyridine – 200 mg/kg orally subcutaneous - highly effective.
- ✰ Fenbendazole – 5 – 20 mg/kg.
- ✰ Oxbendazole - 2.5 mg/kg.

Prevention and Control

- ✰ Improves hygiene.
- ✰ Heavily infected soil should be avoided for several months to allow the natural agencies of sunlight and dryness to kill the eggs.

5.20. Trypanosomosis

***Trypanosomes* of Domestic Animals**

Sl. No.	*Parasite*	*Vertebrate Host*	*Arthropod Vector*	*Trans-mission*	*Develop. Stage in Vertebrate H*
Salivaria (pathogenic)					
1	T. vivax	Cattle, Sheep, Goat and Cattle	*Glossina* spp. (Tse-tse flies)	Cyclical	Trypomastigote
2	*T. congolense* (Nagana)	Cattle, Sheep, Horse and Pig	*Glossina* spp .	Cyclical	Trypomastigote
3	*T. brucei* (Nagana)	Cattle, Sheep, Goat, Horse, Pig, Dog and cat	*Glossina* spp. Tabanids	Cyclical, Also mechanical	Trypomastigote
4	T. evansi	Equines, Dog, Cattle, Sheep, Goat, Cat, camel, Elephant	Tabanids, Stomoxys and other biting flies	Mechanical	Trypomastigote
5	*T. equinum* (Mal-de Caderas)	Equines	Tabanids, Stomoxys and other biting flies	Mechanical	Trypomastigote
6	*T.equiperdum* (Dourine)	Equines	*Coitus* (rarely tabanids)	Mechanical	Trypomastigote
7	*T. simiae*	Pigs, cattle, horses, Sheep and Goat	*Glossina* spp.	Cyclical	Trypomastigote
8	*T. suis*	Pigs, Sheep, Goat and dogs	*Glossina* spp.	Cyclical	Trypomastigote
9	*T. rhodesiense* (Sleeping sickness)	Man, ruminants (domestic and wild) Zoonotic	*Glossina* spp.	Cyclical	Trypomastigote
10	*T. gambiense* (Sleeping sickness)	Man, also animals	*Glossina* spp.	Cyclical	Trypomastigote

Sl. No.	Parasite	Vertebrate Host	Arthropod Vector	Trans-mission	Develop. Stage in Vertebrate H
		Stercoraria (Non-pathogenic)			
1	*T. theileri*	Cattle	Tabanids, *Hippobosca maculata*	Cyclical	Epimastigote
2	*T. melophagium*	Sheep	*Melophagus ovinus* (sheep ked)	Cyclical	Uncertain
3	*T. theodori*	Goat	Hippoboscid	Cyclical	Uncertain
4	*T. cruzi* (Chaga's disease)	Man, Dog and cat	Reduviid bugs	Cyclical	Amastigote

Trypanosoma evansi

Disease: Surra in all hosts

- Tebersa in camels
- Murine in horses
- 1st trypanosome shown to be pathogenic for mammals and is a intercellular parasite in blood and lymph.

Host: Camel, Horses, Donkeys, Cattle, Buffalo, Sheep Goat, Dog, Cat, elephant and other animals (tiger, fox, jackal, hyena, orangutan and mongoose), rodents, rabbits and guinea pig.

Vectors: Tabanids, Stomoxys, Haematopota, Hippobosca, Ornithodorus tick.

Location: Blood and lymph.

Morphology

T. evansi is monomorphic but polymorphism sporadically. Slender, thin, indistinguishable from *T. brucei* and 15-34 μm length. Have sub-terminal kinetoplast, well developed undulating membrane and prominent free flagellum.

Life Cycle

See Figure 5.20.

Epidemiology

Host susceptibility

Increased incidence is in equines and dogs than cattle and buffaloes. Buffaloes greater than cattle; imported dogs greater than native dogs; pups greater than adults.

Transmission

Mechanically biting flies- Tabanus, Stomoxys, Haematopota, Chrysops, Hippobosca and Lyperosia; Ticks-Ornithodorus spp. Interrupted feeding of flies from one host to other.

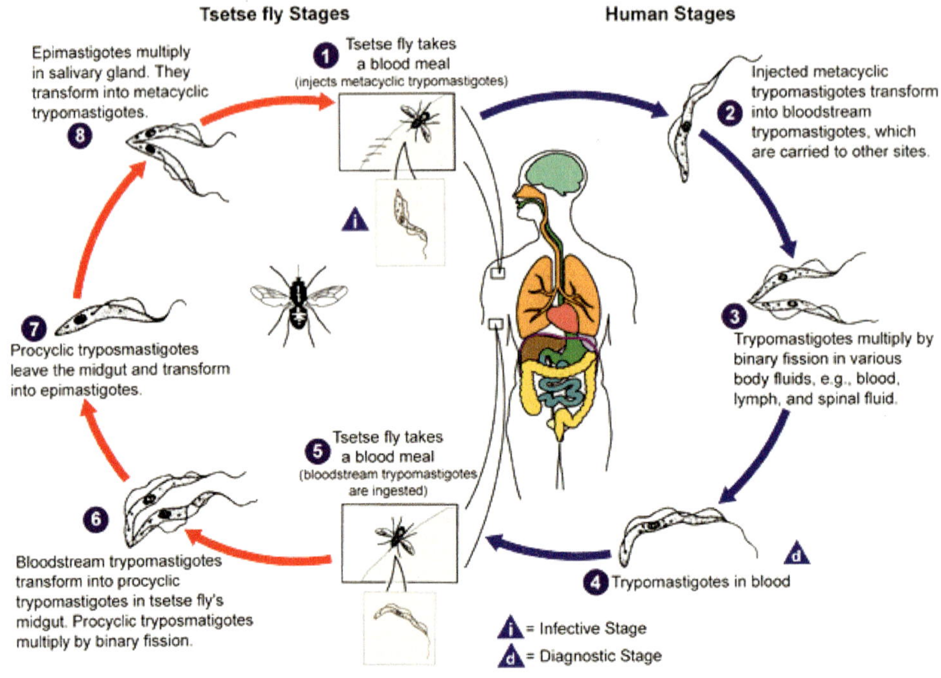

Figure 5.20

During a blood meal on the mammalian host, an infected tsetse fly (genus *Glossina*) injects metacyclic trypomastigotes into skin tissue. The parasites enter the lymphatic system and pass into the bloodstream–1. Inside the host, they transform into bloodstream trypomastigotes–2, are carried to other sites throughout the body, reach other body fluids (*e.g.*, lymph, spinal fluid), and continue the replication by binary fission–3. The entire life cycle of African trypanosomes is represented by extracellular stages. The tsetse fly becomes infected with bloodstream trypomastigotes when taking a blood meal on an infected mammalian host–4, 5). In the fly's midgut, the parasites transform into procyclic trypomastigotes, multiply by binary fission–6, leave the midgut, and transform into epimastigotes–7. The epimastigotes reach the fly's salivary glands and continue multiplication by binary fission–8. The cycle in the fly takes approximately 3 weeks. Humans are the main reservoir for *Trypanosoma brucei gambiense*, but this species can also be found in animals. Wild game animals are the main reservoir of *T. b. rhodesiense*.

Trypanosoma equiperdum

Disease: Dourine, Equine Syphilis, Breeding paralysis.

Distribution: Africa, America and Russia.

Host: All equines (horses are highly susceptible than mules/donkeys).

Epidemiology

Mechanically by coitus, rarely by biting flies. Foals get infected through contamination of nasal/conjunctival membrane with vaginal discharge of infected mare.

Carriers: Jackals.

Pathogenesis

Incubation period - 2 to 12 weeks, phase of edema (4-6 weeks): Mare-edema of genitalia, nymphomania, mucoid vaginal or urethral discharge and ulcers in vaginal mucosa; in severe cases, abortion and frequent micturition. Stallion- Swelling of prepuce and scrotum.

Urticaria phase: Oval or round plaques (3cm dia) under skin on flank are pathognomonic and are called Dollar spots; Anaemia, emaciation, intermittent fever, lymph node enlargement.

Paralytic phase: In coordination, unilateral paralysis of hind limbs, nostrils, ears, lips, recumbency and death (50-70 per cent).

Diagnosis

Clinical signs: Smears from vaginal mucous membrane and urticarial swellings. Laboratory animal inoculation or into a dog.

Treatment: Suramin

Control

Slaughter of infected animals, castration of affected animals, treatment with suramin.

Trypanosoma equinum

Disease: Mal de - caderas or Disease of Hip

Distribution: Central and South America

Host: Horses

Vectors: Tabanid flies and Stomoxys.

Epidemiology: Mechanical transmission by biting flies.

Pathogenesis and Clinical signs

Usually, chronic, rarely acute and death in 2-6 months after infection. Incubation period is 4 to 10 days. Emaciation in early stage followed by weakening of hind quarters in staggering gait and recumbency. Conjunctivitis, keratitis, edema of the eyelids, cutaneous plaques on neck and flank.

Post mortem findings: Spleenomegaly, anaemia, ascites, kidney with petechiae.

Diagnosis

Demonstration of organisms in peripheral blood smear. In chronic cases, animal inoculation test.

Treatment and control: Similar to Trypanosomiasis in horses.

Trypanosoma, Classification, Morphology and Developmental Stages

Classification

Members of the family, the trypanosomes are all parasitic and evolved from alimentary canal of insects. Many are found in blood/tissues of mammals and birds. Members of this genus are found in vertebrates, in the blood stream and tissue fluids and, some in tissue cells. They are transmitted by blood sucking arthropod vectors with below mentioned developmental stages. A few species of this genus are transmitted mechanically by vectors. A few species are overwhelming importance as an serious cause of morbidity in man and animals in tropical regions.

Morphology

They are characteristically leaf like in shape; they have a single flagellum and is attached to the body of the organism by an undulating membrane.

Developmental Stages

Trypomastigote Stage

A blade -like form with the kinetoplast posterior to the nucleus and usually near the posterior extremity. An undulating membrane and free flagellum are present. It is usually present in vertebrate host and also in arthropods.

Epimastigote Stage

- Kinetoplast and axoneme lie anterior to the nucleus with short undulating membrane.
- In few species, it is seen in vertebrate host, but principally in arthropods.

Promastigote Stage

- Kinetoplast and axoneme are at the anterior tip of body with no undulating membrane.
- Seen in arthropods.

Amastigote Stage

- Rounded body with kinetoplast.
- Absence of flagellum (or with short fibrils).
- Found in vertebrate arthropods.

Epidemiology of *Trypanosoma*

Development of Trypanosomes in Vertebrate Host

All trypanosomes in the final host multiply by binary fission or multiple fission (No gamete formation). In Salivaria group, trypanosomes divide chiefly in trypomastigote stage in blood/lymph glands.Intracellular stages have been found in *T. congolense*, *T. brucei*, *T. evansi*, *T. equinum* and *T. equiperdum*. In Stercoraria group, trypanosomes divide in the epimastigote and amastigote stage. In *T. cruzi*, multiplication is intracellular in reticulo-endothelial system (RES) and striated muscles, *e.g.* heart.

Development of Trypanosomes in Vectors (Transmission)

Cyclical Transmission

Salivaria group-- In arthropods, trypanosomes multiply, undergo morphological transformation in digestive tract and proboscis and upon feeding, the new infection is transmitted by inoculation, eg., *T. vivax, T. brucei, T. congolense* by tse-tse flies. Stercoraria group-Multiplication and transformation of trypanosomes occur in gut and migrate to rectum and passed in faeces, *e.g., T. theileri, T. melophagium* by Tabanid spp., *Hippobosca* spp., *Melophagum ovi.*

Mechanical Transmission

Trypanosomes are transferred from one mammalian host to another host by interrupted feeding of biting insects, *e.g.,* Tabanids and Stomoxys.The trypanosomes on the proboscis donot multiply and die quickly so that transmission is possible only for few hours, *e.g., T.evansi* and *T. equinum* by Tabanids/Stomoxys. Vampire bats can also be the vector in the transmission of the *T. evansi* which multiply and survive for a long period. Mechanical transmission can also occur in some salivarian group transmitted cyclically in tse-tse flies, *e.g., T. vivax* and *T. brucei.*

Transmission by Oral Route

Dog, cat and wild carniovores may become infected by eating fresh carcasses or organs of animals died of trypanosomiasis, the parasites penetrating oral abrasions.

Immunity

Trypanosomes are extremely elastic antigenically. Members of subgenus Trypanozoon especially change in antigenic constitution between original infection and the first antigenic relapse and successive relapse. A succession of variation takes place and the parasite manages to survive. However, it reverts to original antigenic structure upon cyclical transmission. As many as 20 or more variants have been reported. The culture forms lack the coating. The destruction of the trypanosomes take place through the complement mediated lysis of trypanosomes/phagocytosis of agglutinated and opsonized trypanosomes by macrophages, monocytes, neutrophils and eosinophils. The immune response (IgM and IgG) is directed against the surface glycoprotein coat. Despite the effective mechanism of host, trypanosomes cause severe and prolonged infection resulting in successive waves of parasitaemia at intervals of few days, each wave representing the multiplication of a new antigenic type. *T. cruzi* evades immunity not by antigenic variation but by intracellular sequestration.

Sexuality

No evidence of sex in trypanosomes.

Cultivation

Relatively easy to cultivate in any artificial media like NNN media.

Trypanosoma, Sections/Group of *Trypanosomes*

Salivaria (Anterior Station/Group B)

Frequently highly pathogenic. Multiplication in vertebrate host is continuous in trypomastigote stage. In arthropod host, metacyclic trypanosomes (epimastigotes) occur in anterior station (anterior/midgut). Transmission is by inoculation.

Stercoraria (Posterior Station/Group A)

Nonpathogenic, Multiplication in vertebrate host is discontinuous, typically taking place in trypomastigote, epimastigote/amastigoteforms. In arthropods, epimastigotes occur in hind gut, accumulate and passed in the faeces, which contaminate skin wounds in vertebrate host thereby transmission of parasite.

Trypanosoma, Pathogenesis and Clinical Signs

Pathogenesis

Course of the disease depends on the factors like genetic constitution of the host, previous exposure to disease and the virulence of the infection, strain of the parasite and species of the host.

Mechanism Responsible for Anaemia-3 Factors

- ☆ Haemolysis of RBCs by trypanosomes.
- ☆ Increased erythrophagocytosis mediated by antibody on antigen with complement.
- ☆ Haemodilution due to increased plasma production.
- ☆ Others- reduced erythropoiesis, intravascular coagulation and death.

Causes of Death

- ☆ Progressive anaemia.
- ☆ Intravascular coagulation.
- ☆ Hypoglycemia due to disturbed metabolism by malfunction of adrenals, pancreas and thyroid and due to direct utilization of glucose by the parasite.

Biochemical Changes

Increase in globulin and decrease in albumin globulin ratio by 14.4 per cent. The infection is severe in dogs and horses than cattle and buffaloes.

Clinical Signs

Equines

- ☆ Incubation Period: 4 to 9 days.
- ☆ Severe in horses.
- ☆ Donkeys are resistant.

- ☆ Death within few days to few months depending on the virulence of strain of the organism.
- ☆ Intermittent fever (44°C) and anaemia are main symptoms.
- ☆ Transient local/urticarial eruptions/plaques on neck/flanks; edema of legs and lower parts of the body.
- ☆ Hemorrhage at the junction of the skin and mucous membrane at nostrils, eyes and anus and petechial haemorrhage on mucous membrane of eye or vulva in mares; pale and dirty yellowish mucous membrane.
- ☆ Staggering gait, paraplegia, laboured breathing.
- ☆ Diarrhoea, constipation, urine with albumin and blood and dark yellowish; Increased thirst, signs of catarrh with yellow tinged nasal discharge.
- ☆ Less common: Enlargement of lymph nodes, keratitis, petechiae in vaginal mucous membrane.

Cattle and Buffaloes

Course varies from a symptomless carrier to per acute infection.

- ☆ Per acute - Death within in 2-3 hour; nervous form and death in convulsion.
- ☆ Acute - Dull, sleepy, staggering gait, encircling movements, nervous excitement, beating head against wall/manger, apparent blindness, stamping of feet, bellowing, groaning, twitching of muscle, shivering of body, coma and death within 6-12 hours.
- ☆ Subacute/Chronic -Parasitaemia is usually low and doesn't coincide with temperature and afebrile animal be positive for parasites, edema of legs, diarrhea, intermittent fever, rapid pulse, dullness, sleepy, bilateral lachrymation, progressive emaciation and death; abortion reported in buffaloes.
- ☆ PM findings: Spleenomegaly, hepatomegaly, enlargement of lymph nodes and kidney, petechial haemorrhage at the junction of skin and mucous membrane.

Dogs

- ☆ Incubation period: 5 to 6 days; untreated dogs die within 12 months, acute and fatal; more serious in pups and imported dogs.
- ☆ Fever, anorexia, edema of head and throat, corneal opacity or blindness.
- ☆ Laryngeal edema resulting in change of voice simulating rabies.
- ☆ Muscular spasm of limb, staggering gait, excitement like biting kennel bars simulating rabies.

Cats: Chronic cases are reported; at times may be fatal.

Sheep and Goats: Rare; intensity of symptoms are also moderate; emaciation and anaemia may be present.

Pigs: Non-pathogenic and low parasitaemia.

Trypanosoma Diagnosis

History of prevalence of *T. evansi* infection and biting flies like tabanids.

Clinical Signs

Differential Diagnosis

Anthrax, Snake bite, Nervous ketosis, Organic and inorganic poisoning, Milk fever, Hypovitaminosis, Milk fever, Brain tumor/cyst.

Direct Examination

In acute cases-demonstration of organisms in blood smears stained freshly with Giemsa stain. Chronic cases- examination of thick and thin blood smear at the height of the temperature will be positive/lymph node puncture smears.

Chemical Tests

- ✰ To detect the changes in the chemical composition of the blood produced by *T. evansi,* like alteration of proteins.
- ✰ Non-specific and less reliable.
    - ✰ Mercuric chloride test, Formal gel test, thymol turbidity test are used for camels.
    - ✰ Stilbamide test-diagnosis of latent infection in bovines in India.
- ✰ Animal inoculation tests
    - ✰ For detection of latent infection of bovines and more reliable than microscopic examination. Albino mice/rat are most suitable for detecting subpatent infection; guinea pigs and rabbits are less susceptible. Injection of 2 ml of blood intraperitoneally into the mice causes organisms appear after 2-3 days in the mice.

Immunodiagnostic Tests

- ✰ IFAT, CFT, ELISA and IHA are most reliable tests.
- ✰ Allergic tests are doubtful- 1ml antigen is injected at the side of the neck with a 2nd dose after 48 hours. Infected cases show hot, edematous, painful swelling and healthy cases show circumscribed, hard, nodular swelling.

Trypanosoma Treatment and Control

Treatment

- ✰ Quinapyramines (Antryside) - Prophylactic (Triquin)- Drug of choice.
    - ❒ Antryside methyl sulphate solution
- ✰ 3mg/kg as 10 per cent aqueous solution, S/C; effective against *T. evansi, T. congolense, T. brucei, T. vivax*.
    - ❒ Antrycide chloride as antrycide prosalt
- ✰ In combination with antrycide methyl sulphate -3 parts of A. M.S + 2 parts A. chloride

- ☆ A solution of 3.5 gm in 15 ml water is given @ 7.4 mg/kg; effective against *T. evansi* and *T.brucei*, for 3 months.
- ☆ Suramins (Sulphonated naphthalamines) - Curative (Naganaol, Antrypol)
  - ❒ Effective against *T. evansi, T. brucei, T. equiperdum*.
- ☆ Cattle: 0.5 g/45 kg followed by half dose after 2 weeks, I/V.
- ☆ Horse: 4g/45 kg as single dose, I/V.
- ☆ Dog: 3.5 ml- 10 per cent solution followed by 2nd dose at 3-4 weeks interval, I/V.
- ☆ Diamidines: Diminazene aceturate (Berenil) - Curative,@ 3.5 mg/kg;
  - ❒ cattle - 10 mg/kg; S/C or deep I/M
  - ❒ Very effective against *T. congolense* and less effective against *T. evansi, T. brucei*, in bovines, ovines and caprines.
  - ❒ Dog and camels react to dogs; resistance may occur to the drug.

Phenanthiridine Compounds

- ☆ Homidium bromide and Homidium chloride- 1-2 per cent sol @ 1gm/kg b. wt, I/M against *T. congolense* and *T.vivax* but not against *T. evansi*.
- ☆ Pyrithridium bromide - 4 per cent sol @ 2mg/kg b. wt, S/C or I/M against *T.congolense* and *T.vivax*.
- ☆ Isometamidium chloride - 0.5 mg/kg b. wt, against *T. simiae* in pigs.

***Trypanosoma* Control**

Control is difficult and the factors responsible for the wide spread existence are:

- ☆ Latent cases of cattle and buffalo,
- ☆ Reservoir wild animals
- ☆ Drug resistant strains and
- ☆ Wide spread prevalence of vectors

Control program consists of

- ☆ Treatment of affected animals
- ☆ Chemoprophylaxis
- ☆ Disposal of manures properly
- ☆ Proper drainage
- ☆ Regular spraying of insecticides: Sprinkling of kerosene oil over water in ponds, ditches, streams or insecticides to kill adults and aquatic larvae.
- ☆ Removal of moist beddings, hay, dung from stable.
- ☆ Keeping animals clean by regular grooming.
- ☆ Segregation of sick animals from healthy during outbreak in flyproof shed.
- ☆ Identification of endemic areas by regular examination of blood of animals for implementation of preventive measures.

Annexure

Annexure

Disease	*Causative Organism*	*Principal Animal Involved*	*Known Distribution*	*Probable Means of Spread to Man*
BACTERIAL DISEASES				
Anthrax	*Bacillus anthracis*	Cattle, sheep, goats, horses, wild herbivorous animals	Worldwide; common in Africa, Asia, South America, eastern Europe	Occupational exposure; food-borne in Africa, Russia, and Asia; occasionally wounds or insect bites; rarely airborne
Borreliosis	*Borrelia* spp	Rodents	Worldwide	Soft ticks (*Ornithodoros* spp)
Lyme disease	*B. burgdorferi*	Deer, wild rodents	Worldwide	Hard ticks (*Ixodes* spp)
Relapsing fever	*B. recurrentis* Louseborne or epidemic	No animal reservoir for the transmitting lice	Epidemic	Crushing infected lice
	Tick-borne or endemic	Wild rodents	Epidemic	Tick bites
Brucellosis	*Brucella abortus*	Cattle, bison, elk, caribou	Worldwide, except North America	Occupational and recreational exposure
	B. melitensis	Goats, sheep	Worldwide	Milk, cheese, contact
	B. suis	Swine, caribou	Northern hemisphere	Rarely airborne
	B. canis	Dogs, coyotes	Rare	
Capnocytophaga infection	*Capnocytophaga canimorsus, C. cynodegmi*	Dogs, cats	USA	Bites or scratches
Campylobacter enteritis	*Campylobacter jejuni*	Domestic animals, dogs, cats, poultry, wild birds	Worldwide	Mainly food-borne, milk, waterborne; occupational; exposure to infected dogs and cats
	C. coli	Nonhuman primates, laboratory animals, domestic pigs	Common	
Cat scratch disease	*Bartonella* (*Rochalimae*) *henselae, B. quintana*	Cats	Worldwide	Scratches, bites, "licks"

Disease	*Causative Organism*	*Principal Animal Involved*	*Known Distribution*	*Probable Means of Spread to Man*
Clostridial diseases	*Clostridium perfringens*, type A	Domestic animals	Worldwide	Food-borne; occasionally wound contaminant
	C. septicum, *C. novyi*	Domestic and wild animals	Worldwide	Wound infection
Coliform diseases Enterohemorrhagic *Escherichia coli* infections (Enterotoxigenic, enteroinvasive, enteropathogenic, and enteroaggressive strains are not considered zoonotic)	*Escherichia coli* 0157: H7; also implicated are types 026:H11, 0111:H8, 0104:H21, and 048:H21	Cattle, man	North and South America, Europe, South Africa, Japan, Australia	Ingestion of undercooked ground beef, or foods or water contaminated with bovine feces
Erysipeloid	*Erysipelothrix rhusiopathiae*	Swine, turkeys, pigeons, sea mammals, fish	Worldwide	Occupational and recreational exposure
Glanders	*Pseudomonas mallei*	Equids	Rare except for some regions in Asia	Occupational exposure
Leptospirosis	*Leptospira interrogans* (200 serovars) in 23 serogroups	Domestic and wild animals, common in rodents, dogs	Worldwide	Occupational and recreational exposure; water- and food-borne
Leprosy	*Mycobacterium leprae*	Armadillos	Southern Texas and Louisiana	Transmission of animal leprosy to man suspected
Listeriosis	*Listeria monocytogenes* types1/2a, 1/2b, 4b	Numerous animals, birds	Worldwide	Food-borne among domestic animals by ensilage and hay; raw contaminated milk, cheese, mud, water, and vegetables are infectious; nosocomial infection in hospitals and institutions
Melioidosis (Pseudo-glanders)	*Pseudomonas pseudomallei*	Rodents, sheep, goats, horses, swine, nonhuman primates, kangaroos, zoo animals	Asia, Africa, Australia, South America, USA; rare	Wound infection and ingestion; organisms live in soil and surface water
Mycobacteriosis	*Mycobacterium avium-intracellulare* complex	Many species of animals, some birds	Worldwide	Rare; reported in AIDS patients

Disease	*Causative Organism*	*Principal Animal Involved*	*Known Distribution*	*Probable Means of Spread to Man*
	Mycobacteria other than tuberculosis	Cattle, other ruminants	Worldwide	
	Mycobacterium paratuberculosis	Cattle, occasionally sheep and other ruminants	Worldwide	Being investigated as cause of Crohn's disease; ingestion exposure
Pasteurellosis	*Pasteurella multocida* and other species	Many species of animals, birds	Worldwide	Wounds, scratches, bites
Plague	*Yersinia pestis*	Rodents, cats, rabbits, squirrels, related animals	Foci in Western USA, South America, Asia, Africa; rare	Fleas, aerosols, handling infected animals
Psittacosis and Ornithosis	*Chlamydia psittaci*	Parakeets, pigeons, parrots, turkeys, ducks, geese, *etc.*; other isolates in cattle, sheep, goats, opossums, *etc.*, rarely cause disease in man	Worldwide; common	Exposure to aerosols
Rat bite fever	*Streptobacillus moniliformis*	Rodents	Worldwide; rare	Bites of rodents; water- or food-borne
	Spirillum minus		Asia	
Salmonellosis	*Salmonella* spp (2000 serotypes, 200 seen in the USA)	Poultry, swine, cattle, horses, dogs, cats, wild mammals and birds, reptiles, amphibians, crustaceans	Worldwide; common	Food-borne infection, especially in the elderly, infants, or immunosuppressed; occupational and recreational exposure
Streptococcal infections	*Streptococcus pyogenes*, other group A streptococci, uncommonly groups B-G	Cattle (*S. agalactiae*), swine (*S. suis*), horses (*S. equi*), occasionally other animals	Worldwide	Ingestion especially of raw milk; direct contact
Tetanus	*Clostridium tetani*	Principally herbivores, but all animals may be carriers	Worldwide	Wound infection and injections
Tuberculosis	*Mycobacterium bovis*	Cattle, rarely other animals	Worldwide; rare in USA, Canada, Europe	Ingestion, inhalation, occupational exposure
	M. tuberculosis	Monkeys, other nonhuman primates, rarely dogs, cats, and other domestic animals	Worldwide	Exposure to animals infected with human type tuberculosis

Disease	*Causative Organism*	*Principal Animal Involved*	*Known Distribution*	*Probable Means of Spread to Man*
Tularemia	*Francisella tularensis* Type A virulent, type B less virulent	Wild animals, rabbits, rodents, cats, sheep	Circumpolar in America, Europe, Asia	Occupational and recreational exposure; insect bites; ingestion; inhalation
Vibrio food infection	*Vibrio parahaemolyticus* (Kanagawa phenomenon)	Marine shellfish	Pacific basin, warm shores of Asia	Ingestion
	V. vulnificus, other non-cholera vibrios		Australia, North America	Ingestion; wound infection
	V. cholerae –nonagglutinating types	Crabs, shrimp, mussels	Worldwide except Europe; epidemic in some developing countries	Ingestion
Yersiniosis	*Yersinia pseudotuberculosis* (6 serotypes)	Animals and birds	Temperate zones	Ingestion; recreational exposure
	Y. enterocolitica (50 serotypes)	Domestic animals especially pigs, dogs, cats		
RICKETTSIAL DISEASES				
Boutonneuse fever	*Rickettsia conorii*, *Rickettsia* spp	Dogs, rodents, other animals	Europe, Asia, Africa	Bite of infected ticks
Ehrlichiosis	*Ehrlichia chaffeensis*,	Deer	USA Japan	Ticks
Sennetsu fever	*E. sennetsu*	Rodents		
Murine typhus	*Rickettsia typhi* (*R. mooseri*) and related species	Rats, cats, opossums	Worldwide	Infected rodent fleas, possibly cat fleas
North Asian tick-borne rickettsiosis	*Rickettsia siberica*	Wild rodents	Siberia, Mongolia, China	Bite of infected ticks
Q fever	*Coxiella burnetii*	Sheep, cattle, goats, cats, other mammals	Worldwide; common	Mainly airborne; exposure to placenta; occasionally ticks and milk
Queensland tick typhus	*Rickettsia australis*	Bandicoots, rodents	Australia	Bite of infected *Ixodes* tick
Rickettsial pox	*Rickettsia akari*	Mice	Eastern USA, Africa, Russia; rare	Bite of infected rodent mites, *Liponyssoides* spp

Disease	*Causative Organism*	*Principal Animal Involved*	*Known Distribution*	*Probable Means of Spread to Man*
Rocky Mountain spotted fever	*Rickettsia rickettsii*	Rabbits, field mice, dogs	Western hemisphere	Bite of infected ticks or their crushing on the skin of *Dermacentor variabilis, D. ndersoni*
Scrub typhus	*Rickettsia*	Rodents	"Typhus islands" in	Bite of infected larval
	tsutsugamushi and related species		Asia, Australia, East Indies	trombiculid mites
Typhus	*Rickettsia prowazekii*	Flying squirrels	Eastern USA	Squirrel fleas or ticks suspected
		FUNGAL DISEASES		
Aspergillosis Allergic bronchopulmonary aspergillosis	*Aspergillus* spp	Birds and mammals; principally environmental indecaying vegetation or grains	Worldwide; sporadic	Environmental exposure
Blastomycosis	*Blastomyces dermatitidis*	Dogs, cats, horses, sea mammals; principally environmental in moist soil	Worldwide	Environmental exposure; also reported by animal exposure
Candidiasis (Moniliasis)	*Candida* spp	Principally human reservoirs, occasionally by birds and mammals	Worldwide	Direct contact; often endogenous in man
Coccidioidomycosis	*Coccidioides immitis*	Cattle, sheep, horses, dogs, wild cats, desert rodents, other animals; principally environmental in specific arid foci	Southwestern USA, Mexico, Central and South America	Environmental exposure
Cryptococcosis	*Cryptococcus neoformans*	Pigeons, mammals; principally environmental	Worldwide	Environmental exposure, especially pigeon nests
Dermatophilosis	*Dermatophilus congolensis*	Cattle, horses, deer, sheep, other mammals	Worldwide	Contact; arthropod vectors
Histoplasmosis	*Histoplasma capsulatum*	Dogs; principally environmental in river valleys	Worldwide	Environmental exposure

Disease	*Causative Organism*	*Principal Animal Involved*	*Known Distribution*	*Probable Means of Spread to Man*
Nocardiosis	*Nocardia asteroides*, *N. brasiliensis, N. caviae*	Cattle, dogs, other mammals, fish; principally environmental in decomposing organic matter	Worldwide	Environmental exposure
Rhinosporidiosis	*Rhinosporidium seeberi*	Horses, cattle, mules, dogs, and birds; unidentified environmental reservoirs	Worldwide, endemic in South Asia	Environmental exposure
Ringworm (Dermatophytosis)	*Microsporum*, *Trichophyton*, and *Epidermophyton* spp	Dogs, cats, cattle, rodents, other animals	Worldwide	Direct contact with infected animals and fomites
Sporotrichosis	*Sporothrix schenckii*	Horses, other domestic and laboratory animals, birds; primarily environmental in vegetation (moss) and wood	Worldwide	Occupational contact, including with animals
PARASITIC DISEASES and PROTOZOAN DISEASES				
Babesiosis	*Babesia microti*, *B. bovis*	Wild rodents, cattle	Worldwide; rare	Bites of infected *Ixodes* ticks
	B. divergens	Cattle, other mammals	Europe	
Balantidiasis	*Balantidium coli*	Swine, rats, nonhuman primates	Worldwide; low incidence	Ingestion, especially of water
Chagas' disease (American trypanosomiasis)	*Trypanosoma cruzi*	Dogs, cats, bats, rodents, armadillos, wild and domestic animals	Western hemisphere, Texas, Mexico, Central and South America	Fecal material of triatoma bug, including Reduviidae (also called cone- nosed, kissing, or assassin bug); contaminates bite wounds, abrasions, or mucous membranes
Cryptosporidiosis	*Cryptosporidium parvum*	Cattle, other animals	Worldwide	Occupational contact; ingestion; waterborne
Giardiasis	*Giardia lamblia*	Beavers, porcupines, dogs, other animals	Worldwide; common	Water and less often food; person to person
Leishmaniasis Visceral (Kala-azar)	*Leishmania donovani* and other species	Wild canids and dogs	Southern Asia, South America, Africa	Bite of infected phlebotomine sandflies

Disease	*Causative Organism*	*Principal Animal Involved*	*Known Distribution*	*Probable Means of Spread to Man*
Cutaneous and mucosal	*L. tropica*, *L. braziliensis* complex	Canids, marsupials, sloths, wild mammals, rodents		
Malaria of nonhuman primates	At least 20 species of *Plasmodium*	Monkeys, chimpanzees	Tropical Americas, Asia, Africa	Anopheline mosquitoes
Pneumocystis pneumonia	*Pneumocystis carinii* (human strain)	Rodents, dogs, cats, cattle (animal strains)	Worldwide; common in AIDS patients	Environmental exposure
Sarcocystosis (Sarcosporidiosis)	*Sarcocystis suihominis*	Swine	Worldwide	Ingestion of raw pork
	S. hominis	Cattle		Ingestion of raw beef
Toxoplasmosis	*Toxoplasma gondii*	Mammals, especially cats, food animals, birds	Worldwide; common	Ingestion of oocysts shed in feces of infected cats or found in meat or raw milk
Trypanosomiasis (African sleeping sickness)	*Trypanosoma brucei*, *T. brucei rhodesiense*, *T. brucei gambiense*	Wild and domestic dogs, ruminants, hyenas, carnivores	Africa; common	Bite of infected tsetse fly (*Glossina* spp.)
TREMATODE (FLUKE) DISEASES				
Clonorchiasis	*Clonorchis sinensis* (Chinese liver fluke)	Dogs, cats, swine, rats, wild animals	Asia	Ingestion of raw or partially cooked infected freshwater fish
Dicrocoeliasis	*Dicrocoelium dendriticum*	Ruminants	Worldwide	Ingestion of infected ants
	D. hospes	Ruminants	Africa	
Echinostomiasis	*Echinostoma ilocanum* and other *Echinostoma* spp	Cats, dogs, rodents, fish	Asia	Ingestion of uncooked fish or shellfish
Fascioliasis	*Fasciola hepatica*	Cattle, sheep, other large ruminants (*e.g.*, water buffalo)	Worldwide	Ingestion of contaminated greens, e.g., watercress
	F. gigantica		Africa and western Pacific	
Fasciolopsiasis	*Fasciolopsis buski*	Swine, dogs	Asian pig-raising regions	Ingestion of raw tubers and nuts of aquatic plants
Gastrodiscoidiasis	*Gastrodiscoides hominis*	Swine, rats	Asia	Snails (metacercariae encyst on plants)

Disease	*Causative Organism*	*Principal Animal Involved*	*Known Distribution*	*Probable Means of Spread to Man*
Heterophyiasis	*Heterophyes* and other heterophids	Cats, dogs, foxes, fish-eating birds	Nile delta, Turkey, the Far East	Ingestion of undercooked fish
Metagonimiasis	*Metagonimus yokogawai*	Cats, dogs, other fish-eating mammals, fish	Asia, Europe, Siberia	Ingestion of undercooked fish
Nanophyetiasis	*Troglotrema salmincola*	Dogs, fish-eating mammals, fish	North America, Siberia	Ingestion of undercooked fish
Opisthorchiasis	*Opisthorchis felineus* (Cat liver fluke)	Cats, dogs, foxes, swine	Eastern Europe, Asia, Siberia	Ingestion of uncooked fish containing encysted larva
	O. viverrini (Small liver fluke)	Dogs, cats, fish- eating mammals	Thailand, Laos	Ingestion of undercooked fish containing encysted larva
	Amphimerus pseudo-felineus	Dogs, cats, coyotes, opossums	USA, Central and South America	Undetermined
Paragonimiasis (Lung fluke disease)	*Paragonimus westermani, P. africanus, P. mexicanus* and other species	Dogs, cats, swine, wild carnivores	China, India, Burma, Africa, tropical America	Ingestion of raw or partially cooked, infected freshwater crustaceans
Schistosomiasis (Bilharziasis)	*Schistosoma japonicum*	Cattle, buffalo, swine, dogs, cats, rodents	Southeast Asia, China, Philippines	Penetration of unbroken skin by cercariae larva from infected snails in water
	S. hematobium	People are the only reservoir	Africa, the Middle East	
	S. mansoni	Baboons, rodents, cattle, dogs	Africa, Arabia, tropical America	
	S. mattbeei S. mekongi	Cattle Dogs, monkeys	Southern Africa Southeast Asia	
Swimmer's itch	Schistosome cercariae	Birds, mammals	Worldwide	Penetration of unbroken skin by cercariae from infected snails in fresh and salt water
CESTODE (TAPEWORM) DISEASES				
Bertielliasis	*Bertiella studeri, B. mucronata*	Primates, oribatid mites	Asia, South America, Africa	Ingestion of infected arthropods

Disease	*Causative Organism*	*Principal Animal Involved*	*Known Distribution*	*Probable Means of Spread to Man*
Coenuriasis	*Taenia multiceps*	Definitive hosts of all species are other canids, sheep, other herbivores	Worldwide in scattered foci	Ingestion of tapeworm eggs in canine feces
	T. serialis	Lagomorphs	Africa, Europe, USA; rare	
	T. brauni	Wild rodents	Africa	
Diphyllobothriasis (Fish tapeworm infection)	*Diphyllobothrium latum* (*Dibothriocephalus latus*), *Diphyllobothrium pacificum*	Man, dogs, bears, fish-eating animals, freshwater fish	Worldwide	Ingestion of raw or partially cooked infected fish
Dipylidiasis (Dog tapeworm infection)	*Dipylidium caninum*	Dogs, cats, fleas	Worldwide	Ingestion of dog or cat fleas
Echinococcosis	*Echinococcus granulosus* *E. multilocularis*	Dogs, sheep, cattle, swine, rodents, deer Foxes, microtine rodents, coyotes, dogs, wolves, cats, voles, lemmings, shrews	Worldwide Alaska, Canada, Asia, Europe	Ingestion of tapeworm eggs Ingestion of tapeworm eggs
	E. vogeli	Bush and hunting dogs, agouti, pacas, spiny rats	Central and South America	Ingestion of tapeworm eggs
Hymenolepiasis (Dwarf tapeworm infection)	*Hymenolepis nana*	Man, rodents	Worldwide	Ingestion of tapeworm eggs or infected insects
Inermicapsifer infection	*Inermicapsifer madagascariensis*	Rodents	Africa, southeast Asia, tropical America	Ingestion of infected arthropods
Mouse or rat tapeworm	*Hymenolepis nana*, *H. diminuta*	Rats, mice	Worldwide	Ingestion of cysticercoids in fleas, mealworms, *etc.*, in food
Pork tapeworm disease	*Taenia solium*	Swine, man	Worldwide where swine are reared (rare in USA, Canada, UK, Scandinavia)	Ingestion of undercooked pork containing *Cysticercus cellulosae*; direct or Autogenous transmission of *T. solium* ova in man may lead to cysticercosis
Asian taeniasis	*Taenia saginata taiwanensis*	Domestic and wild pigs, cattle, monkeys	East and southeast Asia	Ingestion of undercooked meat

Disease	*Causative Organism*	*Principal Animal Involved*	*Known Distribution*	*Probable Means of Spread to Man*
Raillietina infection	*Raillietina* spp	Birds, mammals	Tropical America, east Asia, Australia, Africa	Ingestion of infected arthropods
Sparganosis	*Spirometra* spp (pseudo-phyllidean tapeworms, second larval stage)	Monkeys, cats, pigs, dogs, weasels, rats, chickens, snakes, frogs, mice	Worldwide; common	Ingestion of infected cyclops or raw infected animal flesh
Taeniasis (Beef tapeworm disease) and Cysticercosis	*Taenia saginata*	Cattle, water buffalo	Worldwide	Ingestion of undercooked meat containing *Cysticercus bovis*
NEMATODES (WORM) DISEASES				
Angiostrongyliasis (Visceral larva migrans)	*Angiostrongylus costaricensis*	Cotton rats, slugs	Central and South America, USA, east and southeast Asia	Ingestion of slugs or plants contaminated by their secretions
	A. cantonensis	Rats, snails, slugs		
Anisakiasis (Visceral larva migrans)	Larvae of *Anisakis* and *Pseudoterranova* spp	Marine invertebrates, fish, mammals	Japan, Scandinavia, western South America, western Europe, USA	Ingestion of undercooked marine fish, squid, octopus
Capillariasis Hepatic capillariasis	*Capillaria hepatica*	Rodents, other wild and domestic animals	Worldwide in scattered foci	Ingestion of embryonated eggs in soil
Intestinal capillariasis	*C. philippinensis*	Aquatic birds, freshwater fish	Northern Philippines, Thailand, east Asia, and Egypt	Ingestion of infected fish
Pulmonary capillariasis	*C. aerophila*	Dogs, cats, other carnivores	Worldwide	Ingestion of infective eggs in soil or contaminated food
Dioctophymosis (Giant kidney worm infection) Dracunculiasis (Guinea worm infection)	*Dioctophyma renale*	Dogs, mink, other carnivores, frogs	Europe, Asia, North and South America; rare	Ingestion of infected fish or frog's liver and mesentery
	Dracunculus medinensis	Man	Asia and Africa; common	Ingestion of infected cyclops in water
	D. insignis	Raccoons, mink, dogs	North America	Ingestion of frogs and other paratenic hosts
Dirofilariasis	*Dirofilaria immitis*	Dogs, cats, raccoons, bears, mosquitoes	Worldwide	Bites of infected mosquitoes

Disease	Causative Organism	Principal Animal Involved	Known Distribution	Probable Means of Spread to Man
Malayan filariasis	*Brugia malayi, Brugia pahangi*	Cats, other carnivores, monkeys, mosquitoes	Asia; common	Bites of infected mosquitoes
Tropical eosinophilia Gnathostomiasis	*Gnathostoma spinigerum*	Dogs, cats, wild carnivores, copepods, freshwater fish	East Asia, India, Australia	Ingestion of infected fish or poultry
Gongylonemiasis	*Gongylonema pulchrum*	Ruminants, domestic and wild swine, other mammals; beetles	Worldwide; rare	Ingestion of infected arthropods
Larva migrans, cutaneous	*Ancylostoma braziliense, A. caninum*	Cats, dogs, wild carnivores	Worldwide in tropics and subtropics; common	Contact with infective larvae that penetrate skin
	Strongyloides stercoralis	Cats, dogs, sheep, swine, *etc.*	Worldwide in tropics and subtropics; rare to common	Contact with infective larvae that penetrate skin
Larva migrans, visceral	*Toxocara canis* and *T. cati*	Dogs, cats	Worldwide	Ingestion of embryonated eggs shed in feces of dogs and cats
Angiostrongyliasis	*Baylisascaris procyonis*	Raccoons	North America, Europe	Ingestion of embryonated eggs in soil
Oesophagostomiasis, Ternidensiasis	*Oesophagostomum* spp	Primates	Asia, Africa, South America	Ingestion of infective larvae in soil
	Ternidens diminutus			
Strongyloidiasis	*Strongyloides stercoralis, S. fuelleborni*	Dogs, cats, foxes, primates	Worldwide; rare to common	Contact with infective larvae that penetrate skin
Thelaziasis	*Thelazia* spp.	Dogs, cats, other domestic and wild animals, flies	East and south Asia; rare	Infected insects
Trichinosis (Trichinellosis)	*Trichinella spiralis* and subspecies	Swine, rodents, bears, wild carnivores, marine mammals	Worldwide, especially subarctic region	Ingestion of either pork or flesh of wild animals that contains viable cysts
Trichostrongyliasis	*Trichostrongylus* spp.	Cattle, sheep, wild ruminants	Worldwide	Ingestion of infective larvae on plant foods or in soil
Trichuriasis (Whipworm infection)	*Trichuris trichiura* and other *Trichuris* spp	Man, other primates, domestic and wild canids, swine	Worldwide; common	Ingestion of embryonated eggs on plant foods or in soil

Disease	*Causative Organism*	*Principal Animal Involved*	*Known Distribution*	*Probable Means of Spread to Man*
		ACANTHOCEPHALIASIS		
Macracanthorhynchosis	*Macracanthorhynchus hirudinaceus* and other spp.	Domestic and wild pigs, squirrels, muskrats, arctic foxes, dogs, sea otters, crustaceans, fish	Worldwide; uncommon	Ingestion of infected beetles
		ANNELID (LEECH) DISEASES		
Hirudiniasis	*Limnatis nilotica* and other leeches	Cattle, buffalo, horses, sheep, dogs, pigs	Africa, Asia, Europe, Chile	Direct contact with leeches
		ARTHROPOD DISEASES		
Acariasis (Mange)	Mites of *Sarcoptes*, *Cheyletiella*, *Dermanyssus*, and *Ornithonyssus* spp.	Domestic animals	Worldwide	Contact with infected individuals or animals; contaminated clothing
Myiasis	*Cochliomyia hominivorax* (Screwworm)	Mammals	America	Invasion of living tissues by larvae
	Chrysomyia bezziana		Asia, Africa	
	Cordylobia anthropophaga (Tumbu fly)		Africa	
	Cuterebra spp.		North America	
	Dermatobia hominis (human botfly)		South America, Mexico	
	Gasterophilus spp (equine botfly)		Worldwide	
	Hypoderma lineatum		North America, Europe	
	Hypoderma bovis (warbles)		Asia, North Africa	
	Oestrus ovis, *Rhinoestrus purpurensis*		Worldwide	
	Wohlfahrtia spp.		North America, Europe, north Africa, Asia	

Disease	*Causative Organism*	*Principal Animal Involved*	*Known Distribution*	*Probable Means of Spread to Man*
Pentastomid infections	*Linguatula serrata*, *Armillifer* spp (Tongue vertebrates worms)	Dogs, snakes, other	Northern hemisphere Worldwide	Ingestion of infected animal tissues
Tick paralysis	Envenomization of ticks *Dermacentor andersoni*, *D. variabilis* and sometimes *Ixodes*, *Haemaphysalis*, *Rhinocephalus*, and *Argas* spp.	Various animals	North America, Australia, South Africa, Ethiopia	Direct contact (attachment) with tick
Tunga infections	*Tunga penetrans* (Sand fleas, jiggers)	Man, dogs, pigs, other mammals	Subtropical Africa, Americas, south Asia	Contact with contaminated soil
VIRAL DISEASES				
African hemorrhagic fever	Marburg and Ebola viruses	African green monkeys	Central and southern Africa	Contact with infected tissues
Filovirus infections	Ebola-related Filoviruses	Cynomolgus monkeys	Southeast Asia	Person to person
Argentinean hemorrhagic fever	Junin virus (arenavirus)	Rodents	Argentina	Rodent excretions and secretions
Bolivian hemorrhagic fever	Machupo virus (arenavirus)	Rodents	Bolivia	Rodent excretions
Brazilian hemorrhagic fever	Sabiá virus (arenavirus)	Rodents are suspected	Brazil	Rodent excretions suspected; other aerosols
California group infections LaCross encephalitis	California group of bunya-viruses	Ground squirrels, other rodents	USA, Canada	Bites of mosquitoes (*Aedes* spp.)
Tahyna fever		Hares, rodents, other mammals	Europe, Africa	
Central European tick-borne encephalitis	Central European ence-phalitis virus (flavivirus)	Rodents, hedgehogs, birds, goats, sheep	Europe	Bites of *Ixodes* ticks; may be milk-borne
Colorado tick fever	Colorado tick fever virus	Ground squirrels, chipmunks, porcupines, small rodents	Western USA; common	Bites of ticks (*Dermacentor andersoni*)
Contagious ecthyma (Orf)	Orf virus (parapox)	Sheep, goats, wild ruminants	Worldwide; common	Occupational exposure

Disease	*Causative Organism*	*Principal Animal Involved*	*Known Distribution*	*Probable Means of Spread to Man*
Cowpox	Cowpox virus	Cattle, rodents, cats, zoo cats	Worldwide; rare, no recent cases	Contact exposure
Crimean-Congo hemorrhagic fever	Crimean-Congo hemorrhagic fever virus (bunyavirus)	Cattle, rodents, sheep, goats, hares, birds	Southern Russia, eastern Europe, Africa, the Middle East, Asia	Bites of ticks (*Hyalomma* and *Boophilus* spp)
Eastern equine encephalomyelitis	EEE virus (alphavirus) Wild birds, domestic	Fowl, horses, mules, donkeys	Western hemisphere	Mosquitoes (*Culiseta melanura* and *Aedes* spp)
Encephalomyocarditis	Encephalomyocarditis virus (picornavirus)	Rats, mice, squirrels, swine, nonhuman primates	Worldwide	Environmental contamination
Far eastern tick-borne encephalitis (Russian spring-summer encephalitis)	Far eastern (Russian encephalitis) virus (flavivirus)	Birds, small mammals, sheep	Asia, Europe; rare	Bites of ticks (*Ixodes persulcatus* and *Ixodes ricinus*)
Foot-and-mouth disease	Foot-and-mouth disease virus (aphthovirus types A, O, C, SAT, and Asia)	Cattle, swine, related cloven-hoofed animals	Europe, Asia, Africa, South America	Contact exposure; people quite resistant but can be carriers
Hantaviral diseases	Hantaviruses (bunyavirus)	Rodents	Worldwide	Aerosols from rodent excretions and secretions
Hantaviral pulmonary syndrome	Sin Nombre virus Black Creek Canal virus	*Peromyscus* spp., *Sigmodon hispidus*	USA, may be more widespread	
Hemorrhagic fever with renal syndrome (Korean hemorrhagic fever)	Hemorrhagic fever with renal syndrome virus (Hantaan virus)	*Apodemus* spp.	China, Siberia, Korea, Manchuria, Japan	
Other hantaviral diseases	Dobrava virus Pnumala virus Seoul virus	*Apodemus* spp., *Clethrionomys* spp., *Rattus* spp.	Balkan countries Europe Worldwide	
Simian herpes B virus disease	Simian B virus	Old World monkeys; cell cultures	Worldwide; rare	Bites of monkeys; occupational exposure
Influenza including type A (swine and equine)	Influenza virus (myxovirus)	Swine, ducks	Worldwide; common	Contact exposure; animals rarely a source

Disease	*Causative Organism*	*Principal Animal Involved*	*Known Distribution*	*Probable Means of Spread to Man*
Japanese B encephalitis	Japanese encephalitis virus (flavivirus)	Swine, wild birds, horses	Asia, Pacific Islands from Japan to the Philippines	Bites of mosquitoes (*Culex tritaeniorhynchus*, other *Culex* spp.)
Kyasanur forest disease	Kyasanur forest virus (flavivirus)	Rodents, monkeys	India	Bites of ticks(*Haemaphysalis spinigera*)
Lassa fever	Lassa virus (arenavirus)	Wild rodents	Africa	Rodent excretions and secretions; contact in hospitals and laboratories
Louping ill	Louping ill virus (flavivirus)	Sheep, goats, grouse, small rodents	Great Britain, Northern Ireland; rare	Bites of ticks (*Ixodes ricinus*)
Lymphocytic choriomeningitis	Lymphocytic choriomeningitis virus (arenavirus)	House mice, dogs, monkeys, guinea pigs, hamsters	Worldwide	Host excretions and secretions
Milker's nodules (Pseudocowpox)	Pseudocowpox virus (parapoxvirus)	Cattle	Worldwide; common	Occupational exposure
Monkeypox	Monkeypox virus	Nonhuman primates	West Africa; very rare	Contact; aerosols
Murray Valley encephalitis	Murray Valley encephalitis virus(flavivirus)	Wild birds	Australia, New Guinea; rare	Bites of mosquitoes (*Culex annulirostris*)
Newcastle disease	Newcastle disease virus (Paramyxovirus)	Fowl, wild birds	Worldwide; common	Occupational exposure
Omsk hemorrhagic fever	Omsk hemorrhagic fever virus (flavivirus)	Rodents, muskrats	Omsk, Siberia; rare	Bites of ticks (*Dermacentor* spp)
Rabies and rabies- related infections	Lyssaviruses Rabies virus	Wild and domestic canids, mustelidae,	Worldwide except Australia, New	Bites of diseased animals; aerosols in closed environments
Lyssaencephalitis	Duvenhage virus Mokola virus, Ibadan shrew virus, Obodhiang virus	viverridae, vampire and insectivorous bats	Zealand, UK, Ireland, Scandinavia, Japan, Taiwan; many smaller islands are also free, including Hawaii	
Rift Valley fever	Rift Valley fever virus (phlebovirus)	Sheep, goats, cattle, camels	Africa; common to rare	Bites of mosquitoes (*Aedes* spp); contact on necropsy or handling fresh meat

Disease	*Causative Organism*	*Principal Animal Involved*	*Known Distribution*	*Probable Means of Spread to Man*
St. Louis encephalitis	St. Louis encephalitis virus (flavivirus)	Wild birds, domestic fowl	Western hemisphere	Bites of mosquitoes (*Culex tarsalis*, *C. pipiens- quinquefasciatus* complex, *C. nigripalpus*)
Sindbis virus disease	Sindbis virus (alphavirus)	Birds	Eastern hemisphere; rare	Bites of mosquitoes (*Culex* spp)
Ross River fever	Ross River virus (alpha-virus)	Undetermined	Australia, South Pacific Islands	Bites of mosquitoes (*Culex annulirostris* and *Aedes* spp.)
Tanapox	Tanapox virus	Asian and African monkeys	Asia, Africa, and in colonies of monkeys	Contact; aerosols
Venezuelan hemorrhagic fever	Gnanarito virus (arenavirus)	Rodents	Venezuela	Rodent excretions
Venezuelan equine encephalomyelitis	VEE virus (alphavirus)	Rodents, equids	Western hemisphere; common	Bites of mosquitoes (*Monsonia*, *Aedes*, *Culex* spp.)
Vesicular stomatitis	Vesicular stomatitis virus (Indiana and New Jersey strains)	Swine, cattle, horses, bats, rodents, other wild mammals	North and South America	Contact exposure and insect bites, including mosquitoes and biting flies (*Phlebotomus* spp.)
Wesselsbron fever	Wesselsbron virus (flavivirus)	Sheep	Southern Africa, southeast Asia	Bites of mosquitoes (*Aedes*, *Mansonia*, *Culex* spp.)
West Nile fever	West Nile virus (flavivirus)	Wild birds, horses	Eastern hemispher; common	Bites of mosquitoes (*Culex univittatus*, *C. pipiens*, *C. modestus*)
Western equine encephalomyelitis	WEE virus (alphavirus)	Wild birds, domestic fowl, horses, mules, donkeys, bats, reptiles, amphibians	Western and central USA, Canada, South America	Mosquitoes (*Culex tarsalis* in USA, other *Culex* and *Aedes* spp outside USA)
Yabapox	Yabapox virus	African monkeys	Africa; rare	Contact; aerosols
Yellow fever	Yellow fever virus (flavivirus)	Monkeys, baboons	Tropical America, Africa; sporadic	Bites of mosquitoes (*Aedes aegypti* in urban cycles, *Haemagogus* spp. in jungle cycles in South America, *Aedes* spp. in jungle cycles in Africa)

References

Aiello, Susan E. [and others], eds. *The Merck Veterinary Manual.* 8th ed. Whitehouse Station, NJ: Merck and Company, in cooperation with Merial, 1998. $32.00. Also CD-ROM.

Anderson, Roy C. *Nematode Parasites of Vertebrates: Their Development and Transmission.*2nd ed. Wallingford, UK: CABI Publishing, c2000. $185.00.

Baker, Anne S. *Mites and Ticks of Domestic Animals: An Identification Guide and Information Source.* London, UK: NHM Publishing, 1999. £32.50.

Blowey, R. W., and Weaver, A. David. *Color Atlas of Diseases and Disorders of Cattle.* 2nd ed. New York, NY: Mosby, 2003. $110.00.

Bowman, Dwight D. [and others]. *Feline Clinical Parasitology.* Ames, IA: Iowa State University Press, 2002. $84.99.

Bowman, Dwight D. [and others]. *Georgis' Parasitology for Veterinarians.* 8th ed. St. Louis, MO: Saunders, c2003. $64.95.

Buergelt, Claus D. *Color Atlas of Reproductive Pathology of Domestic Animals.* St. Louis, MO: Mosby, c1997. $125.00.

Campbell, Terry W. *Avian Hematology and Cytology.* 2nd ed. Ames, IA: Iowa State University Press, 1995. $89.99.

Capen, Charles C. [and others], eds. *Pathobiology of the Aging Dog.* Ames, IA: Iowa State University Press, 2001. $599.99. 2 volumes.

Cheville, Norman F. *Introduction to Veterinary Pathology.* 2nd ed. Ames, IA: Iowa State University Press, c1999. $74.99. Also CD-ROM.

Cheville, Norman F. *Ultrastructural Pathology: An Introduction to Interpretation.* Ames, IA: Iowa State University Press, 1994. $199.99.

Colahan, Patrick T. [and others]. *Equine Medicine and Surgery.* 5th ed. St. Louis, MO: Mosby, 1998. $250.00. 2 volumes.

Cook, Gordon C., and Zumla, Alimuddin I., eds. *Manson's Tropical Diseases.* 21st ed. London, UK: Saunders, c2003. $179.00. Biomedical title.

Cotran, Ramzi S. [and others], eds. *Robbins Pathologic Basis of Disease.* 6th ed. Philadelphia, PA: Saunders, c1999. $87.95. Biomedical title.

Cowart, Ross P., and Casteel, Stan W. *An Outline of Swine Diseases: A Handbook.* 2nd ed. Ames, IA: Iowa State University Press, c2001. $34.99.

Cowell, Rick L. [and others], eds. *Diagnostic Cytology and Hematology of the Dog and Cat.* 2nd ed. St. Louis, MO: Mosby, c1999. $99.00.

Cowell, Rick L., and Tyler, Ronald D. *Diagnostic Cytology and Hematology of the Horse.*2nd ed. St. Louis, MO: Mosby, c2002. $125.00.

Feldman, Bernard F. [and others], eds. *Schalm's Veterinary Hematology.* 5th ed. Philadelphia, PA: Lippincott Williams and Wilkins, c2000. $159.00.

Fletcher, Robert H. [and others]. *Clinical Epidemiology: the Essentials.* 3rd ed. Baltimore, MD: Williams and Wilkins, c1996. $32.95. Biomedical title.

Foreyt, William J. *Veterinary Parasitology Reference Manual.* 5th ed. Ames, IA: Iowa State University Press, c2001. $39.99.

Goldschmidt, Michael H., and Shofer, Francis. *Skin Tumors of the Dog and Cat.* Woburn, MA: Butterworth-Heinemann, 1998. $74.95.

Gopinath, C. [and others]. *Atlas of Experimental Toxicological Pathology.* Lancaster, UK: MTP Press, c1987. $467.00.

Griner, Lynn A. *Pathology of Zoo Animals: A Review of Necropsies Conducted Over a Fourteen-Year Period at the San Diego Zoo.* San Diego, CA: Zoological Society of San Diego, c1983. $25.00.

Howard, Jimmy L., and Smith, Robert, eds. *Current Veterinary Therapy: Food Animal Practice.* 4th ed. Philadelphia, PA: W. B. Saunders Company, 1999. $149.00.

Jones, Thomas Carlyle [and others]. *Veterinary Pathology.* 6th ed. Baltimore, MD: Williams and Wilkins, c1997. $99.95.

Jubb, K.V.F. [and others], eds. *Pathology of Domestic Animals.* 4th ed. San Diego, CA: Academic Press, c1993. $311.95. 3 volumes.

Kaufmann, Johannes. *Parasitic Infections of Domestic Animals: A Diagnostic Manual.* Basel, Switzerland: Birkhauser Verlag, c1996. $69.50.

Kettle, D.S., ed. *Medical and Veterinary Entomology.* 2nd ed. Wallingford, UK: CAB International, c1995. $80.00.

Knottenbelt, Derek C., and Pascoe, Reg R. *A Color Atlas of Diseases and Disorders of the Horse.* St. Louis, MO: Mosby-Year Book, c1994. $155.00.

Kumar, V. *Trematode Infections and Diseases of Man and Animals.* Dordrecht, The Netherlands: Kluwer; Antwerp Institute of Tropical Medicine, c1999. $214.50.

Kumar, Vinay [and others], eds. *Robbins Basic Pathology.* 7th ed. Philadelphia, PA: Saunders, c2003. $64.95. Biomedical title.

Latimer, Kenneth S. [and others], eds. *Duncan and Prasse's Veterinary Laboratory Medicine: Clinical Pathology.* 4th ed. Ames, IA: Iowa State University Press, 2003. $49.99.

Maronpot, Robert, ed. *Pathology of the Mouse.* Vienna, IL: Cache River Press, 1999. $137.50.

Marquardt, William C. [and others]. *Parasitology and Vector Biology.* 2nd ed. San Diego, CA: Academic Press, c2000. $94.95. Biomedical title.

Martin, S. Wayne [and others]. *Veterinary Epidemiology: Principles and Methods.* Ames, IA: Iowa State University Press, 1987. $69.99. Biomedical title.

Martin, W. B., and Aitken, I.D., eds. *Diseases of Sheep.* 3rd ed. Malden, MA: Blackwell Science, 1999. $152.99.

Mcentee, Kenneth. *Reproductive Pathology of Domestic Mammals.* San Diego, CA: Academic Press, c1990. $179.95.

Mcgavin, M. Donald [and others], eds. *Thomson's Special Veterinary Pathology.* 3rd ed. St. Louis, MO: Mosby, 2001. $105.00.

Mehlhorn, Heinz, ed. *Encyclopedic Reference of Parasitology: Diseases, Treatment, Therapy.*2nd ed. New York, NY: Springer, 2001. $199.00. 2 volumes. Also CD-ROM. Biomedical title.

Meuten, Donald J., ed. *Tumors in Domestic Animals.* 4th ed. Ames, IA: Iowa State University Press, c2002. $179.99.

Mullen, Gary, and Durden, Lance, eds. *Medical and Veterinary Entomology.* San Diego, CA: Academic Press, c2002. $99.95.

Noordhuizen, J.P.T.M. [and others], eds. *Application of Quantitative Methods in Veterinary Epidemiology.* 2d rev. reprint. Wageningen, The Netherlands: Wageningen Press, 2001. $93.00.

Percy, Dean H., and Barthold, Stephen W. *Pathology of Laboratory Rodents and Rabbits.*2nd ed. Ames, IA: Iowa State University Press, 2001. $99.99.

Pond, Wilson G., and Mersmann, Harry J., eds. *Biology of the Domestic Pig.* Ithaca, NY: Comstock Publishing Associates, Cornell University Press, 2001. $75.00.

Pugh, D.G., ed. *Sheep and Goat Medicine.* Philadelphia, PA: Saunders, c2002. $92.95.

Radostits, Otto M. [and others], eds. *Veterinary Medicine: A Textbook of the Diseases of Cattle, Sheep, Pigs, Goats and Horses.* 9th ed. New York, NY: Saunders, c2000. $159.00.

Radostits, Otto M. *Herd Health: Food Animal Production Medicine.* 3rd ed. Philadelphia, PA: Saunders, c2001. $139.00.

Radostits, Otto. M. [and others]. *Veterinary Clinical Examination and Diagnosis.* London, UK: W. B. Saunders, 2001. $89.95.

Raskin, Rose E., and Meyer, Denny J. *Atlas of Canine and Feline Cytology*. Philadelphia, PA: W. B. Saunders, c2001. $89.95.

Reed, Stephen M. [and others], eds. *Equine Internal Medicine*. 2nd ed. Philadelphia, PA: Saunders, 2004. $159.00.

Roberts, Ronald J., ed. *Fish Pathology*. 3rd ed. New York, NY: W. B. Saunders, 2001. $175.00.

Rose, Reuben J., and Hodgson, David R. *Manual of Equine Practice*. 2nd ed. Philadelphia, PA: Saunders, c2000. $95.00.

Rothman, Kenneth J., and Greenland, Sander, eds. *Modern Epidemiology*. 2nd ed. Philadelphia, PA: Lippincott-Raven, c1998. $79.95. Biomedical title.

Samuel, William S. [and others], eds. *Parasitic Diseases of Wild Mammals*. 2nd ed. Ames, IA: Iowa State University Press, 2001. $94.99. Also CD-ROM.

Slauson, David O., and Cooper, Barry J. *Mechanisms of Disease: A Textbook of Comparative General Pathology*. 3rd ed. St. Louis, MO: Mosby, c2002. $64.95.

Sloss, Margaret W. [and others]. *Veterinary Clinical Parasitology*. 6th ed. Ames, IA: Iowa State University Press, 1994. $44.99.

Smith, Bradford P., ed. *Large Animal Internal Medicine*. 3rd ed. St. Louis, MO: Mosby, c2002. $169.00.

Smith, Mary C., and Sherman, David M. *Goat Medicine*. Malvern, PA: Lea and Febiger, c1994. $80.00.

Smith, Ronald D. *Veterinary Clinical Epidemiology: A Problem-Oriented Approach*. 2nd ed. Boca Raton, FL: CRC Press, c1995. $99.95.

Stockham, Steven L., and Scott, Michael A. *Fundamentals of Veterinary Clinical Pathology*.Ames, IA: Iowa State Press, 2002. $74.99.

Straw, Barbara E. [and others], eds. *Diseases of Swine*. 8th ed. Ames, IA: Iowa State University Press, 1999. $174.99. Also CD-ROM.

Summers, Brian A. [and others]. *Veterinary Neuropathology*. St. Louis, MO: Mosby, c1995. $160.00.

Thrusfield, Michael. *Veterinary Epidemiology*. 2nd ed. Oxford, UK: Blackwell, 1995. $64.99.

Urquhart, G.M. [and others]. *Veterinary Parasitology*. 2nd ed. Cambridge, UK: Blackwell Science, 1996. $79.99.

Veterinary Clinics of North America: Equine Practice. Philadelphia, PA: W. B. Saunders Company, 1985–.

Veterinary Clinics of North America: Food Animal Practice. Philadelphia, PA: W. B. Saunders Company, 1985–.

Wall, Richard, and Shearer, David. *Veterinary Ectoparasites: Biology, Pathology and Control*. 2nd ed. Malden, MA: Blackwell Science, c2001. $66.99.

Ward, Jerrold Michael [and others], eds. *Pathology of Genetically Engineered Mice.* Ames, IA: Iowa State University Press, c2000. $199.99.

West, D.M. [and others]. *The Sheep, Health, Disease, and Production: Written for Veterinarians and Farmers.* 2nd ed. Palmerston, NZ: Veterinary Continuing Education, Massey University, 2002. $59.50 AUD.

Whittemoore, Colin. *Science and Practice of Pig Production.* 2nd ed. Malden, MA: Blackwell Science, 1998. $139.99.

World Health Organization. *International Histological Classification of Tumours of Domestic Animals.* Geneva, Switzerland: World Health Organization. Multiple volumes.

Index

M

N

O

P

Q

R

S

T

U

V

Z

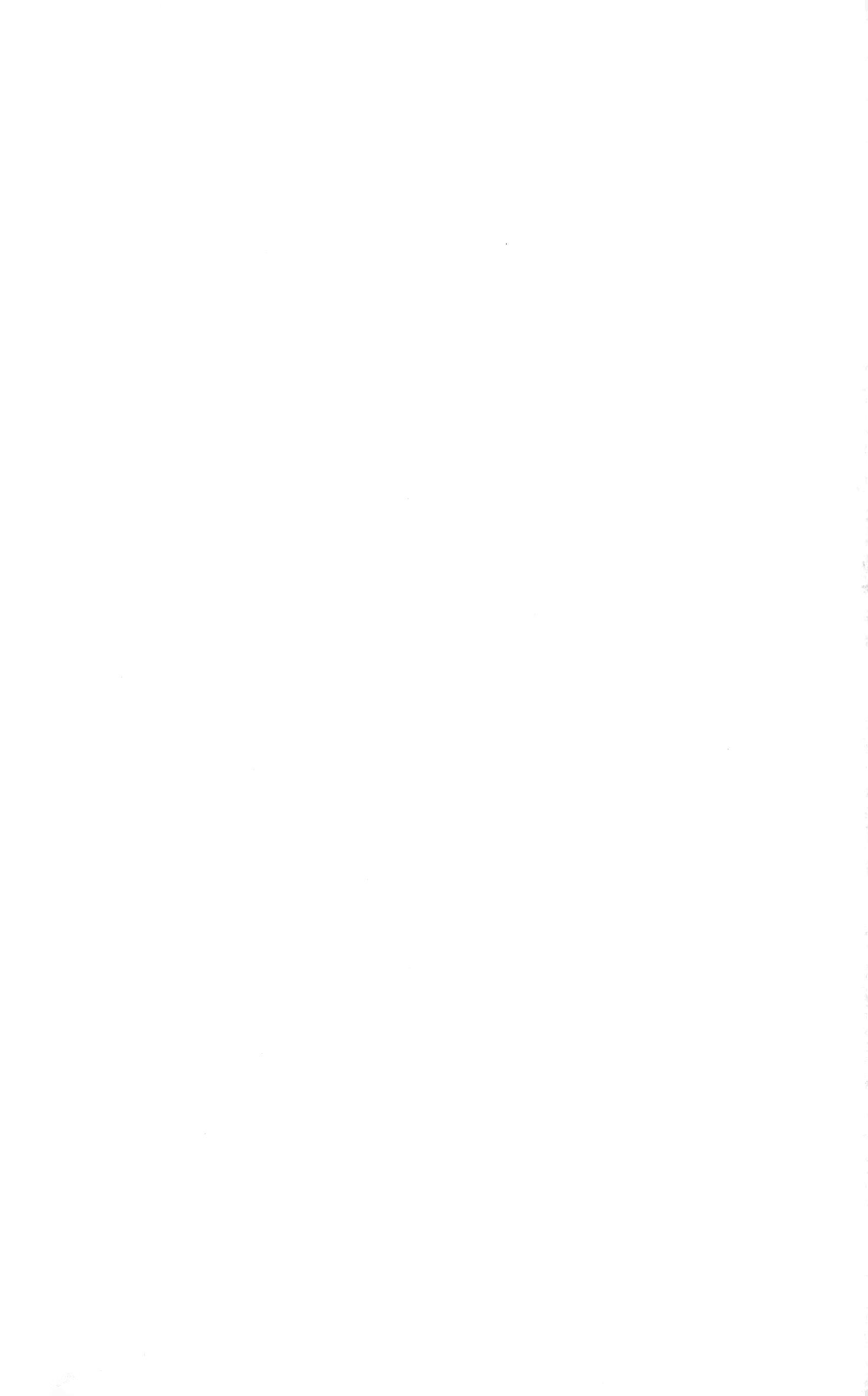